Perimenopause

Guest Editor

NANETTE SANTORO, MD

OBSTETRICS AND GYNECOLOGY CLINICS OF NORTH AMERICA

www.obgyn.theclinics.com

Consulting Editor
WILLIAM F. RAYBURN, MD, MBA

September 2011 • Volume 38 • Number 3

SAUNDERS an imprint of ELSEVIER, Inc.

W.B. SAUNDERS COMPANY
A Division of Elsevier Inc.

Elsevier, Inc. • 1600 John F. Kennedy Blvd. • Suite 1800 • Philadelphia, PA 19103-2899

http://www.theclinics.com

OBSTETRICS AND GYNECOLOGY CLINICS OF NORTH AMERICA Volume 38, Number 3
September 2011 ISSN 0889-8545, ISBN-13: 978-1-4557-1047-8

Editor: Stephanie Donley

Obstetrics and Gynecology Clinics (ISSN 0889-8545) is published quarterly by Elsevier Inc., 360 Park Avenue South, New York, NY 10010-1710. Months of issue are March, June, September, and December. Periodicals postage paid at New York, NY, and additional mailing offices. Subscription price per year is $275.00 (US individuals), $474.00 (US institutions), $137.00 (US students), $331.00 (Canadian individuals), $598.00 (Canadian institutions), $201.00 (Canadian students), $402.00 (foreign individuals), $598.00 (foreign institutions), and $201.00 (foreign students). To receive student/ resident rate, orders must be accompanied by name of affiliated institution, date of term, and the signature of program/ residency coordinator on institution letterhead. Orders will be billed at individual rate until proof of status is received. Foreign air speed delivery is included in all *Clinics* subscription prices. All prices are subject to change without notice. POSTMASTER: Send address changes to *Obstetrics and Gynecology Clinics*, Elsevier Health Sciences Division, Subscription Customer Service, 3251 Riverport Lane, Maryland Heights, MO 63043. **Customer Service: Telephone: 1-800-654-2452 (U.S. and Canada); 314-447-8871 (outside U.S. and Canada). Fax: 314-447-8029. E-mail: journalscustomerservice-usa@elsevier.com (for print support); journalsonlinesupport-usa@ elsevier.com (for online support).**

Reprints. For copies of 100 or more of articles in this publication, please contact the Commercial Reprints Department, Elsevier Inc., 360 Park Avenue South, New York, New York 10010-1710. Tel.: 212-633-3818; Fax: 212-462-1935; E-mail: reprints@elsevier.com.

Obstetrics and Gynecology Clinics of North America is also published in Spanish by McGraw-Hill Interamericana Editores S.A., P.O. Box 5-237, 06500, Mexico; in Portuguese by Reichmann and Affonso Editores, Rio de Janeiro, Brazil; and in Greek by Paschalidis Medical Publications, Athens, Greece.

Obstetrics and Gynecology Clinics of North America is covered in *MEDLINE/PubMed (Index Medicus)*, *Excerpta Medica*, *Current Concepts/Clinical Medicine*, *Science Citation Index*, *BIOSIS*, *CINAHL*, and *ISI/BIOMED*.

Printed and bound by CPI Group (UK) Ltd, Croydon, CR0 4YY

Transferred to Digital Print 2011

GOAL STATEMENT

The goal of *Obstetrics and Gynecology Clinics of North America* is to keep practicing physicians up to date with current clinical practice in OB/GYN by providing timely articles reviewing the state of the art in patient care.

ACCREDITATION

The *Obstetrics and Gynecology Clinics of North America* is planned and implemented in accordance with the Essential Areas and Policies of the Accreditation Council for Continuing Medical Education (ACCME) through the joint sponsorship of the University of Virginia School of Medicine and Elsevier. The University of Virginia School of Medicine is accredited by the ACCME to provide continuing medical education for physicians.

The University of Virginia School of Medicine designates this enduring material activity for a maximum of 15 *AMA PRA Category 1 Credit*(s)™ for each issue, 60 credits per year. Physicians should only claim credit commensurate with the extent of their participation in the activity.

The American Medical Association has determined that physicians not licensed in the US who participate in this CME enduring material activity are eligible for a maximum of 15 *AMA PRA Category 1 Credit*(s)™ for each issue, 60 credits per year.

Credit can be earned by reading the text material, taking the CME examination online at http://www.theclinics.com/home/cme, and completing the evaluation. After taking the test, you will be required to review any and all incorrect answers. Following completion of the test and evaluation, your credit will be awarded and you may print your certificate.

FACULTY DISCLOSURE/CONFLICT OF INTEREST

The University of Virginia School of Medicine, as an ACCME accredited provider, endorses and strives to comply with the Accreditation Council for Continuing Medical Education (ACCME) Standards of Commercial Support, Commonwealth of Virginia statutes, University of Virginia policies and procedures, and associated federal and private regulations and guidelines on the need for disclosure and monitoring of proprietary and financial interests that may affect the scientific integrity and balance of content delivered in continuing medical education activities under our auspices.

The University of Virginia School of Medicine requires that all CME activities accredited through this institution be developed independently and be scientifically rigorous, balanced and objective in the presentation/discussion of its content, theories and practices.

All authors/editors participating in an accredited CME activity are expected to disclose to the readers relevant financial relationships with commercial entities occurring within the past 12 months (such as grants or research support, employee, consultant, stock holder, member of speakers bureau, etc.). The University of Virginia School of Medicine will employ appropriate mechanisms to resolve potential conflicts of interest to maintain the standards of fair and balanced education to the reader. Questions about specific strategies can be directed to the Office of Continuing Medical Education, University of Virginia School of Medicine, Charlottesville, Virginia.

The faculty and staff of the University of Virginia Office of Continuing Medical Education have no financial affiliations to disclose.

The authors/editors listed below have identified no professional or financial affiliations for themselves or their spouse/partner:

Nancy E. Avis, PhD; Joyce T. Bromberger, PhD; Claudia U. Chae, MD, MPH; Sybil Crawford, PhD; Sheila Dugan, MD; Joel S. Finkelstein, MD; Ellen B. Gold, PhD; Robin Green, PSYD; Gail A. Greendale, MD; Siobán D. Harlow, PhD; Carla Holloway, (Acquisitions Editor); William Irvin, MD (Test Author); Howard M. Kravitz, DO, MPH; Bill L. Lasley, PhD; Pauline M. Maki, PhD; Daniel S. McConnell, PhD; Pangaja Paramsothy, MPH; John F. Randolph, Jr., MD; William F. Rayburn, MD, MBA (Consulting Editor); MaryFran R. Sowers, PhD; Barbara Sternfeld, PhD; Kim Sutton-Tyrrell, PhD; Rebecca C. Thurston, PhD; and Rachel P. Wildman, PhD.

The authors/editors listed below identified the following professional or financial affiliations for themselves or their spouse/partner:

Sherri-Ann M. Burnett-Bowie, MD, MPH is an industry funded research/investigator for Amgen.
Carol A. Derby, PhD is an industry funded research/investigator for Bristol Meyers-Squibb.
Hadine Joffe, MD, MSc is an industry funded research/investigator for Bayer HealthCare Pharmaceuticals, Forest Laboratories, and GlaxoSmithKline, and is a consultant for Pfizer.
Joan C. Lo, MD is an industry funded research/investigator for Amgen, Johnson and Johnson, and GlaxoSmithKline.
Nanette Santoro, MD (Guest Editor) is a stock and patent holder with Menogenix.

Disclosure of Discussion of Non-FDA Approved Uses for Pharmaceutical Products and/or Medical Devices:

The University of Virginia School of Medicine, as an ACCME provider, requires that all faculty presenters identify and disclose any off-label uses for pharmaceutical and medical device products. The University of Virginia School of Medicine recommends that each physician fully review all the available data on new products or procedures prior to clinical use.

TO ENROLL

To enroll in the Obstetrics and Gynecology Clinics of North America Continuing Medical Education program, call customer service at 1-800-654-2452 or visit us online at www.theclinics.com/home/cme. The CME program is available to subscribers for an additional fee of $180.00.

Contributors

CONSULTING EDITOR

WILLIAM F. RAYBURN, MD, MBA
Randolph Seligman Professor and Chair, Department of Obstetrics and Gynecology; Chief of Staff, University Hospital, University of New Mexico Health Science Center, Albuquerque, New Mexico

GUEST EDITOR

NANETTE SANTORO, MD,
Professor and E Stewart Taylor Chair, Obstetrics & Gynecology University of Colorado School of Medicine, Anschutz Medical Campus, Aurora, Colorado

AUTHORS

NANCY E. AVIS, PhD
Professor, Department of Social Sciences and Health Policy, Division of Public Health Sciences, Wake Forest University School of Medicine, Winston-Salem, North Carolina

JOYCE T. BROMBERGER, PhD
Associate Professor, Departments of Epidemiology and Psychiatry, University of Pittsburgh, Pittsburgh, Pennsylvania

SHERRI-ANN M. BURNETT-BOWIE, MD, MPH
Assistant Professor of Medicine, Harvard Medical School; Physician, Massachusetts General Hospital, Boston, Massachusetts

CLAUDIA U. CHAE, MD, MPH
Instructor in Medicine, Harvard Medical School, Division of Cardiology, Massachusetts General Hospital, Boston, Massachusetts

SYBIL CRAWFORD, PhD
Department of Medicine, Division of Preventive and Behavioral Medicine, University of Massachusetts, Worcester, Massachusetts

CAROL A. DERBY, PhD
Associate Professor, Departments of Neurology, Epidemiology and Population Health, Albert Einstein College of Medicine, Bronx, New York

SHEILA DUGAN, MD
Associate Professor, Department of Physical Medicine and Rehabilitation and Preventive Medicine, Rush University Medical Center, Chicago, Illinois

JOEL S. FINKELSTEIN, MD
Associate Professor of Medicine, Harvard Medical School; Physician, Massachusetts General Hospital, Boston, Massachusetts

ELLEN B. GOLD, PhD
Professor of Epidemiology and Chair, Department of Public Health Sciences, School of Medicine, University of California, Davis, California

ROBIN GREEN, PSYD
Assistant Professor of Obstetrics, Gynecology and Women's Health, Department of Obstetrics, Gynecology and Women's Health, Albert Einstein College of Medicine, Bronx, New York

GAIL A. GREENDALE, MD
Division of Geriatrics, David Geffen School of Medicine, University of California, Los Angeles, Los Angeles, California

HADINE JOFFE, MD, MSc
Assistant Professor, Director of Research, Department of Psychiatry, Center for Women's Mental Health, Massachusetts General Hospital, Harvard Medical School, Boston, Massachusetts

SIOBÁN D. HARLOW, PhD
Professor, Department of Epidemiology, University of Michigan, Ann Arbor, Michigan

HOWARD M. KRAVITZ, DO, MPH
Professor, Departments of Psychiatry and Preventive Medicine, Rush University Medical Center, Chicago, Illinois

BILL L. LASLEY, PhD
Professor Emeritus, Center for Population Health and the Environment, University of California at Davis, Davis, California

JOAN C. LO, MD
Research Scientist, Division of Research, Kaiser Permanente Northern California, Oakland; Associate Clinical Professor of Medicine, University of California San Francisco, San Francisco, California

PAULINE M. MAKI, PhD
Associate Professor of Psychiatry and Psychology, Department of Psychiatry and Psychology, Center for Cognitive Medicine, University of Illinois at Chicago, College of Medicine, Chicago, Illinois

DANIEL S. McCONNELL, PhD
Department of Epidemiology, University of Michigan, Ann Arbor, Michigan

PANGAJA PARAMSOTHY, MPH
Doctoral Candidate, Department of Epidemiology, University of Michigan, Ann Arbor, Michigan

JOHN F. RANDOLPH JR, MD
Professor, Director, Department of Obstetrics and Gynecology, Division of Reproductive Endocrinology, University of Michigan, Ann Arbor, Michigan

NANETTE SANTORO, MD
Professor and E Stewart Taylor Chair, Obstetrics & Gynecology University of Colorado School of Medicine, Anschutz Medical Campus, Aurora, Colorado

†MARYFRAN R. SOWERS, PhD
John G. Searle Professor of Public Health; Adjunct Professor, Internal Medicine; Adjunct Professor, Obstetrics/Gynecology; Professor, Epidemiology, Director, Center for Integrated Approaches to Complex Diseases, University of Michigan School of Public Health, Ann Arbor, Michigan

BARBARA STERNFELD, PhD
Senior Research Scientist, Division of Research, Kaiser Permanente, Oakland, California

KIM SUTTON-TYRRELL, PhD
Professor and Vice-Chair for Academics, Department of Epidemiology, University of Pittsburgh, Pittsburgh, Pennsylvania

REBECCA C. THURSTON, PhD
Assistant Professor, Department of Psychiatry, University of Pittsburgh School of Medicine; Assistant Professor, Department of Epidemiology, University of Pittsburgh Graduate School of Public Health, Pittsburgh, Pennsylvania

RACHEL P. WILDMAN, PhD
Associate Professor, Department of Epidemiology & Population Health, Albert Einstein College of Medicine, Jack and Pearl Resnick Campus, Bronx, New York[1]

[†] Deceased.

Contents

Reproductive health can be a reflection of overall health. It follows that abnormalities of reproductive milestones may be a manifestation of unhealthy aging. Since 1994, the Study of Women's Health Across the Nation (SWAN) has assessed how menopause and the process of that transition may affect future health. Themes have emerged from SWAN associating patterns of hormones and symptoms with metabolic status. The nature of these relationships vary as women traverse the menopause and ovarian hormone production ceases. This review describes these cross-cutting themes and their possible meaning for the health of the mid-life woman.

The timing of natural menopause is a clinically important indicator of longevity and risk of morbidity and mortality. Demographic, menstrual, reproductive, familial, genetic, and lifestyle factors seem to be important in this timing. Smoking, lower parity and poor socioeconomic status are associated with earlier menopause. However, a number of relationships have been inconsistent; others remain largely unexplored. Much remains to be learned about factors that affect follicular atresia and the onset and duration of perimenopause and the timing of the natural menopause. Knowledge about these relationships offers women and their health care providers enhanced understanding and choices to deal with menopause.

This review summarizes the published literature on the potentially circular relationship between adiposity and the menopause. Although

---

† Deceased.

data are limited, current information suggests there are substantial effects of obesity and adiposity on the magnitude of hormone changes experienced during the transition, as well as on the risks of chronic disease resulting from the menopause transition. However, evidence regarding the reverse, namely, effects of the menopause transition and its associated hormone changes on weight gain and redistribution of body fat, are inconclusive.

The hormonal correlates of reproductive aging and the menopause transition reflect an initial loss of the follicle cohort, while a responsive ovary remains, and an eventual complete loss of follicle response, with persistent hypergonadotropic amenorrhea. The physiology of the process is described, along with key findings of relevant studies, with an emphasis on the Study of Women's Health Across the Nation. A clinical framework is provided to help clinicians to forecast the major milestones of the menopausal transition and to predict potential symptoms or disease.

The concept that adrenal androgen production gradually declines with age has changed after analysis of longitudinal data from the Study of Women's Health Across the Nation (SWAN). It is now recognized that 4 adrenal androgens rise during the menopausal transition in most women. Ethnic and individual differences in sex steroids are more apparent in circulating adrenal steroids than in either estradiol or cyclic ovarian steroid hormone profiles, particularly during the early and late perimenopause. Thus, adrenal steroid production may play a larger role in the occurrence of symptoms and the potential for healthier aging than previously recognized.

The incidence of cardiovascular disease, which is the leading single cause of death among women, increases substantially after menopause. This may be related to adverse changes in cardiovascular risk factors that occur during the menopausal transition. Proatherogenic changes in lipid and apolipoprotein profiles seem to be specifically related to ovarian aging; unfavorable changes in other cardiovascular risk factors may be influenced more by chronologic aging. Whether these changes are due to aging or to menopause itself, increased attention to risk factor modification in the pre- and perimenopausal years will help reduce future cardiovascular disease risk among women.

> Vasomotor symptoms (VMS), or hot flashes and night sweats, are often considered the cardinal symptoms of menopause. SWAN, one of the largest and most ethnically diverse longitudinal studies of the menopausal transition, has allowed unique insights into VMS. Specifically, SWAN has helped yield important information about the prevalence of, racial/ethnic differences in, risk factors for, and implications of VMS for midlife women's mental and physical health. We have reviewed the literature on VMS, emphasizing findings that have emerged from SWAN and new areas of inquiry in the area of VMS.

> Loss of ovarian function has a profound impact on female skeletal health. Bone mineral density findings from the Study of Women's Health Across the Nation demonstrate an accelerated rate of bone loss during the menopausal transition. The greatest reduction occurs in the year before the final menstrual period and the first 2 years thereafter. Clinical management includes maintenance of adequate dietary calcium and vitamin D intake, attention to modifiable risk factors, and osteoporosis screening. Indications, benefits, and risks of pharmacologic osteoporosis therapy should be assessed individually; there are currently no established guidelines addressing the treatment and prevention of osteoporosis in perimenopausal women.

> The impact of perimenopause on cognition seems to be characterized by an absence of improved scores rather than a decline. In the SWAN, the perimenopausal decrement in cognitive performance was not accounted for; however, increases in anxiety and depressive symptoms had independent, unfavorable effects on performance. Estradiol has been found to protect against changes resulting from serotonin withdrawal and defend against changes from cholinergic depletion. There is support for the critical timing hypothesis—that estrogen benefits cognitive function when instituted early, but not later. The menopausal transition may affect cognitive function in older age owing to worsened cardiovascular risk factors.

> The benefits of regular physical activity are well established, but evidence for a protective effect against the adverse health conse-

quences accompanying the menopausal transition is limited. This article reviews that evidence, concluding that more physical activity is generally associated with fewer somatic and mood symptoms. Physical activity seems to minimize weight gain and changes in body composition and fat distribution experienced at midlife and might attenuate the rapid bone density loss that occurs. Given these benefits, clinicians treating perimenopausal women should encourage their patients to follow guidelines for physical activity (≥150 minutes a week of moderate intensity activity).

Is there evidence for a perimenopausal sleep disorder? We address this question in our presentation of the Study of Women's Health Across the Nation (SWAN) "sleep story," in which we summarize and discuss data addressing sleep quality, objective measures of sleep patterns, and sleep disorders that have been published to date by the SWAN and the ancillary SWAN Sleep Study. We describe what has been learned about sleep during the perimenopause. Analyses exploring racial/ethnic diversity and the role of hot flashes and mood disturbance in sleep—perimenopause associations are described. Implications for clinical practice are considered.

Sexual functioning is an important component of women's lives. Sexual functioning, however, declines with age, and there is much debate about the contribution of menopause to sexual activity and functioning. The present article covers cross-sectional and longitudinal community-based research on sexual functioning during the perimenopause. The article addresses the relative contributions of perimenopause and other factors (eg, relationship with partner, previous sexual enjoyment, psychosocial factors and health) to sexual functioning.

This paper characterizes changes in menstrual bleeding during perimenopause, including bleeding changes that represent markers of the menopausal transition. Recent results from the Study of Women's Health Across the Nation and other cohort studies are reviewed. Emerging data describing subpopulation differences in the transition experience are highlighted. When treating women in the midlife, clinicians should pay careful attention to medical factors, including both conditions and treatments, that may increase menstrual blood loss or alter menstrual cycle characteristics sufficiently to obscure the onset of the menopausal transition or the final menstrual period.

Women are twice as likely as men to suffer from depressive symptoms/disorder. Research has focused on physiologic and psychosocial differences between men and women; an important target of study has been periods of reproductive changes. Controversy has existed regarding the extent to which the menopausal transition or postmenopause increases the risk for depressive symptoms/disorders. This paper presents findings from analyses of data from the SWAN study and an ancillary study on mental health. We found that risk for high depressive symptoms and disorder is greater during and possibly after the menopausal transition. Other factors contribute to risk for depression.

THE CLINICS ARE NOW AVAILABLE ONLINE!

Access your subscription at:
www.theclinics.com

Foreword
Perimenopause

This issue of the *Obstetrics and Gynecology Clinics*, edited by Nanette Santoro, MD, provides an important update about the perimenopause and its impact on American women. A clearer picture of this transition period is provided by the authors using survey results from women through the National Institutes of Health's funded Study of Women's Health Across the Nation (SWAN). Menopause is the permanent cessation of any vaginal bleeding. Those years before menopause that encompass the change from normal ovulatory cycles to the cessation of menses are known as the perimenopause or the menopausal transition. The median age for the onset of the perimenopause process is 47–48 years, while this transition period from reproductive to postreproductive status lasts between 2 to 8 years for most women.

Throughout the perimenopause, vaginal bleeding results from an increasing dysfunction of ovulation with a proliferating endometrium from estrogen effects not fully modulated by progesterone. Most women report hot flushes for up to several years that range daily from less than 1 to more than 15 episodes. In addition to this nuisance, women have frequent concerns about the relation between a lack of estrogen and any potential harm on their mental health, metabolism, coronary artery function, cancer risk, and bone integrity.

This *Obstetrics and Gynecology Clinics* issue addresses many of these health issues common to an aging female population. For example, the perimenopause and menopause are not supported by the medical literature to have a deleterious effect on mental health. Emotional stability during this transition period may be disrupted by impaired sleep resulting from hot flushes. Supplemental estrogen may improve sleep quality by shortening the time to sleep onset and by increasing the proportion of sleep that is rapid eye movement. Estrogen is also believed to protect against neuronal cytotoxicity by several mechanisms. Beneficial effects from estrogen supplementation have been reported on cognition, especially verbal memory. Any positive influences are likely only in select populations and of very limited value, especially among healthy women.

Reproductive-age women lag behind men in the incidence of coronary heart disease and by 20 years for myocardial infarction and sudden death. After menopause, the risk of coronary heart disease doubles for women, with atherogenic lipid levels rising to levels that are equivalent to or above those in men. A strong correlation exists between the magnitude of weight gained during the perimenopause and a worsening of cardiovascular risk factors (lipid and lipoprotein changes, blood pressure, and insulin levels). Close attention to weight gain is, therefore, a major component of good preventive health care.

The density of bone reflects a balance between osteoclastic and osteoblastic cell activities. Aging and a loss of estrogen are believed to lead to greater osteoclastic activity with a subsequent risk of bone loss. Fractures from osteoporosis depend on peak bone mass and this rate of bone loss after menopause.

As described in this issue, much of what women know about their health is gathered

Obstet Gynecol Clin N Am 38 (2011) xv–xvi
doi:10.1016/j.ogc.2011.07.003
0889-8545/11/$ – see front matter © 2011 Elsevier Inc. All rights reserved.

from the mass media and not from the scientific literature. Common medications available for menopausal women include hormone preparations; selective estrogen receptor modulators; and other compounds such as bisphosphonates, tibolone, human parathyroid hormone 1-34, phytoestrogens, and bioidentical hormones. Subsequent care involves no one hormonal regimen for all but individualization to accommodate a woman's preferences. The symptoms, patient's risk factors, and any family history for certain diseases need to be considered.

Information in this issue represents the opinions of experts in reproductive endocrinology and related fields. Their contributions are noteworthy, especially in addressing patient's preconceived impressions and in providing certain articles that contain useful educational materials. Views expressed here are not absolute, however, but flexible guidelines based on evidence-based medical advice and available local resources.

William F. Rayburn, MD, MBA
Department of Obstetrics and Gynecology
University of New Mexico School of Medicine
MSC 10 5580; 1 University of New Mexico
Albuquerque, NM 87131-0001, USA

E-mail address:
wrayburn@salud.unm.edu

Preface

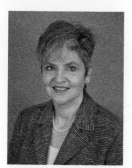

Nanette Santoro, MD
Guest Editor

The Study of Women's Health Across the Nation (SWAN) was begun in 1994 to assess the impact of the menopausal process on American women. It's hard to believe our SWAN is now 17 years old! The SWAN Study is the largest cohort of its kind in the world, and the hours of time and hundreds of thousands of surveys and samples the women in our cohorts have provided are a tremendous gift to science.

In this issue of *Obstetrics and Gynecology Clinics*, we feature the principal findings of the SWAN Study to date. Since the women who entered the longitudinal study were as young as 42 at the onset of recruitment, and recruitment was completed in December of 1997, the youngest women in the cohort at this time are now 56 years old and virtually all have completed their menopausal transition.

The value of the data our dedicated SWAN women have given us are displayed in this issue, which encompasses as much of the breadth and depth of our study as possible. Each group of investigators represented in each article has worked collaboratively with all of the other groups to provide you, the reader, with the clearest picture possible of the menopausal transition. The journey we, the investigators, have taken has often been one of surprise, sometimes incorrect hypotheses, and always deepening insight. I sincerely hope that you share some of our journey and gain new clarity about this incompletely understood process that is universal to all women. This issue is dedicated to the women of SWAN, who have stood up and been counted and continue to participate, year after year.

The SWAN Study has grant support from the National Institutes of Health (NIH), Department of Health and Human Services (DHHS), through the National Institute on Aging (NIA), the National Institute of Nursing Research (NINR), and the NIH Office of Research on Women's Health (ORWH) (Grants NR004061, AG012505, AG012535, AG012531, AG012539, AG012546, AG012553, AG012554, AG012495). The content

doi:10.1016/j.ogc.2011.07.002
0889-8545/11/$ – see front matter © 2011 Elsevier Inc. All rights reserved.
obgyn.theclinics.com

of this article is solely the responsibility of the author and does not necessarily represent the official views of the NIA, NINR, ORWH, or NIH.

Nanette Santoro, MD
University of Colorado School of Medicine
Anschutz Medical Campus
12631 East 17th Avenue
Mail Stop B-198
Academic Office 1, Room 4010
Aurora, CO 80045, USA

E-mail address:
Nanette.santoro@ucdenver.edu

Dedication

This issue is dedicated to the memory of MaryFran Sowers, PhD.

The SWAN Song: Study of Women's Health Across the Nation's Recurring Themes

Nanette Santoro, MD[a],*, Kim Sutton-Tyrrell, PhD[b]

KEYWORDS

- Menopause • Menopause transition • Metabolic syndrome
- Hot flashes • Estrogen • Progesterone

Menopause transects the aging process in women and presents an immediate dilemma for health care providers, who are often prevailed upon to determine whether or not a specific symptom or problem is attributable to the ovarian hormonal changes associated with menopause or simply to the aging process. Whereas the former is sometimes treatable with hormone therapy or other nonhormonal remedy that addresses the lack of ovarian function, the latter problems are often irreversible and only addressed by strategies designed to treat or delay the development of a chronic condition. It is therefore important for clinicians to have as clear as possible a categorization of the menopausal process and attribution of symptoms. In addition, the development of chronic diseases of aging should be predicted and addressed in mid-life women. This preface discusses the overall impact of menopause and the menopausal transition on women's health, and identifies the impacts of common modifiable (obesity, lifestyle) and nonmodifiable (ethnicity) conditions on the process of menopause and subsequent health and risks for disease, principally cardiovascular disease.

DOES AGE AT MENOPAUSE INFLUENCE THE LIFESPAN?

It is tempting to speculate that reproductive health is a reflection of overall health. If so, it follows that women who experience early menopause are likely to be less

Dr Nanette Santoro holds stock options in Menogenix.

The Study of Women's Health Across the Nation (SWAN) has grant support from the National Institutes of Health (NIH), DHHS, through the National Institute on Aging (NIA), the National Institute of Nursing Research (NINR) and the NIH Office of Research on Women's Health (ORWH) (Grants NR004061; AG012505, AG012535, AG012531, AG012539, AG012546, AG012553, AG012554, AG012495). The content of this manuscript is solely the responsibility of the authors and does not necessarily represent the official views of the NIA, NINR, ORWH or the NIH.

[a] Department of Obstetrics and Gynecology, University of Colorado School of Medicine, Anschutz Medical Campus, 12631 East 17th Avenue, Mail Stop B-198, Academic Office 1, Room 4010, Aurora, CO 80045, USA

[b] Department of Epidemiology, 505A Parran Hall, University of Pittsburgh, Pittsburgh, PA 15261, USA

* Corresponding author.

E-mail address: Nanette.Santoro@ucdenver.edu

healthy and women with late menopause are more likely to be healthy. Although there are limited data to support this concept, it is at best an oversimplification. Cooper and Sandler,[1] using data from the National Health and Nutrition Examination Study, observed an increased adjusted mortality rate ratio of 1.50 (95% confidence interval [CI], 0.97–2.34) for women with a natural menopause earlier than age 40, with an increased risk of cancer-related mortality (adjusted rate ratio, 2.34; 95% CI, 1.20–4.58). Data from the Women's Ischemia Syndrome Evaluation indicates that hypogonadotropic, hypoestrogenic amenorrhea before the age of natural menopause is strongly related to cardiovascular disease risk (odds ratio [OR], 7.4; 95% CI, 1.7–33.3).[2] Another recent evaluation of 2509 women from the Multi-Ethnic Study of Atherosclerosis observed an association between early menopause (age ≤45 years) and cardiovascular disease, stroke, and coronary heart disease-related death.[3]

These studies have been based on association, and cannot determine causality. Data from the Framingham study of cardiovascular risk imply that the widely accepted causal inference that loss of estrogen owing to menopause results in increased heart disease may be incorrect, or is at least an oversimplification. These investigators studied 695 women who were premenopausal at the onset of the Framingham study and who underwent menopause during follow-up. They found that each premenopausal 1% increase in Framingham score was associated with a decrease in menopausal age of 1.8 years.[4] Thus, it is possible that adverse cardiovascular risk predisposes women to earlier loss of ovarian function.

Ethnicity is also related to timing of menopause and the risk for surgical menopause. African-American women are more likely to undergo hysterectomy and surgical menopause,[5] whereas Hispanic women are more likely to undergo early or premature natural menopause.[6]

If early menopause predicts early mortality, then it may follow that late menopause predicts longevity. In one study that has examined this question, the life expectancy for a woman who underwent menopause at age 55 was 2 years longer than a woman who underwent menopause at age 40.[7] Women who underwent later menopause seemed to be at greater risk for breast and endometrial cancers, but an overall lesser risk of coronary heart disease. This observation implies that a prolonged reproductive life span results in risks that must be balanced against the acquired (or preexisting) risks that predispose a woman to earlier menopause. Thus, there may be an optimal window for menopause that balances these 2 competing risks. It is interesting that, despite dramatic increases in overall health and longevity in industrialized populations over the past century, there has only been a small delay in the age at menopause. Taken together, these data imply that age at menopause is not a major predictor of the life span.

In contrast with women who have undergone natural menopause, women with surgical removal of their ovaries seem to suffer increased morbidity from a number of causes. In an ongoing cohort study of more than 1000 women who underwent premenopausal bilateral oophorectomy, more congestive heart failure, stroke, fracture, Parkinsonism, cognitive impairment, dementia, depression and anxiety were observed compared to 2400 controls.[8] Interestingly, when mortality was examined within this cohort, the only group that seemed to have significantly increased mortality was women who underwent prophylactic bilateral oophorectomy before age 45.[9] Use of hormone therapy did not uniformly prevent subsequent morbidities.

A BRIEF DESCRIPTION OF THE STUDY OF WOMEN'S HEALTH ACROSS THE NATION

The Study of Women's Health Across the Nation (SWAN) is a multicenter, multi-ethnic, longitudinal study designed to characterize the physiologic and psychosocial

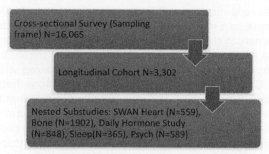

Fig. 1. SWAN Cohort Assembly. A cross-sectional survey of 16,065 women was conducted, from which most sites drew their samples for the longitudinal study (3302 women at baseline). The various substudies within SWAN are listed in this figure, with their initial sample sizes. Details of the SWAN cohort assembly and design are available through reference.[32]

changes that occur during the menopausal transition and to observe their effects on subsequent health and risk factors for age-related diseases. A total of 3302 women were enrolled at 7 clinical sites between 1996 and 1997. At the time of enrollment, women were premenopausal, not taking hormones, and between 42 and 52 years of age. Participants self-identified as African American (28%), Caucasian (47%), Chinese (8%), Hispanic (8%), or Japanese (9%). Women were followed annually for 10 years and are now being followed every other year with the year 14 visit set to begin in the fall of 2011 (**Fig. 1**).

SWAN has a multidisciplinary focus and thus has repeated measures of bone health, cardiovascular risk factors, psychosocial factors, and ovarian hormones. Thus, SWAN is compiling the most comprehensive characterization to date of the health and the physiologic and psychosocial changes of women from premenopause to postmenopause in a community-based sample. SWAN is now poised to study the effects of these menopause-related changes on subsequent healthy aging and on age-related diseases in the post-reproductive period; we are focusing on outcomes such as fractures, depression, subclinical cardiovascular disease, cardiovascular events, and physical and cognitive functioning.

ETHNICITY IS RELATED TO MANY OUTCOMES

The SWAN cohort includes Caucasian women at all sites, African-American women at 4 sites, and non-Mexican Hispanic, Chinese-American, and Japanese-American women each from a single site. Because ethnic minority groups were not recruited from all sites, there is the potential for site-to-site variation that can influence risks and outcomes. Indeed, SWAN outcomes vary by site as well as by ethnicity. Site variation is even observed among the Caucasian and African-American groups. SWAN data are therefore often presented with statistical adjustments for these site and ethnic associations.

African-American women are more likely to report heavy menstrual bleeding and to undergo hysterectomy.[5] Hispanic women are more likely to develop metabolic syndrome and incident type 2 diabetes mellitus. When bone density is examined as a function of ethnicity, and statistical adjustments are made for body mass index (BMI), non-Hispanic Caucasian women have been found to have the lowest bone density in the cohort.[10] These key findings of SWAN will be presented along with each contribution to this issue.

There are also several nuances within the ethnic groups in SWAN. The Hispanic subgroup, for example, is a mixture of Central/South American, Cuban, Puerto Rican, and Dominican women. Within the group of Hispanic women, there is also evidence of variation. Puerto Rican women had the highest rate of the metabolic syndrome, anxiety, and depression[11,12] and trouble sleeping[13] compared with other Hispanic women, whereas Central American women reported more frequent vasomotor symptoms than other subgroups.[13] This was despite the fact that the Puerto Rican participants in SWAN were more likely to report greater acculturation.[12]

A second complication arises when there is little or no overlap between traits found in different ethnic groups. BMI is such an example. African-American women have the highest mean BMI in SWAN, and in the highest BMI categories, there are few to no Chinese and/or Japanese Americans. Yet BMI clearly modifies several key SWAN-related outcomes. Among these are hot flashes. African-American and Hispanic women are the 2 highest BMI groups in SWAN and reported more frequent and severe hot flashes than other ethnic groups at baseline.[14] Separating the ethnic contribution from the BMI-associated contribution to hot flashes becomes challenging when the between group differences are large.

SOCIOECONOMIC STATUS IS RELATED TO MANY OUTCOMES

A second theme that has emerged from SWAN is that relative economic well-being, education, and financial security (or lack thereof) are related to outcomes and risks. SWAN utilizes several methods for determining socioeconomic status (SES). Educational level is one variable. Economic strain is assessed by a question that addresses the degree of difficulty the participant experiences in paying for the basic necessities of life (food, clothing, shelter). Adverse life events are also assessed. Primary outcomes of SWAN are related to SES. Women of low SES are more likely to experience early menopause.[15,16] Factors associated with low SES (financial strain, adverse life events, poor social support) are also related to increased depressive symptoms[17] and to menopausal symptoms.[18]

Women of lower SES who are not within the SWAN cohort are more likely to experience early menopause, and seem to have more and worse symptoms. This is consistent with other studies that have evaluated the effects of SES on the menopause transition. In a cohort study of perimenopausal women in the Bronx, half of whom were HIV infected and half of whom used street drugs, the median age at menopause was found to be 46 to 47 years, substantially younger than 51.4 years, the median age at the final menstrual period in SWAN.[16,19] Thus, the menopausal experience is likely to be more difficult for women in vulnerable groups.

BMI IS ASSOCIATED WITH HORMONE LEVELS AND STUDY OUTCOMES

Weight gain has long been observed to occur in conjunction with the menopausal transition, but studies before SWAN have concluded that weight gain is driven primarily by age. SWAN has been able to identify specific aspects of the transition that contribute to weight gain over and above age. We have found that higher androgens, lower sex hormone binding globulin, surgical menopause, and early hormone therapy use are all key factors associated with the development of obesity and/or severe obesity. Results also underscore the importance of physical activity as a preventive strategy for weight gain.[20]

The link between body weight and hormone levels is another interesting phenomenon that SWAN has been able to shed light on. The median adjusted BMI of the women in SWAN was 27.3 kg/m^2 at the study baseline visit.[21] Higher BMI is associated with worse vasomotor symptoms as women traverse the menopause,[22] but this relationship may change once women become postmenopausal.[23] High BMI is also related to the trajectory of reproductive hormones across the transition. Women of high BMI have lower gonadotropin and estradiol levels before the menopause, and have a lesser decline in estradiol associated with the transition.[24] BMI is related to mood, symptoms, and hormones as well as the metabolic syndrome and cardiovascular risk factors in SWAN.

The relationship of BMI and several key SWAN outcomes seems to change as women complete the transition into menopause. This is explainable by the fact that adipose tissue causes increased peripheral estrogen production from hormone precursors. When the ovary is still producing estrogen, before menopause, the contribution of adiposity to the total body estrogen pool is minimal. However, once the ovary becomes essentially inactive after menopause, the adipose contribution to the total body estrogen pool becomes biologically significant. This may account for the greater risk of vasomotor symptoms in obese women before menopause (owing perhaps to increased insulation of the body by fat), and a loss of this relationship after menopause (owing to a contribution of peripheral conversion to estrogens by adipose tissue).

The metabolic syndrome was present in almost 14% of the women in SWAN by the time of the final menstrual period.[25] Incident metabolic syndrome is predicted by stage of perimenopause, androgens, and the testosterone to estradiol ratio—an index of relative androgen excess.[25,26] After menopause, the risk of developing metabolic syndrome seems to decrease. There thus seems to be a contribution of menopause apart from aging per se on the development of the metabolic syndrome.

LATE PERIMENOPAUSE AS A CRITICAL TIME WHEN THE BIOLOGICAL EFFECTS OF THE TRANSITION ARE CONSISTENTLY OBSERVED

One of the most consistent findings across SWAN has been that late perimenopause (3 months of amenorrhea) seems to be the time frame that coincides most strongly with both symptoms and measureable physiologic changes across all health areas. Transition to late perimenopause was the strongest predictor of vasomotor symptoms.[14] From a bone health perspective, SWAN has shown that bone loss accelerates substantially in the late perimenopause to an average loss of $0.018g/cm^2$ per year in the spine and $0.010 g/cm^2$ per year in the hip.[27] From a psychosocial perspective, women with a low Center for Epidemiologic Studies Depression Scale score at baseline had significantly higher odds of depressive symptoms when they reached the late perimenopause.[28] In addition, in an evaluation of depression and inflammatory markers, late perimenopausal women had elevated factor VIIC, fibrinogen, and tissue type plasminogen activator antigen levels, suggesting that the late perimenopause may be uniquely associated with alterations in hemostasis.[29] The prevalence of sleep difficulty was also found to be greatest in the late perimenopausal stage. Most important, this finding was independent of the effects of vasomotor symptoms.[30] Finally, from a cardiovascular perspective, late perimenopausal and postmenopausal women were found to have larger common carotid artery lumen and adventitial diameters than premenopausal and early perimenopausal women. This suggests that declining estrogen levels are associated with remodeling or adaptation of the vasculature.[31]

SUMMARY

The SWAN study has provided a tremendous amount of insight into the many determinants and interactions that predict health and wellness as well as disease risk in midlife women. Major factors that influence risk include race/ethnicity, SES, adverse life events, and BMI—particularly metabolically unhealthy obesity. Because most of the cohort has now completed the transition into menopause, we anticipate that there will be changes in the risk factors for disease and that we will be able to track health outcomes in greater numbers.

REFERENCES

1. Cooper GS, Sandler DP. Age at natural menopause and mortality. Ann Epidemiol 1998;8:229–35.
2. Bairey Merz CN, Johnson BD, Sharaf BL, et al. Hypoestrogenemia of hypothalamic origin and coronary artery disease in premenopausal women: a report from the NHLBI-sponsored WISE study. J Am Coll Cardiol 2003;41:413–9.
3. Wellons MD, Vaidya MD, Herrington D, et al. Early menopause is associated with cardiovascular disease events: the Multi-Ethnic Study of Atherosclerosis (MESA). The Endocrine Society, Annual Meeting, San Diego, CA, 2010.
4. Kok HS, van Asselt KM, van der Schouw YT, et al. Heart disease risk determines menopausal age rather than the reverse. J Am Coll Cardiol 2006;47:1976–83.
5. Powell LH, Meyer P, Weiss G, et al. Ethnic differences in past hysterectomy for benign conditions. Womens Health Issues 2005;15:179–86.
6. Luborsky JL, Meyer P, Sowers MF, et al. Premature menopause in a multi-ethnic population study of the menopause transition. Hum Reprod 2003;18:199.
7. Ossewaarde ME, Bots ML, Verbeek AL, et al. Age at menopause, cause-specific mortality and total life expectancy. Epidemiology 2005;16:556–62.
8. Parker WH, Jacoby V, Shoupe D, et al. Effect of bilateral oophorectomy on women's long-term health. Womens Health (Lond Engl) 2009;5:565–76.
9. Rocca WA, Grossardt BR, de Andrade M, et al. Survival patterns after oophorectomy in premenopausal women: a population-based cohort study. Lancet Oncol 2006;7:821–8.
10. Finkelstein JS, Lee ML, Sowers M, et al. Ethnic variation in bone density in premenopausal and early perimenopausal women: effects of anthropometric and lifestyle factors. J Clin Endocrinol Metab 2002;87:3057–67.
11. Derby CA, Wildman RP, McGinn AP, et al. Cardiovascular risk factor variation within a Hispanic cohort: SWAN, the Study of Women's Health Across the Nation. Ethn Dis 2010;20:396–402.
12. Green R, Santoro NF, McGinn AP, et al. The relationship between psychosocial status, acculturation and country of origin in mid-life Hispanic women: data from the Study of Women's Health Across the Nation (SWAN). Climacteric 2010;3:534–43.
13. Green R, Polotsky AJ, Wildman RP, et al. Menopausal symptoms within a Hispanic cohort: SWAN, the Study of Women's Health Across the Nation. Climacteric 2010;13:376–84.
14. Gold EB, Colvin AB, Avis N, et al. Longitudinal analysis of the association between vasomotor symptoms and race/ethnicity across the menopausal transition: Study of Women's Health Across the Nation. Am J Public Health 2006;96:1226–35.
15. Luoto R, Kaprio J, Uutela A. Age at natural menopause and sociodemographic status in Finland. Am J Epidemiol 1994;139:64–76.
16. Schoenbaum EE, Hartel D, Lo Y, et al. HIV infection, drug use, and onset of natural menopause. Clin Infect Dis 2005;41:1517–24.
17. Bromberger JT, Harlow S, Avis N, et al. Racial/ethnic differences in the prevalence of depressive symptoms among middle-aged women: The Study of Women's Health Across the Nation (SWAN). Am J Public Health 2004;94:1378–85.

18. Gold EB, Block G, Crawford S, et al. Lifestyle and demographic factors in relation to vasomotor symptoms: baseline results from the Study of Women's Health Across the Nation. Am J Epidemiol 2004;159:1189–99.

19. Gold EB, Bromberger J, Crawford S, et al. Factors associated with age at natural menopause in a multiethnic sample of midlife women. Am J Epidemiol 2001;153: 865–74.

20. Sutton-Tyrrell K, Zhao X, Santoro N, et al. Reproductive hormones and obesity: 9 years of observation from the Study of Women's Health Across the Nation. Am J Epidemiol 2010;171:1203–13.

21. Santoro NF. What a SWAN can teach us about menopause. Contemporary Ob/Gyn 2004;49:69.

22. Greendale GA, Gold EB. Lifestyle factors: are they related to vasomotor symptoms and do they modify the effectiveness or side effects of hormone therapy? Am J Med 2005;118(Suppl 12B):148–54.

23. Hyde Riley E, Inui TS, Kleinman K, et al. Differential association of modifiable health behaviors with hot flashes in perimenopausal and postmenopausal women. J Gen Intern Med 2004;19:740–6.

24. Randolph JF Jr, Zheng H, Sowers MR, et al. Change in follicle-stimulating hormone and estradiol across the menopausal transition: effect of age at the final menstrual period. J Clin Endocrinol Metab 2011;96:746–54.

25. Janssen I, Powell LH, Crawford S, et al. Menopause and the metabolic syndrome: the Study of Women's Health Across the Nation. Arch Intern Med 2008;168:1568–75.

26. Torrens JI, Sutton-Tyrrell K, Zhao X, et al. Relative androgen excess during the menopausal transition predicts incident metabolic syndrome in midlife women: study of Women's Health Across the Nation. Menopause 2009;16:257–64.

27. Finkelstein JS, Brockwell SE, Mehta V, et al. Bone mineral density changes during the menopause transition in a multiethnic cohort of women. J Clin Endocrinol Metab 2008;93:861–8.

28. Bromberger JT, Kravitz HM, Matthews KA, et al. Lifetime episodes of major and minor depression in midlife women. Psychol Med 2008;39:55–64.

29. Matthews KA, Schott LL, Bromberger J, et al. Associations between depressive symptoms and inflammatory/hemostatic markers in women during the menopausal transition. Psychosom Med 2007;69:124–30.

30. Kravitz HM, Ganz PA, Bromberger J, et al. Sleep difficulty in women at midlife: a community survey of sleep and the menopausal transition. Menopause 2003;10: 19–28.

31. Wildman RP, Colvin AB, Powell LH, et al. Associations of endogenous sex hormones with vasculature in menopausal women: the Study of Women's Health Across the Nation (SWAN). Menopause 2008;15:414–21.

32. Sowers M, Crawford S, Sternfeld B, et al. Design, survey sampling and recruitment methods of SWAN: a mutli-center, multi-ethnic, community-based cohort study of women and the menopausal transition. In: Kelsey J, Lobo RA, Marcus R, editors. Menopause: biology and pathobiology. San Diego: Academic Press; 2000. p. 175.

The Timing of the Age at Which Natural Menopause Occurs

Ellen B. Gold, PhD

KEYWORDS

- Menopause • Smoking • Parity • Race/ethnicity
- Socioeconomic status • Age • Genetics • Family history
- Diet

The age at the final menstrual period holds intrinsic clinical and public health interest because the age at which natural menopause occurs may be a marker of aging and health.[1–3] Later age at natural menopause has been associated with:

- longer overall survival and greater life expectancy[4] and reduced all-cause mortality[5];
- reduced risk of cardiovascular disease[4,6–11] and mortality from cardiovascular[12] and ischemic heart disease,[13] stroke,[14] angina after myocardial infarction,[15] and atherosclerosis[16];
- less loss of bone density,[17] and a reduced risk of osteoporosis[18] and fracture[19];
- but an increased risk of breast,[20,21] endometrial, and ovarian[4,22–25] cancers.

In addition, women who have undergone bilateral oophorectomy under the age of 45 years have been observed to be at increased risk of mortality from cardiovascular disease, particularly if they were not treated with estrogen.[26] However, women who underwent natural menopause before age 45 years had an increased risk of ischemic heart disease that was not attenuated by use of hormone therapy.[27] Further, early menopause has been associated with earlier decline in cognitive function.[28–30] Because 40 million women in the United States alone and several hundred million worldwide[31] experienced the menopausal transition between 1990 and 2010 due to the aging of the baby boomer generation,[32] millions of women are undergoing or have recently undergone the menopause transition, and the timing of their final natural menstrual periods could have important clinical and health implications, because one third of women's lives is spent postmenopause.

Although menopause is a universal phenomenon among women, the timing of the onset and the duration of the menopausal transition and the timing of the final menstrual period are not.[33] Most of our knowledge and perceptions of menopause

Department of Public Health Sciences and Division of Epidemiology, School of Medicine, University of California, Davis, One Shields Avenue, Med Sci 1C, Davis, CA 95616 USA
E-mail address: ebgold@ucdavis.edu

Obstet Gynecol Clin N Am 38 (2011) 425–440
doi:10.1016/j.ogc.2011.05.002
0889-8545/11/$ – see front matter © 2011 Elsevier Inc. All rights reserved.

obgyn.theclinics.com

have been based largely on studies of white women, and many have been studies of clinic-based, rather than population-based, samples of women. Thus, until recently, much of the knowledge about the timing of the natural final menstrual period has been affected by the nature of the samples of women studied and a number of other methodologic differences in the studies of this phenomenon, which must be considered in comparing and summarizing their results.

METHODOLOGIC CONCERNS

Most studies of the menopausal transition have been cross-sectional, rather than longitudinal, in design, providing an opportunity for distortion of the true picture of the timing of the final natural menstrual period, particularly for understanding factors that precede and may affect the timing of menopause. Further, definitions of menopause or the final menstrual period have varied from study to study in terms of the number of months of amenorrhea considered to represent in retrospect the final menstrual period. Studies have also varied with regard to which factors have been included in multivariable analyses that control simultaneously for the effects of multiple variables, which also makes the studies not directly comparable.

The analysis of age at natural menopause in a number of studies has been calculated as a simple mean, rather than using the less-biased survival or multivariable time-to-event analytic approaches. These last two approaches include more information and observations for every woman studied, because all women are included but withdrawn or censored when they experience surgical menopause, start using menopausal hormone therapy or oral contraceptives (OC; which generally masks the natural cessation of menses), or are still premenopausal.[34] Also, the accuracy of reporting of age at menopause can vary by whether menopause was natural and by duration from the time of the final menstrual period to the time of the interview about menopause, the latter being directly affected by the age group of the study sample.[35] Further, in some studies that have reported age at menopause, it is unclear if the age at the final menstrual period is being reported, the more frequent approach, or if the age at cessation of menses plus 1 year of amenorrhea, the World Health Organization's definition of menopause.[31] is what is reported, a more rare occurrence.[36] Most studies do not use a hormonally based definition of menopause.

Recently, more information has been published regarding differences in the timing of menopause experienced by samples of women of different socioeconomic, racial/ethnic, and lifestyle backgrounds, and standardization of instruments and definitions has increased, resulting in a fuller, clearer, and more insightful picture regarding the underlying physiology.

SUMMARY OF UNDERLYING PHYSIOLOGY

Menopause is defined as the cessation of menstruation which reflects cessation of ovulation owing to a loss of ovarian follicles, which in turn results in reduced ovarian production of estradiol, the most biologically active form of estrogen,[37,38] as well as increased circulating concentrations of follicle-stimulating hormone (FSH) and decreased concentrations of inhibin, which inhibits the release of FSH.[37] Age at menopause may be more sensitive to varying rates of atresia of ovarian follicles[39] than to the absolute number of oocytes depleted,[40] but menopause is reached when depletion of follicles reaches approximately 1000 (from a peak of 5 million follicles at mid-gestation and 2 million at birth).[41,42] The age at which sufficient depletion of follicles occurs is affected by the number of follicles achieving migration to the gonadal ridge during gestation, their mitotic abilities until mid-gestation, and the rate of follicular atresia.[42,43]

As circulating estrogen concentrations decline during the menopausal transition, variations in the regularity, timing, and nature of menstrual bleeding may occur.[44] As menstrual cycles become increasingly irregular, bleeding may occur after an inadequate luteal phase or without ovulation,[44] usually indicated by a short luteal phase, characteristic of women over the age of 40 years.[45,46] Such cycles may be associated with insufficient FSH (or insufficient FSH responsiveness of the follicle) in the follicular phase, in turn resulting in lower luteal phase estrogen and progesterone secretion. Lack of a corpus luteum, resulting in estrogen secretion (even hyperestrogenicity[45,47]) unopposed by progesterone, may lead to profuse bleeding.

The nature and timing of bleeding may vary both within and between women. What is known about the host, environmental, or lifestyle factors that may affect such variation is summarized herein. Although some factors have been identified that are associated with early age at natural menopause, the relation of many has not been examined, and most have not been examined in relation to duration of the perimenopause.

Factors Related to Timing of Menopause

Results from cross-sectional studies have indicated that endocrine changes characteristic of the onset of the perimenopause begin at around age 45.[48] The median age at menopause among white women from industrialized countries ranges between 50 and 52 years and at onset of the perimenopause is 47.5 years,[49-53] with slight evidence of increasing age at menopause over time.[53-57] These onsets seem to vary by race and ethnicity[58-60] and are affected by demographic and lifestyle factors.[50,51,55,57-69] Although some studies have reported no familial relationship, 1 study has reported that age at menopause was positively associated with maternal age at menopause,[61] and 1 recent study has shown genetic control of age at menopause in a study of twins.[70] However, a number of potentially modifiable factors which may affect estrogen metabolism, including body mass index (BMI), diet (particularly calories and alcohol intake), and passive smoke exposure have not been examined, nor has the time-varying effect of these and of the other factors that have been previously identified been examined in longitudinal analyses of sufficiently large and diverse study populations.

Sociodemographic Differences

International and geographic differences
Several studies have indicated that women living in developing countries (including Latin America, Indonesia, Singapore, Pakistan, Chile, and Peru) experience natural menopause several years earlier than those in developed countries.[71-76] Some work has also indicated that women living in urban areas have a later natural menopause than women in rural areas.[62] Women living at high altitude in the Himalayas or in the Andes of Peru undergo natural menopause 1 to 1.5 years earlier than those living at lower altitudes or in less rural areas.[72,77-79] It is unclear whether these geographic and international differences in the age at natural menopause reflect genetic, socioeconomic, environmental, racial/ethnic, or lifestyle differences and whether and how these affect physiology.

Racial/ethnic differences

Some studies have reported that African American[59] and Latina[58,60] women have natural menopause about 2 years earlier than white women. However, 1 small study in Nigeria reported the average age at menopause to be 52.8 years,[80] over 1 year later than that generally reported for white women in industrialized nations. Mayan women, despite their high parity (see Reproductive History), have been reported to experience natural menopause fairly early, at about age 45.[81] In contrast, Asian women tend to have similar age at menopause to Caucasian women,[58,82] although Thai women have been reported to have a lower median age at menopause, at age 49.5 years, despite their high parity,[83] and Filipino Malay women have been reported to have an earlier average age at natural menopause at 47 to 48 years.[84]

Differences by socioeconomic status

A number of studies have observed that lower social class, as measured by the woman's educational attainment or by her own or her husband's occupation, is associated with an earlier age at natural menopause.[51–54,57,58,61,71,85,86] However, results from a British birth cohort indicated that early life socioeconomic status (SES) was more strongly associated than adult status with age at natural menopause,[87] although even the relation of early life SES was greatly attenuated when adjusted for childhood cognitive ability and having been breastfed.[88] One study found that education was more strongly associated with age at natural menopause than occupation.[52] Most studies that have examined the relation of marital status have found that single women undergo an earlier natural menopause, and this association cannot be explained by nulliparity.[52,89,90]

Health-Related Influences

Menstrual and reproductive history

The age at which the final natural menstrual period occurs may be a marker for hormonal status or changes earlier in life.[91] In the landmark Treloar longitudinal study of largely white, well-educated women, those whose median menstrual cycle length between the ages of 20 and 35 years was fewer than 26 days underwent natural menopause 1.4 years earlier than women with cycle lengths between 26 and 32 days, whereas a later natural menopause (mean = 0.8 year later) was observed in women with cycle lengths of 33 days or longer.[92] In addition, 9 or more days of variability in cycle length has been associated with a later age at natural menopause in this and other studies,[52,59] although 1 study reported an earlier natural menopause in women with irregular menses.[53]

Increasing parity, particularly among women of higher SES, has also been associated with later age at natural menopause,[50–52,55,57,58,61,90,91,93–96] consistent with the theory that natural menopause occurs after oocytes have been sufficiently depleted.[93] Although some studies have reported no familial relationship, 1 study reported that women's age at natural menopause was positively associated with their mother's age at natural menopause,[61] and 1 study of twins showed genetic control of age at natural menopause.[70] Age at menarche has been fairly consistently observed not to be associated with age at menopause, after adjusting for parity and cycle length,[52,53,55,83,89,97,98] as have prior spontaneous abortion, age at first birth, and history of breastfeeding.[52,97,98]

A number of studies have reported that women who have used OCs have a later age at natural menopause.[52,58,61,63,72,98] an observation that is also consistent with the theory that OCs delay depletion of oocytes. However, the finding has not been wholly consistent across studies, because 1 study reported that this delay became nonsignificant after a time-dependent adjustment for when OCs were used,[52] and another study reported that OC users had a significantly earlier natural menopause than nonusers, although this association was not consistent across 5-year age groups.[50]

Body mass and composition

Several studies have examined the relation of body mass to age at menopause, with inconsistent findings. Some studies have reported that both increased BMI (indicated by weight over height squared) and upper body fat distribution (indicated by waist-to-hip ratio) were associated with later age at natural menopause[50,57,96,99,100] and increased sex hormone concentrations.[100] However, at least as many other studies have reported no significant association of BMI with age at natural menopause.[51,52,54,59,101,102] Some studies have found a relationship between lower weight[69] or increased upper body fat distribution[101] and earlier age at natural menopause, particularly among smokers. One study reported earlier natural menopause in women on weight reduction programs or who had gained more than 26 pounds between the ages of 20 and 45 years.[59]

Some of these apparently inconsistent findings may be explained by differences in study design (cross-sectional or retrospective vs prospective) or analysis (eg, inadequate or varying control of confounding variables or survival analysis vs. comparison of crude means). In general, the better designed and analyzed studies have shown no relation of body mass or body fat distribution to age at the final natural menstrual period. Although body mass and composition may be related to age at natural menopause, they are also related inversely to physical activity, alcohol consumption, and education, and positively related to infertility and parity.[103] Further research is needed in which all of these potentially confounding variables are simultaneously controlled in the statistical analyses of data from large study samples to be able to assess adequately the independent contribution or interactive effect of body mass and composition and these other factors on the age at the natural final menstrual period and duration of menopause transition, using appropriate longitudinal study design and data analysis techniques.

Familial, genetic, and early childhood factors

In recent years, studies of factors related to age at natural menopause have begun to focus on genetic factors that may be related. Results of family and twin studies suggest that familial and genetic factors may play an important role, with estimates of heritability ranging from 30% to 85%.[70,104,105] In 1 relatively large cross-sectional study and 1 large longitudinal British birth cohort study, a strong association was found between mothers' and daughters' ages at natural menopause,[88,106] which have also been found in a few other smaller studies,[107–109] but few longitudinal studies have investigated this relationship. One European genome-wide association study of nearly 3000 women identified 6 single nucleotide polymorphisms in 3 loci on chromosomes 13, 19, and 20 associated with age at natural menopause.[110] A Dutch study showed that polymorphisms of an estrogen receptor gene were associated with earlier natural and surgical menopause.[111] Results of genome-wide association studies, using samples from thousands of women in the Nurses' Health Study and the Women's Genome Health Study, identified 13 single nucleotide polymorphisms on 4 chromosomes that were associated with age at menopause.[112] Analyses of candidate genes from 9 biologically plausible pathways, using the same samples from the same women in these 2 studies, indicated that the steroid hormone metabolism and biosynthesis pathways were associated with age at natural menopause and that genes involved in premature ovarian failure were also significantly associated with age at menopause.[113] Two single nucleotide polymorphisms of the tumor necrosis factor receptor family have also been shown to be significantly associated with age at natural menopause.[114]

A number of analyses have been conducted on prospective data collected across the lifespan from a nationally representative birth cohort of nearly 1600 British women born in 1946 and followed to age 53 years, the Medical Research Council National Survey of Health and Development. These analyses have revealed that women who had a low weight at 2 years of age had an earlier natural menopause,[115] whereas those who were heaviest at 2 years of age had a later natural menopause.[89] Those who were breastfed had a later natural menopause.[115] Another cohort study in England also found that low weight at 1 year of age was associated with earlier natural menopause.[116] However, an Australian twin study and the English cohort study found no association of birth weight with age at natural menopause.[116,117] The British birth cohort and other cohort studies have shown that poorer cognitive ability in childhood was associated with earlier natural menopause,[118–120] suggesting that perhaps markers in early life may determine not only age at natural menopause, but may also predict the adverse health outcomes that are associated with early age at menopause. Further, additional findings from the British birth cohort indicate that women whose parents divorced early in their lives had an earlier natural menopause than other women, suggesting that early life stressors may also be related to early menopause.[87,88]

Environmental Influences

Active and passive smoke exposure

Perhaps the single most consistently shown environmental effect on age at menopause is that women who smoke stop menstruating 1 to 2 years earlier than comparable nonsmokers.[50,51,55,57–59,61,63–68,86,96,121] and have a shorter perimenopause.[122] Some studies have shown a dose–response effect on atrophy of ovarian follicles, in that heavy smokers have an earlier natural menopause than light smokers.[61,67,69,123,124] Former smokers have only a slightly earlier age at natural menopause than those who never smoked, and increased time since quitting diminishes the difference.[123,125] The latter observation of only a slightly earlier natural menopause in former smokers is inconsistent with the presumed toxic effect of smoking on ovarian follicles, resulting in their atrophy and thus earlier menopause, because such an effect should be nonreversible so that former smokers would also experience the earlier natural menopause observed in current smokers. If the dose–response effect is a true effect, the apparent paradox might partly be explained by fewer years of smoking and thus toxic exposure to the ovaries in former smokers than in current smokers of similar age.

The polycyclic aromatic hydrocarbons in cigarette smoke are known to be toxic to ovarian follicles[126,127] and thus could result in premature loss of ovarian follicles and early natural menopause among smokers. Because drug metabolism is enhanced in smokers,[128] estrogen also may be more rapidly metabolized in the livers of smokers, which could lead to an earlier reduction of estrogen levels.[99] Further, smoking has also been observed to have antiestrogenic effects.[129] Greater prevalence of hysterectomy among premenopausal smokers than nonsmokers[100,123] apparently does not account for smokers having an earlier natural menopause.[130] Only 1 study has shown that nonsmoking women whose spouses smoked had an age at natural menopause resembling that of smokers[131]; thus, very little is known about the effect of passive or secondhand smoke exposure on the age at which the final natural menstrual period is experienced.

Occupational/environmental factors

Although almost nothing is known about the relations of occupational or other environmental factors to age at the final natural menstrual period and duration of the menopausal transition, occupational exposures and stressors (such as shift work, hours worked, hours spent standing, and heavy lifting) have been related to increased risk of adverse pregnancy outcomes[132–135] and changes in menstrual cycle length and variability as well as fecundability.[136–139] In addition, such environmental exposures as dichlorodiphenyltrichloroethane and polychlorinated biphenyls have been shown to have estrogenic activity and to be associated with an increased risk of breast cancer,[140,141] although this association has not been consistently observed.[142,143] Thus, the presumed endocrine effects of such exposures make it reasonable to expect that occupational and environmental exposures may be related to endocrine disruption that is reflected in altered age at natural menopause. One study showed a modest effect on age at natural menopause in women in Seveso, Italy, who were exposed to 2,3,7,8-tetrachlorobenzo-p-dioxin, a halogenated compound that may affect ovarian function, during a chemical plant explosion in 1976.[144] Another study showed that exposure to 1,1-dichloro-2,2-bis(p-chlorophenyl) ethylene was also associated with earlier natural menopause.[145]

Physical activity Physical activity is associated with a number of changes in hormonal parameters [estradiol, progesterone, prolactin, luteinizing hormone (LH), and FSH), both during and after intense physical activity.[146–148] The concentrations of these hormones tend to be lower at rest among women who are physically active.[146,147,149,150] Also, athletes tend to have a later age at menarche and increased occurrences of anovulation[151] and amenorrhea[152] and, among those who menstruate, a shortened luteal phase and reduced mean and peak progesterone levels.[104,149] Although physical activity is associated with decreased concentrations of reproductive hormones and frequency of ovulation, few studies have examined the effect of exercise on age at natural menopause, although 1 modestly sized study reported no relationship,[59] and 1 large study of Chinese women showed a later age at natural menopause associated with leisure time physical activity during adolescence and adulthood.[94]

Diet One early study from Papua, New Guinea, suggested that malnourished women ceased menstruation about 4 years earlier than well-nourished women,[153] consistent with other studies showing that women with greater weight[62,69] and height[89] may have a later age at natural menopause. Findings regarding the relationship of specific dietary patterns to age at menopause have been inconsistent. For example, vegetarians were observed to have an earlier age at natural menopause in 1 study,[154] whereas another study in Japan reported that higher green and yellow vegetable intake was significantly associated with later age at natural menopause.[155] Further, a large cross-sectional study of Japanese women found that higher intakes of fat, cholesterol, and coffee were significantly associated with earlier natural menopause after controlling for age, total energy, parity, menarche age, and relative weight.[156] A longitudinal study of nearly 5000 German women observed that high carbohydrate consumption and high intake of vegetable, fiber, and cereal products were related to an earlier age at natural menopause, whereas higher intake of total fat, protein, and meat were associated with a later natural menopause.[157] The large, prospective

Shanghai Women's Health Study found that higher total intake of calories, fruits, and protein was significantly associated with later age at natural menopause, whereas vegetable, fat, soy, and fiber intakes were not significantly related to age at menopause.[94] Inclusion of meat in the diet of vegetarians has been observed to increase the episodic releases of LH and FSH and the length of the menstrual cycle.[158] Thus, meat may modify the interaction of hormones along the hypothalamic–pituitary–ovarian axis. A couple of studies have reported that increased meat or alcohol consumption is significantly associated with later age at menopause, after adjusting for age and smoking.[61,121] Dietary fiber (whose intake tends to be inversely related to meat intake) may interrupt enterohepatic circulation of sex hormones, leading to the lower circulating estrogen concentrations among vegetarian women.[159] Nonetheless, a low-fat, high-carbohydrate intervention diet to prevent breast cancer in over 2600 women with extensive mammographic density followed for an average 7 years did not influence the timing of natural menopause, except a significantly earlier natural menopause was observed in those with low BMI who were on the intervention diet.[160]

Premenopausal women administered soy have shown increased plasma estradiol concentrations and follicular phase length, delayed menstruation, and suppressed midcycle surges of LH and FSH.[161] Among postmenopausal women fed soy, FSH and LH did not decrease significantly, nor did sex hormone-binding globulin increase, and little change occurred in endogenous estradiol or body weight, although a small estrogenic effect on vaginal cytology was observed.[162] However, the role of dietary fiber, phytoestrogens, fat, protein, and other nutrients in affecting age at menopause and duration of the perimenopause remains to be systematically studied, but has potentially important implications for prevention of chronic disease in midlife and older women.

CONCLUSION

Despite important methodologic differences, the limitations in the study designs used and the populations studied in the accumulating literature regarding factors that affect the age at which the natural final menstrual period is experienced, an interesting and complex picture is emerging. A number of demographic (eg, education, employment, race/ethnicity), menstrual and reproductive (eg, parity and OC use), familial and genetic, and lifestyle (eg, smoking, weight, physical activity and diet) factors seem to be important determinants of the age at which natural menopause occurs. Smoking, lower parity, and lower SES have been found fairly consistently to be associated with earlier menopause, an indicator of reduced longevity. However, the relationships with African American and Latina race/ethnicity, vegetarian diet, and undernutrition, body mass and composition, and physical activity have been inconsistent, possibly owing to varying methodologic approaches and limitations (**Table 1**).

Other relationships remain largely unexplored (eg, passive smoke exposure and occupational and other environmental exposures). Therefore, much remains to be learned about how these factors affect follicular atresia and hormone levels and thus determine the onset and potentially the duration of the perimenopause and the timing of the final menstrual period. Furthermore, increased understanding of the underlying physiologic mechanisms of these influences needs to include potential genetic, metabolic, and racial/ethnic differences in physiologic responses to lifestyle factors and other environmental exposures and the interaction of genetic factors with these lifestyle and environmental factors. Increasing knowledge about these relationships ultimately offers women and their health care providers enhanced understanding and

Table 1	
Factors related to earlier and later age at natural menopause	
Factors Consistently Related to Earlier Age at Natural Menopause (References)	Factors Inconsistently Related to Age at Natural Menopause (References)
Low socioeconomic status[51–54,57,58,61,71,85–88]	Race/ethnicity[58–60,80–84]
Low parity[50–52,55,57,58,61,90,91,93,96]	Body mass index or body composition[50–52,54,57,59,62,69,98–101]
Not using oral contraceptives[50,52,58,61,63,72,98]	Physical activity[59,94]
Active smoking[50,51,55,57–59,61,63–69,86,96,121,124–126]	Dietary (vegetable, meat, fat, fiber) intake[61,121,153–157,160]

choices, based on greater knowledge, to deal with the individual presentations of menopause.

ACKNOWLEDGMENTS

The Study of Women's Health Across the Nation (SWAN) has grant support from the National Institutes of Health (NIH), DHHS, through the National Institute on Aging (NIA), the National Institute of Nursing Research (NINR) and the NIH Office of Research on Women's Health (ORWH) (Grants NR004061; AG012505, AG012535, AG012531, AG012539, AG012546, AG012553, AG012554, AG012495). Dr Gold was supported by AG012554. The content of this article is solely the responsibility of the author and does not necessarily represent the official views of the NIA, NINR, ORWH or the NIH.

REFERENCES

1. Cooper GS, Sandler DP. Age at natural menopause and mortality. Ann Epidemiol 1998;8:229–35.
2. Wise AM, Krajnak KM, Kashon ML. Menopause: the aging of multiple pacemakers. Science 1996;273:67–70.
3. Snowdon DA, Kane RL, Beeson WL, et al. Is early natural menopause a biologic marker of health and aging? Am J Public Health 1989;79:709–14.
4. Ossewaarde ME, Bots ML, Verbeek ALM, et al. Age at menopause, cause-specific mortality and total life expectancy. Epidemiology 2005;16:556–62.
5. Jacobsen BK, Heuch I, Kvale G. Age at natural menopause and all-cause mortality: a 37-year follow-up of 19,731 Norwegian women. Am J Epidemiol 2003;157:923–9.
6. De Kleijn MJ, van der Schouw YT, Verbeek AL, et al. Endogenous estrogen exposure and cardiovascular mortality risk in postmenopausal women. Am J Epidemiol 2002; 155:339–45.
7. Van der Schouw YT, van der Graaf Y, Steyerberg EW, et al. Age at menopause as a risk factor for cardiovascular mortality. Lancet 1996;347:714–8.
8. Jacobsen BK, Nilssen S, Heuch I, et al. Does age at natural menopause affect mortality from ischemic heart disease? J Clin Epidemiol 1997;50:475–9.
9. Hu FB, Grodstein F, Hennekens CH, et al. Age at natural menopause and risk of cardiovascular disease. Arch Intern Med 1999;159:1061–6.
10. Atsma F, Bartelink ML, Grobbec DE, et al. Postmenopausal status and early menopause as independent risk factors for cardiovascular disease: a meta-analysis. Menopause 2006;13:265–79.
11. Cui R, Iso H, Toyoshima H, et al, JACC Study Group. Relationships of age at menarche and menopause, and reproductive year with mortality from cardiovascular

disease in Japanese postmenopausal women: the JACC study. J Epidemiol 2006;16:177–84.

12. Jansen SC, Temme EH, Schouten EG. Lifetime estrogen exposure versus age at menopause as mortality predictor. Maturitas 2002;43:105–12.

13. Jacobsen BK, Knutsen SF, Fraser GE. Age at natural menopause and total mortality and mortality from ischemic heart disease: the Adventist Health Study. J Clin Epidemiol 1999;52:303–7.

14. Lisabeth LD, Beiser AS, Brown DL, et al. Age at natural menopause and risk of ischemic stroke The Framingham Heart Study. Stroke 2009;40:1044–9.

15. Parashar S, Reid KJ, Spertus JA, et al. Early menopause predicts angina after myocardial infarction. Menopause 2010;17:938–45.

16. Joakimsen O, Bonaa KH, Stensland-Bugge E, et al. Population-based study of age at menopause and ultrasound assessed carotid atherosclerosis: the Tromso Study. J Clin Epidemiol 2000;53:525–30.

17. Parazzini F, Bidoli E, Franceschi S, et al. Menopause, menstrual and reproductive history, and bone density in northern Italy. J Epidemiol Community Health 1996;50: 519–23.

18. Kritz-Silverstein D, Barrett-Connor E. Early menopause, number of reproductive years, and bone mineral density in postmenopausal women. Am J Public Health 1993;83:983–8.

19. Van Der Voort DJ, Van Der Weijer PH, Barentsen R. Early menopause: increased fracture risk at older age. Osteoporos Int 2003;14:525–30.

20. Kelsey JL, Gammon MD, John EM. Reproductive factors and breast cancer. Epidemiol Rev 1993;15:36–47.

21. Monninkhof EM, van der Schouw YT, Peeters PH. Early age at menopause and breast cancer: are leaner women more protected? A prospective analysis of the Dutch DOM cohort. Breast Cancer Res Treat 1999;55:285–91.

22. De Graaff J, Stolte LA. Age at menarche and menopause of uterine cancer patients. Eur J Obstet Gynecol Reprod Biol 1978;8:187–93.

23. Franceschi S, La Vecchia C, Booth M, et al. Pooled analysis of 3 European case-control studies of ovarian cancer: II. Age at menarche and at menopause. Int J Cancer 1991;49:57–61.

24. Kaaks R, Lukanova A, Kurzer MS. Obesity, endogenous hormones, and endometrial cancer risk: a synthetic review. Cancer Epidemiol Biomarkers Prev 2002;11:1531–43.

25. Xu WH, Xiang YB, Ruan ZX, et al. Menstrual and reproductive factors and endometrial cancer risk: results from a population-based case-control study in urban Shanghai. Int J Cancer 2004;108:613–9.

26. Rivera CM, Grossardt BR, Rhodes DJ, et al. Increased cardiovascular mortality after early bilateral oophorectomy. Menopause 2009;16:15–23.

27. Lokkegaard E, Jovanovic Z, Heitmann BL, et al. The association between early menopause and risk of ischaemic heart disease: influence of hormone therapy. Maturitas 2006;53:226–33.

28. Woods NF, Mitchell ES, Adams C. Memory functioning among midlife women: observations for the Seattle Midlife Women's health Study. Menopause 2000;7: 257–65.

29. Halbreich U, Piletz J, Halaris A. Influence of gonadal hormones on neurotransmitters, receptor, cognition and mood. Clin Neuropharmacol 1992;15(Suppl A):590A–1A.

30. Kok HS, Kuh D. Cooper R, et al. Cognitive function across the life course and the menopausal transition in a British birth cohort. Menopause 2006;13:19–27.

31. World Health Organization. Research on the menopause in the 1990s. Geneva (Switzerland): World Health Organization; 1996.

32. Skolnick AA. At third meeting, menopause experts make the most of insufficient data. JAMA 1992;268:2483–5.

33. Avis NE, Kaufert PA, Lock M, et al. The evolution of menopausal symptoms. Baillieres Clin Endocrinol Metab 1993;7:17–32.

34. Cramer DW, Xu H. Predicting age at menopause. Maturitas 1996;23:319–26.

35. Hahn RA, Eaker E, Rolka H. Reliability of reported age at menopause. Am J Epidemiol 1997;146:771–5.

36. Sowers MF, LaPietra MT. Menopause: its epidemiology and potential association with chronic diseases. Epidemiol Rev 1995;17:287–302.

37. Gosden RG. Biology of the menopause: the causes and consequences of ovarian ageing. London: Academic Press; 1985.

38. Burger HG, Dudley EC, Hopper JL. The endocrinology of the menopausal transition: a cross-sectional study of a population-based sample. J Clin Endocrinol Metab 1995;80:3537–45.

39. Soule MR, Bremner WJ. The menopause and climacteric: endocrinologic basis and associated symptomatology. J Am Geriatrics Soc 1982;30:547.

40. Thomford PJ, Jelovsek FR, Mattison DR. Effect of oocyte number and rate of atresia on the age of menopause. Repro Toxicol 1987;1:41–51.

41. Faddy MJ, Gosden RG, Gougeon A, et al. Accelerated disappearance of ovarian follicles in mid-life: implications for forecasting menopause. Hum Reprod 1992;7: 1342–6.

42. Ginsberg J. What determines the age at the menopause. BMJ 1991;302:1288–9.

43. Aydos SE, Elhan AH, Tukun A. Is telomere length one of the determinants of reproductive life span? Arch Gynecol Obstet 2005;2727:113–6.

44. Sherman BM, West JH, Korenman SG. The menopausal transition: analysis of LH, FSH, estradiol and progesterone concentrations during menstrual cycles of older women. J Clin Endocrinol Metab 1976;42:629–36.

45. Santoro N, Rosenberg-Brown J, Adel T, et al. Characterization of reproductive hormonal dynamics in the perimenopause. J Clin Endocrinol Metab 1996;81:1495–1501.

46. Upton GV. The perimenopause: physiologic correlates and clinical management. J Reprod Med 1982;27:1–28.

47. Shideler SE, DeVane GW, Kalra PS, et al. Ovarian pituitary hormone interactions during the menopause. Maturitas 1989;11:331–9.

48. Trevoux R, DeBrux J, Castaneir M, et al. Endometrium and plasma hormone profile in the peri-menopause and post-menopause. Maturitas 1986;8:309–26.

49. McKinlay SM, Brambilla DJ, Posner JG. The normal menopause transition. Maturitas 1992;14:103–15.

50. Greendale G, Hogan P, Kritz-Silverstein D, et al. (for the PEPI trial investigators). Age at menopause in women participating in the postmenopausal estrogen/progestins interventions (PEPI) trial: an example of bias introduced by selection criteria. Menopause 1995;2:27–34.

51. Luoto R, Laprio J, Uutela A. Age at natural menopause and sociodemographic status in Finland. Am J Epidemiol 1994;139:64–76.

52. Stanford JL, Hartge P, Brinton LA, et al. Factors influencing the age at natural menopause. J Chron Dis 1987;40:995–1002.

53. Magursky V, Mesko M, Sokolik L. Age at the menopause and onset of the climacteric in women of Martin district, Czechoslovakia. Int J Fertil 1975;20:17–23.

54. Gold EB, Sternfeld B, Brown C, et al. The relation of demographic and lifestyle variables to symptoms in a multi-racial/ethnic population of women aged 40-55 years. Am J Epidemiol 2000;152:463–73.
55. van Noord PAH, Dubas JS, Dorland M, et al. Age at natural menopause in a population-based screening cohort: the role of menarche, fecundity, and lifestyle factors. Fertil Steril 1997;68:95–102.
56. Flint M. Is there a secular trend in age of menopause. Maturitas 1978;1:133–9.
57. Rodstrom K, Bengtsson C, Milsom I, et al. Evidence for a secular trend in menopausal age: a population study of women in Gothenburg. Menopause 2003;10:538–43.
58. Gold EB, Bromberger J, Crawford S, et al. Factors associated with age at menopause in a multi-ethnic population of women. Am J Epidemiol 2001;153:865–74.
59. Bromberger JT, Matthews KA, Kuller LH, et al. Prospective study of the determinants of age at menopause. Am J Epidemiol 1997;145:124–33.
60. Alvarado G, Rivera R, Ruiz R, et al. Characteristicas del patron de sangrado menstrual en un grupo de mujeres normales de Durango. Ginecol Obstetr Mex 1988;56:127–33.
61. Torgerson DJ, Avenell A, Russell IT, et al. Factors associated with onset of menopause in women aged 45–49. Maturitas 1994;19:83–92.
62. MacMahon B, Worcester J. Age at menopause, United States 1960–1962. Vital Health Stat 1966;19:1–19.
63. Palmer JR, Rosenberg L, Wise LA, et al. Onset of natural menopause in African American women. Am J Public Health 2003;93:299–306.
64. McKinlay SM, Bifano NL, McKinlay JB. Smoking and age at menopause in women. Ann Intern Med 1985;103:350–6.
65. Andersen FS, Transbol I, Christiansen C. Is cigarette smoking a promoter of the menopause. Acta Med Scand 1982;212:137–9.
66. Hiatt RA, Fireman BH. Smoking, menopause, and breast cancer. J Natl Cancer Inst 1986;76:833–8.
67. Hartz AJ, Kelber S, Borkowf H, et al. The association of smoking with clinical indicators of altered sex steroids—a study of 50,145 women. Pub Health Rep 1987;102:254–9.
68. Brambilla DJ, McKinlay SM. A prospective study of factors affecting age at menopause. J Clin Epidemiol 1989;42:1031–9.
69. Willett W, Stampfer MJ, Bain C, et al. Cigarette smoking, relative weight and menopause. Am J Epidemiol 1983;117:651–8.
70. Snieder H, MacGregor AJ, Spector ID. Genes control cessation of a woman's reproductive life: a twin study of hysterectomy and age at menopause. J Clin Endocrinol Met 1998;83:1875–80.
71. Castelo-Branco C, Blümel JE, Chedraui P, et al. Age at menopause in Latin America. Menopause 2006;13:706–12. Erratum in: Menopause 2006;13:850.
72. Gonzales GF, Villena A. Age at menopause in central Andean Peruvian women. Menopause 1997;4:32–8.
73. McCarthy T. The prevalence of symptoms in menopausal women in the Far East: Singapore segment. Maturitas 1994;19:199–204.
74. Samil RS, Wishnuwardhani SD. Health of Indonesian women, city-dwellers of perimenopausal age. Maturitas 1994;19:191–7.
75. Wasti S, Robinson SC, Akhtar Y, et al. Characteristics of menopause in three groups in Karachi, Pakistan. Maturitas 1993;16:61–9.
76. Blumel J, Cubillos M, Brandt A, et al. Some clinical aspects of menopause. Rev Chil Obstet Ginecol 1988;53:278–82.

77. Kapoor AK, Kapoor S. The effects of high altitude on age at menarche and menopause. J Biometeor 1986;30:21–6.
78. Beall CM. Ages at menopause and menarche in a high altitude Himalayan population. Ann Hum Biol 1983;10:365–70.
79. Flint MP. Menarche and menopause in Rajput women. PhD dissertation, City University of New York, 1974.
80. Otolorin EO, Adeyefa I, Osotimehin BO, et al. Clinical, hormonal and biochemical features of menopausal women in Ibadan, Nigeria. Afr J Med Sci 1989;18:251–5.
81. Beyene Y. Cultural significance and physiological manifestations of menopause, a bicultural analysis. Culture Med Psychiatr 1986;10:47–71.
82. Boulet M. The menopause and the climacteric in seven Asian countries. In: Sixth International Congress on the Menopause. New Jersey: Parthenon; 1990.
83. Chompootweep S, Tankeyoon M, Yamarat K, et al. The menopausal age and climacteric complaints in Thai women in Bangkok. Maturitas 1993;17:63–71.
84. Ramoso-Jalbuena J. Climacteric Filipino women: a preliminary survey in the Philippines. Maturitas 19:183–90.
85. Lawlor DA, Ebrahim S, Smith GD. The association of socio-economic position across the life course and age at menopause: the British Women's Heart and Health Study. Br J Obstet Gynecol 2003;110:1078–87.
86. Santoro N, Brockwell S, Johnston J, et al. Helping midlife women predict the onset of the final menses: SWAN, the Study of Women's Health Across the Nation. Menopause 2007;14:415–24.
87. Hardy R, Kuh D. Social and environmental conditions across the life course and age at menopause in a British birth cohort study. BJOG 2005;112:346–54.
88. Mishra G, Hardy R, Kuh D. Are the effects of risk factors for timing of menopause modified by age? Results from a British birth cohort study. Menopause 2007;14:717–24.
89. Brand PC, Lehert PH. A new way of looking at environmental variables that may affect the age at menopause. Maturitas 1978;1:121–32.
90. McKinlay S, Jefferys M, Thompson B. An investigation of the age at menopause. J Biosoc Sci 1972;4:161–73.
91. Whelan EA, Sandler DP, McConnaughey DR, et al. Menstrual and reproductive characteristics and age at natural menopause. Am J Epidemiol 1990;131:625–32.
92. Treloar AE, Boynton RE, Behn BG, et al. Variation of the human menstrual cycle through reproductive life. Int J Fertil 1966;12 (Pt 2):77–126.
93. Soberon J, Calderon JJ, Goldzieher JW. Relation of parity to age at menopause. Am J Obstet Gynecol 1966;96:96–100.
94. Dorjgochoo T, Kallianpur A, Gao Y-T, et al. Dietary and lifestyle predictors of age at natural menopause and reproductive span in the Shanghai Women's Health Study. Menopause 2008;15:924–33.
95. Loh FH, Khin LW, Saw SM, et al. The age of menopause and the menopause transition in a multiracial population: a nation-wide Singapore study. Maturitas 2005;52:169–80.
96. Reynolds RF, Obermeyer CM. Age at natural menopause in Spain and the United States: results from the DAMES project. Am J Hum Biol 2005;17:331–40.
97. Parazzini F, Negri E, LaVecchia C. Reproductive and general lifestyle determinants of age at menopause. Maturitas 1992;15:141–9.
98. van Keep PA, Brand PC, Lehert PH. Factors affecting the age at menopause. J Biosoc Sci Suppl 1979;6:37–55.
99. Lindquist O, Bengtsson C. Menopausal age in relation to smoking. Acta Med Scand 1979;205:73–7.

100. Daniell HWP. Smoking, obesity, and the menopause. Lancet 1978;2:373.
101. den Tonkelaar I, Seidell J. Fat distribution in relation to age, degree of obesity, smoking habits, parity and estrogen use: a cross-sectional study of 11,825 Dutch women participating in the DOM project. Int J Obesity 1990;14:753–61.
102. Kaufman DW, Slone D, Rosenberg L, et al. Cigarette smoking and age at natural menopause. Am J Public Health 1980;70:420–2.
103. Kaye S, Folsom A, Prineas RJ, et al. The association of body fat distribution with lifestyle and reproductive factors in a population study of postmenopausal women. Int J Obesity 1990;14:583–91.
104. Kok HS, van Asselt KM, van der Schouw YT, et al. Genetic studies to identify genes underlying menopause age. Hum Reprod Update 2005;11:483–93.
105. Van Asselt KM, Kok HS, Pearson PL, et al. Heritability of menopausal age in mothers and daughters. Fertil Steril 2004;82:1348–51.
106. Torgerson DJ, Thomas RE, Reid DM. Mothers and daughters menopausal ages: is there a link? Eur J Obstet Gynecol Reprod Biol 1997;74:63–6.
107. Cramer DW, Xu H, Harlow BL. Family history as a predictor of early menopause. Fertil Steril 1995;64:740–5.
108. De Bruin JP, Bovenhuis H, Van Noord PA, et al. The role of genetic factors in age at natural menopause. Hum Reprod 2001;16:2014–8.
109. Murabito JM, Yang Q, Fox C, et al. Heritability of age at natural menopause in the Framingham Heart Study. J Clin Endocrinol Metab 2005;90:3427–30.
110. Stolk L, Zhai G, Van Meurs JB, et al. Loci at chromosomes 13, 19 and 20 influence age at natural menopause. Nat Genet 2009;41:645–7.
111. Weel AE, Uitterlinden AG, Westendorp IC, et al. Estrogen receptor polymorphism predicts the onset of natural and surgical menopause. J Clin Endocrinol Metab 1999;84:3146–50.
112. He C, Kraft P, Chen C, et al. Genome-wide association studies identify loci associated with age at menarche and age at natural menopause. Nat Genet 2009;41: 724–8.
113. He C, Kraft P, Chasman DI, et al. A large-scale candidate gene association study of age at menarche and age at natural menopause. Hum Genet 2010;128:515–27.
114. Lu Y, Liu P, Recker RR, et al. *TNFRSF11A* and *TNFSF11* are associated with age at menarche and natural menopause in white women. Menopause 2010;17:1048–54.
115. Hardy R, Kuh D. Does early growth influence timing of the menopause? Evidence from a British birth cohort. Hum Reprod 2002;17:2474–9.
116. Cresswell JL, Egger P, Fall CH, et al. Is the age of menopause determined in-utero? Early Hum Dev 1997;49:143–8.
117. Treloar SA, Sadrzadeh S, Do KA, et al. Birth weight and age at menopause in Australian female twin pairs: exploration of the fetal origin hypothesis. Hum Reprod 2000;15:55–9.
118. Kuh D, Butterworth S, Kok H, et al. Childhood cognitive ability and age at menopause: evidence from two cohort studies. Menopause 2005;12:475–82.
119. Richards M, Kuh D, Hardy R, et al. Lifetime cognitive function and timing of the natural menopause. Neurology 1999;53:308–14.
120. Whalley LJ, Fox HC, Starr JM, et al. Age at natural menopause and cognition. Maturitas 2004;49:148–56.
121. Kinney A, Kline J, Levin B. Alcohol, caffeine and smoking in relation to age at menopause. Maturitas 2006;54:27–38.
122. McKinlay SM, Brambilla DJ, Posner JG. The normal menopause transition. Maturitas 1992;14:103–15.

123. Adena MA, Gallagher HG. Cigarette smoking and the age at menopause. Ann Human Biol 1982;9:121–30.

124. Jick H, Porter J, Morrison AS. Relation between smoking and age of natural menopause. Lancet 1977;1:1354–5.

125. Midgett AS, Baron JA. Cigarette smoking and the risk of natural menopause. Epidemiol 1990;1:464–80.

126. Mattison DR, Thorgierssen SS. Smoking and industrial pollution and their effects on menopause and ovarian cancer. Lancet 1978;1:187–8.

127. Essenberg JM, Fagan L, Malerstein AJ. Chronic poisoning of the ovaries and testes of albino rats and mice by nicotine and cigarette smoke. West J Surg Obstet Gynecol 1951;59:27–32.

128. Hart P, Farrell GC, Cooksley WGE, et al. Enhanced drug metabolism in cigarette smokers. Br Med J 1976;3:147–9.

129. Michnovicz J, Hershcopf R, Naganuma H, et al. Increased 2-hydroxylation of estradiol as a possible mechanism for the anti-estrogenic effect of cigarette smoking. N Engl J Med 1986;315:1305–9.

130. Krailo MD, Pike MC. Estimation of the distribution of the age at natural menopause from prevalence data. Am J Epidemiol 1983;117:356–61.

131. Everson RB, Sandler DP, Wilcox AJ, et al. Effect of passive exposure to smoking on age at natural menopause. Br Med J 1986;293:792.

132. Mamelle N, Laumon B, Lazar P. Prematurity and occupational activity during pregnancy. Am J Epidemiol 1984;119:309–22.

133. McDonald AD, McDonald JC, Armstrong B, et al. Fetal death and work in pregnancy. Br J Ind Med 1988;45:148–57.

134. Beaumont JJ, Swan SH, Hammond SK, et al. Historical cohort investigation of spontaneous abortion in the Semiconductor health Study: methods and analyses of risk in fabrication overall and in fabrication work groups. Am J Ind Med 1995;28:735–50.

135. Swan SH, Beaumont JJ, Hammond SK, et al. Historical cohort study of spontaneous abortion among fabrication workers in the Semiconductor Health Study; agent-level analysis. Am J Ind Med 1995;28:751–70.

136. Ng TP, Foo SC, Young T. Menstrual function in workers exposed to toluene. Br J Ind Med 1992;49:799–803.

137. Messing K, Saurel-Cubizolles MG, Bourgine M, et al. Menstrual cycle characteristics and work condition of workers in poultry slaughterhouses and canneries. Scand J Work Environ Health 1992;18:302–9.

138. Eskenazi B, Gold EB, Samuels SJ, et al. Prospective assessment of fecundability of female semiconductor workers. Am J Ind Med 1995;28:817–32.

139. Gold EB, Eskenazi B, Hammond SK, et al. Prospectively assessed menstrual cycle characteristics in female wafer-fabrication and nonfabrication semiconductor employees. Am J Ind Med 1995;28:799–816.

140. Falck F Jr, Ricci A Jr, Wolff MS, et al. Pesticides and polychlorinated biphenyl residues in human breast lipids and their relation to breast cancer. Arch Environ Health 1992;47:143–6.

141. Wolff MS, Toniolo PG, Lee EW, et al. Blood levels of organochlorine residues and risk of breast cancer. J Natl Cancer Inst 1993;85:648–52.

142. Krieger N, Wolff MS, Hiatt RA, et al. Breast cancer and serum organochlorines: a prospective study among white, black and Asian women. J Natl Cancer Inst 1994;86:589–99.

143. Hunter DJ, Hankinson SE, Laden F, et al. Plasma organochlorine levels and risk of breast cancer. N Engl J Med 1997;337:1253–8.

144. Eskenazi B, Warner M, Marks AR, et al. Serum dioxin concentrations and age at menopause. Environ Health Perspect 2005;113:858–62.

145. Cooper GS, Savitz DA, Millikan R, et al. Organochlorine exposure and age at natural menopause. Epidemiol 2002;13:729–33.

146. Cummings SR, Kelsey J, Nevitt MC, et al. Epidemiology of osteoporosis and osteoporotic fractures. Epidemiol Rev 1985;7:178–208.

147. Bonen A, Ling WH, Belcastro AN, et al. Profiles of selected hormones during menstrual cycles of teenage athletes. J Appl Physiol 1981;50:545–51.

148. Jurkowski JE, Joanes NL, Walker C, et al. Ovarian hormonal responses to exercise. J Appl Physiol 1978;44:109–14.

149. Loucks AB, Mortola LF, Girtoon L, et al. Alterations in the hypothalamic-pituitary-ovarian and the hypothalamic-pituitary-adrenal axes in athletic women. J Clin Endocrinol Metab 1989;68:402–11.

150. Jasienska G, Ziomkiewicz A, Thune I, et al. Habitual physical activity and estradiol levels in women of reproductive age. Eur J Cancer Prev 2006;15:439–45.

151. Bernstein L, Ross RK, Lobo RA, et al. The effects of moderate physical activity on menstrual cycle patterns in adolescence: implications for breast cancer prevention. Br J Cancer 1987;55:681–5.

152. Loucks AB, Horvath SM. Athletic amenorrhea: a review. Med Sci Sports Exer 1985;17:56–72.

153. Scragg RFR. Menopause and reproductive span in rural Nuigini. Proc Ann Symp Papua New Guinea Med Soc 1973;126–44.

154. Baird DD, Trlavsky FA, Anderson JJB. Do vegetarians have earlier menopause? Proc Soc Epidemiol Res 1988;907–8.

155. Nagata C, Takatsuka N, Kawakami N, et al. Association of diet with the onset of menopause in Japanese women. Am J Epidemiol 2000;152:863–7.

156. Nagata C, Takatsuka N, Inaba S, et al. Association of diet and other lifestyle with onset of menopause in Japanese women. Maturitas 1998;29:105–13.

157. Nagel G, Altenburg HP, Nieters A, et al. Reproductive and dietary determinants of the age at menopause in EPIC-Heidelberg. Maturitas 2005;52:337–47.

158. Hill PB, Garbaczewski L, Daynes G, et al. Gonadotrophin release and meat consumption in vegetarian women. Am J Clin Nutr 1986;43:37–41.

159. Adlercreutz H, Mousavi Y, Loukovaara M, et al. Lignans, isoflavones, sex hormone metabolism and breast cancer. In: Hochberg R, Naftolin F, editors. The new biology of steroid hormones. New York: Raven Press; 1992. p. 145–54.

160. Martin LJ, Greenberg CV, Kriukov V, et al. Intervention with a low-fat, high-carbohydrate diet does not influence the timing of menopause. Am J Clin Nutr 2006;84:920–8.

161. Cassidy A, Bingham S, Setchell KDR. Biological effects of a diet of soy protein rich in isoflavones on the menstrual cycle of premenopausal women. Am J Clin Nutr 1994;60:333–40.

162. Baird DD, Umbach DM, Lansdell L, et al. Dietary intervention study to assess estrogenicity of dietary soy among postmenopausal women. J Clin Endocrinol Metab 1995;80:1685–90.

Adiposity and the Menopausal Transition

Rachel P. Wildman, PhD[a],*, MaryFran R. Sowers, PhD[b],†

KEYWORDS

• Obesity • Adiposity • Abdominal obesity • Menopause

The prevalence of obesity has reached epidemic proportions in the United States and other developed countries, and is rapidly becoming a primary public health concern in developing countries. In the United States, the frequency of obesity [body mass index (BMI) ≥ 30 kg/m^2) is higher among women than men; grade 2 or 3 obesity (BMI ≥ 35 kg/m^2 and ≥ 40 kg/m^2, respectively) is especially prevalent among women (17.8% in women vs 10.7% in men in recent U.S. National Health and Nutrition Examination Survey data).[1] In the United States, which is relatively far along in the obesity epidemic, obesity rates among women are stabilizing; however, there is no evidence that rates are decreasing.[1] The prevalence of abdominal obesity, the depot more strongly associated with negative health consequences, is almost double that of general obesity, at 65.5% in women aged 40 to 59 years and 73.8% in women aged 60 years or more in 2008.[1]

Weight gain among midlife women has been frequently reported, but the interrelationships between obesity, weight gain, and the menopausal transition remain incompletely understood. The purpose of this review is to summarize the published literature on this topic from 3 primary vantage points: (1) The potential influence of adiposity and weight gain on the timing and characteristics of the menopausal transition, (2) the potential influence of the menopausal transition on adiposity and weight gain, and (3) the potential modification of menopausal transition effects on health outcomes by adiposity.

WHAT DO STUDIES OF REPRODUCTIVE AGING REVEAL ABOUT POTENTIAL EFFECTS OF ADIPOSITY ON THE MENOPAUSE TRANSITION?
Adiposity and Menstrual Cycle Characteristics

Although there has been considerable research into the effects of weight and obesity on the timing of menarche and on menstrual cycle characteristics in women of

[a] Department of Epidemiology & Population Health, Albert Einstein College of Medicine, 1300 Morris Park Avenue, Belfer Building, Room 1309, Bronx, NY 10461, USA
[b] Department of Epidemiology, Center for Integrated Approaches to Complex Diseases, University of Michigan, 1846 SPH I, 1415 Washington Heights, Ann Arbor, MI 48109-2029, USA
†Deceased.
* Corresponding author.
E-mail address: rachel.wildman@einstein.yu.edu

Obstet Gynecol Clin N Am 38 (2011) 441–454
doi:10.1016/j.ogc.2011.05.003
0889-8545/11/$ – see front matter © 2011 Elsevier Inc. All rights reserved.
obgyn.theclinics.com

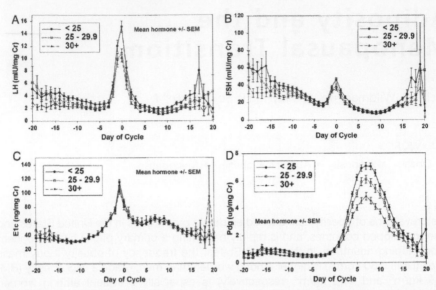

Fig. 1. Mean ± standard error of the mean daily levels of urinary hormones by BMI category (<25, 25–29.9, and ≥30 kg/m²). All hormone values normalized for creatinine (*Cr*). Note that women with BMIs (>25 kg/m²) are more likely to have lower LH, FSH, and progesterone metabolite pregnanediol glucuronide. (*From* Santoro N, Lasley B, McConnell D, et al. Body size and ethnicity are associated with menstrual cycle alterations in women in the early menopausal transition: The Study of Women's Health across the Nation (SWAN) Daily Hormone Study. J Clin Endocrinol Metab 2004;89:2626; with permission.)

reproductive age, a relative paucity of data exists about whether obesity contributes to menstrual cycle alterations associated with the menopause transition. Data from the Study of Women's Health Across the Nation (SWAN), a multicenter, multiethnic, prospective cohort study tracking changes in biological, psychological, and psycho-social parameters across the menopause transition, has been one of the few studies to explore the influence of obesity on diminishing ovarian function and menstrual cycle characteristics among midlife women. In addition to the annual follow-up visits conducted among the approximately 3300 SWAN enrollees, daily urinary hormones were collected on a subset of approximately 850 SWAN women for 1 complete menstrual cycle or for 50 days once per year, forming the basis of the Daily Hormone Ancillary Study. Data from the SWAN Daily Hormone Ancillary Study suggest that obese women may have fewer cycles with evidence of luteal activity than their normal weight counterparts (BMI <25 kg/m²; 78.3% vs 84.7%, respectively).[2] SWAN data also suggest that among women with evidence of luteal activity, obesity is associated with altered menstrual cycle length and hormone patterns. Obese women tended to have longer total cycle lengths, apparently attributable to longer follicular phases and significantly shorter luteal phases.[2] Furthermore, within the single characterized menstrual cycle, obese women tended to have lower total cycle gonadotropin levels and luteal phase progesterone metabolites, as evidenced by lower values of urinary follicle-stimulating hormone (FSH), urinary luteinizing hormone, and pregnanediol glucuronide (**Fig. 1**).[2] Therefore, as the authors note, hormonal dynamics are altered by obesity even during an ovulatory cycle.[2] This finding in perimenopausal women echoes findings among younger cycling obese women,[3–5] and recent evidence among younger ovulatory female candidates for bariatric surgery suggests that weight loss improves, although does not completely ameliorate, these hormone deficiencies.[6]

Adiposity and the Timing of Menopause

Although cycling obese women were less likely to have evidence of luteal activity and to have altered menstrual cycle lengths when there was evidence of luteal activity, it is not clear whether age at menopause is different among obese women. A number of studies have reported that obese women have a later age at menopause than nonobese women,[7–11] and cite this as consistent with higher circulating estrogen (estrone) levels arising from aromatization of androgens in expanded adipose beds in obese women. However, other studies have found a similar age at menopause among obese and nonobese women,[12–14] and 1 study has even found obese women to have an earlier age at menopause.[15] Among women in cross-sectional analyses of the SWAN study, obesity was not related to age at natural menopause, but was related to the likelihood of surgical menopause, with premenopausal obese women more likely to undergo surgical menopause.[13] This had the effect of lessening the number of obese women in the premenopausal category, whereas the percent of obese women in the perimenopausal and postmenopausal categories were similar.[13] Both SWAN and the Penn Ovarian Aging Study (POAS), a longitudinal study of midlife African-American and Caucasian women, have evaluated whether obesity influences time to menopause, apart from age at menopause. Among perimenopausal women, SWAN did not observe an association between obesity and time to the final menstrual period (FMP),[16] whereas in the POAS, there was a positive association between BMI and the odds of transitioning from premenopause to perimenopause, but no association between BMI and transition from perimenopause to postmenopause.[17] This latter finding may relate to the findings of a greater likelihood for obese women to be anovulatory and have either very short or very long cycles, which may result in their meeting definitions for early perimenopausal more readily than normal weight women, but not necessarily experiencing the FMP sooner.

Adiposity and Hormone Changes During the Transition

A number of investigations have reported the magnitude or pattern of hormone changes across the menopausal transition in obese versus nonobese women. In both SWAN and POAS, obese and nonobese women had different estradiol and FSH levels, and in the POAS, different luteinizing hormone and inhibin B levels as well.[18–21] The POAS suggested that findings were similar when measures of central adiposity, such as waist circumference and waist:hip ratio, were utilized to categorize obese and nonobese women.[17] More recently, a number of more rigorous analyses have tracked changes in hormone levels across the time before and after the FMP in obese versus nonobese women. These investigations have revealed similar differences in absolute hormone levels in obese versus nonobese women with respect to earlier investigations cited above, with lower estradiol levels in obese women before the FMP, and the reverse after the FMP (**Fig. 2**).[22] In addition, although the pattern of observed hormone changes in estradiol and FSH were similar in obese and nonobese women until approximately 2 years before the FMP, after this point there was a blunted hormone change surrounding the FMP in obese versus nonobese women. Data from the Michigan Bone Health and Metabolism Study (MBHMS), a prospective study of Caucasian midlife women living in the Detroit area, also demonstrate this blunted estradiol decline in obese women.[23] The lesser estradiol decline observed in obese women may result from enhanced aromatization rates given their excess adipose

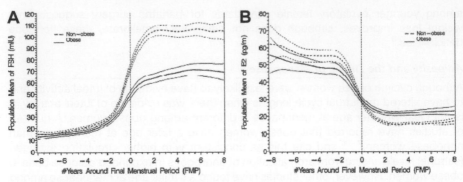

Fig. 2. Mean and 95% confidence interval for FSH and estradiol (E2) in obese versus nonobese women in relation to the FMP. (*From* Randolph JF Jr, Zheng H, Sowers MR, et al. Change in follicle-stimulating hormone and estradiol across the menopausal transition: effect of age at the final menstrual period. J Clin Endocrinol Metab 2011;96:749, with permission.)

tissue. In SWAN, the rate of estradiol decline during the critical transition period around the FMP seemed to be determined by both obesity and single nucleotide polymorphisms for aromatase and type 1 β17HSD genes (the enzyme associated with the potentially bidirectional conversion of estrone and estradiol).[24] The blunted decline observed in estradiol among obese women observed in the MBHMS and SWAN data is physiologically corroborated by a similarly blunted FSH rise surrounding the FMP in obese versus nonobese women (**Fig. 2**).[22]

Summary

The literature clearly supports that the magnitude of reproductive hormone changes experienced within individual menstrual cycles as the transition approaches, as well as during the transition itself, are altered in obese women, seeming to be blunted in comparison with nonobese women. The published literature also finds that the pattern of the difference in hormone levels between obese and nonobese women changes at some point late in the menopause transition. One mechanism likely underlying these findings relates to the change in the primary source of circulating estradiol as the menopause transition progresses; the primary source of circulating estradiol premenopausally is the ovary, whereas in postmenopause, the primary source of circulating estradiol is aromatization of androgens within adipose tissue. This change in estradiol source provides postmenopausal obese women with a nonovarian reservoir of estrogen that normal weight women do not have, which may blunt the gonadotropin rises and mitigate ovarian estrogen loss with menopause. These hormonal alterations may also blunt menopause-associated adverse health effects. What mechanisms underlie the lower estradiol levels in obese versus nonobese women premenopausally are presently unclear. Some have posited low ovarian reserve. However, this is not supported by recent ultrasound data identifying no difference in antral follicle count between obese and normal weight late reproductive-age women (40–52 years),[25] as well as the lack of evidence (cited above) suggesting that obese women have an earlier menopause. Follicular dysfunction and alterations in central nervous system regulation of hormonal levels among obese women may be factors, but additional research in this area is needed.

WHAT DO STUDIES OF REPRODUCTIVE AGING REVEAL ABOUT POTENTIAL EFFECTS OF THE MENOPAUSE TRANSITION ON ADIPOSITY?
Chronological Aging Versus the Menopause Transition

Much of the early work examining the possible link between adiposity and the menopausal transition focused on whether women gained weight during the menopausal transition. Although it is commonly thought that menopause is associated with weight gain, longitudinal analyses with careful accounting of chronologic versus ovarian aging are inconclusive. Studies using body weight suggest that weight gain in midlife among women is more consistent with a pattern of chronologic aging, and not uniquely due to the menopausal transition,[26–29] whereas a study using actual fat mass measures finds otherwise. Wing and colleagues[28] were among the first to attempt to tease this apart by following women over time and comparing weight gain among women who remained premenopausal over follow-up to weight gain among women who experienced a natural menopause by the end of follow-up. Weight gain was similar in the 2 groups, and perhaps even a bit greater among women who remained premenopausal (+2.07 vs +1.35 kg).[28] Similarly, in a comparison of premenopausal and postmenopausal women matched for age, premenopausal women actually had a higher mean body weight.[30] Weight gain during midlife may be an ambiguous measure, because it represents not only increasing fat tissue, but also potential declines in bone mass and skeletal muscle. Body composition analyses within a SWAN ancillary study demonstrated a positive, linear slope of fat mass by study year as a proxy for chronologic aging (**Fig. 3**, *bottom left*), but a curvilinear increase in fat mass was seen surrounding the FMP, whereby fat mass increased to a greater degree before menopause and thereafter leveled off (**Fig. 3**, *bottom right*), suggesting that accumulation of fat mass slowed after the FMP.[31]

Menopause Transition Effects on Body Fat Distribution

The literature also suggests that ovarian aging may influence where fat is distributed, with a central redistribution of fat. Cross-sectional analyses comparing premenopausal women with postmenopausal women have reported that adjustment for age eliminates significant differences in total body fat and subcutaneous adipose tissue, but that abdominal adiposity measures remain higher in postmenopausal women.[32,33] However, other cross-sectional analyses have failed to show differences in waist circumference between premenopausal and postmenopausal women.[30,34]

Three reports all using longitudinal analyses to track patterns of body fat distribution measures across the menopausal transition anchored by the FMP have produced inconclusive results. In a study of women aged 43 years and older at baseline, changes in body weight, percent fat mass, and abdominal subcutaneous fat seemed linear from 4 years before the start of postmenopause (12 months without a period and FSH >30 mIU/mL) through the first 2 years of postmenopause, whereas abdominal visceral adipose tissue seemed to change quickly during perimenopause, leveling off approximately at the FMP (**Fig. 4**).[35] A similar pattern was reported using waist circumference change tracked around the FMP in the SWAN body composition ancillary study among African-American and Caucasian women (**Fig. 3**, *top right*), although these results were less pronounced, perhaps because waist circumference represents changes in both subcutaneous and visceral adipose tissue.[31] However, in subsequent SWAN longitudinal analyses with longer follow-up (9 vs 6 years) and including Japanese and Chinese women, change in waist seemed to be linear in relation to the FMP (**Fig. 5**).[36]

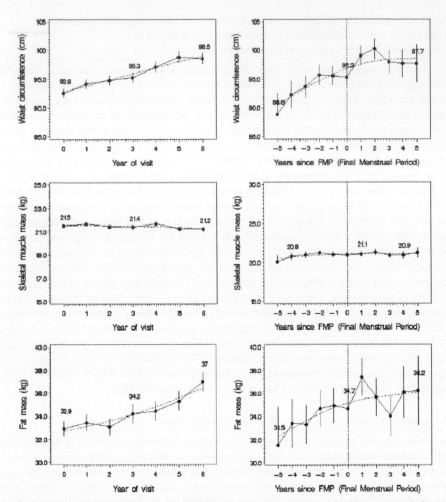

Fig. 3. Mean waist circumference and body composition values in relation to time (*left side*) and the FMP (*right side*). (*From* Sowers M, Zheng H, Tomey K, et al. Changes in body composition in women over six years at midlife: ovarian and chronological aging. J Clin Endocrinol Metab 2007;92:898; with permission.)

Reproductive Hormone Effects on Adiposity

In addition to analyses of the associations between weight or weight change and the menopause transition, the question of whether ovarian aging may cause weight gain has also been addressed from the perspective of sex hormones. In the SWAN study, neither changes in circulating estradiol nor FSH levels were associated with incident obesity or severe obesity over 9 years of follow-up.[37] Similarly, null findings were reported in relation to central adiposity in cross-sectional analyses of a SWAN ancillary study relating estradiol levels to computed tomography-determined abdominal visceral adipose tissue levels,[38] and in longitudinal analyses of the Melbourne Women's Midlife Health Project relating baseline estradiol and change in estradiol from baseline with central fat measurements 5 years later derived from dual energy x-ray absorptiometry.[39]

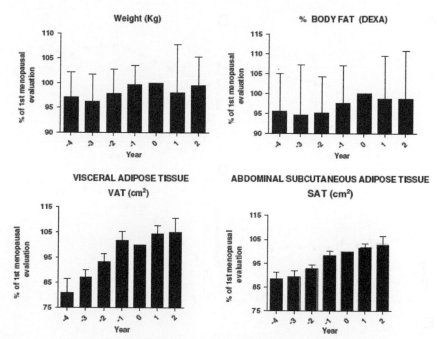

Fig. 4. Longitudinal changes in body composition and body fat distribution in relation to the FMP. (*From* Lovejoy JC, Champagne CM, de Jonge L, et al. Increased visceral fat and decreased energy expenditure during the menopausal transition. Int J Obes (Lond) 2008;32:953, with permission.)

Summary

Although the published literature is quite convincing of an effect of obesity on the magnitude of menopause-associated hormonal changes, it does not clearly support a relationship in the opposite direction, namely an effect of the menopause transition or its associated hormonal changes on either overall weight gain or central redistribution of body fat. There is some evidence that the perimenopause is associated with more rapid increases in fat mass and redistribution of fat to the abdomen, but published findings are conflicting, and additional longitudinal investigations are needed.

DOES OBESITY MODIFY THE EFFECTS OF THE MENOPAUSE TRANSITION ON THE EXPERIENCE OF MENOPAUSAL SYMPTOMS OR HEALTH OUTCOMES?

A fairly large body of literature has assessed the influence of obesity on the experience of vasomotor symptoms associated with the menopausal transition. It was initially hypothesized that obese women would experience fewer vasomotor symptoms owing to an assumption that obese women would have higher estradiol levels resulting from peripheral conversion of androgens to estrogens in the adipose tissue. As discussed, however, estradiol levels are not higher; rather, they are lower in obese women early in the transition. It is only by the late transition and postmenopause that the peripheral conversion of androgens to estrogen have an impact on circulating estradiol. Evidence suggests that obese women actually experience more vasomotor symptoms and more bothersome symptoms, at least in the relatively earlier stages of the

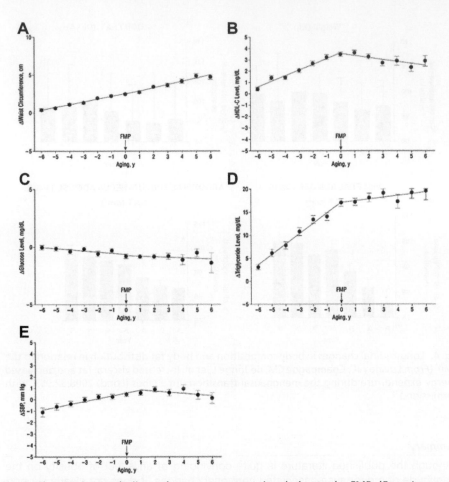

Fig. 5. Changes in metabolic syndrome components in relation to the FMP. (*From* Janssen I, Powell LH, Crawford S, Lasley B, et al. Menopause and the metabolic syndrome: the Study of Women's Health Across the Nation. Arch Intern Med 2008;168:1572; with permission.)

menopausal transition. Among SWAN enrollees, a higher percent body fat, a higher mass of abdominal subcutaneous fat, and greater weight gain are each associated with more frequent hot flashes.[40–42] Similarly, the MBHMS has reported that the bothersomeness of symptoms is greater with increasing BMI.[43] These findings have been interpreted as suggestive that adipose tissue acts as an insulator, increasing hot flashes and their intensity.[42] Although these findings were not altered by menopausal stage among SWAN participants, other studies have demonstrated that such findings are strongest earlier in the menopause transition.[44] This raises the potential that the relatively higher circulating estradiol levels in obese women later in the menopausal transition may somewhat counteract symptoms.

There has been less work examining whether obesity modifies the menopause-associated increased risks of various chronic diseases. The SWAN study was the first to examine the influence of body weight on the increases in lipids associated with the menopausal transition. Examination of lipid and lipoprotein changes across menopause status categories revealed that the gradual increase in lipids observed from

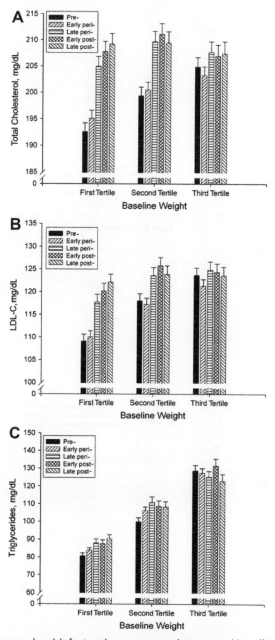

Fig. 6. Mean cardiovascular risk factors by menopausal status and baseline weight category. (*From* Derby CA, Crawford SL, Pasternak RC, et al. Lipid changes during the menopause transition in relation to age and weight: the Study of Women's Health Across the Nation. Am J Epidemiol 2009;169:1358; with permission.)

premenopause to perimenopause to postmenopause, independent of aging, was blunted in heavier women (**Fig. 6**); this effect was partially explained by the higher estradiol levels among heavier postmenopausal women.[45] Consistent with these findings, a subsequent SWAN analysis, limited to women with a natural menopause,

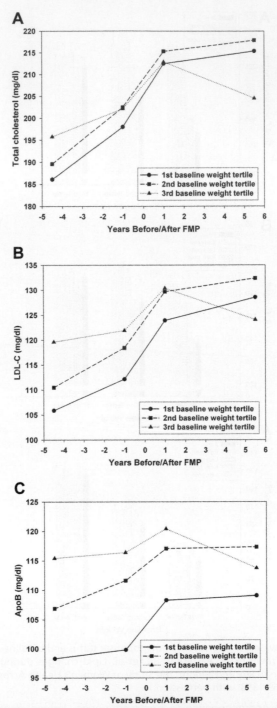

Fig. 7. Annual mean lipids in relation to the FMP by baseline weight. (*From* Matthews KA, Crawford SL, Chae CU, et al. Are changes in cardiovascular disease risk factors in midlife women due to chronological aging or to the menopausal transition? J Am Coll Cardiol 2009;54:2372; with permission.)

identified that body size did not seem to influence the pattern of lipid changes leading up to the FMP (all body weight groups experienced a sharp increase in lipids leading up to the FMP), but did seem to alter postmenopausal lipid changes (**Fig. 7**).[46] Among the heaviest women, adverse lipid and lipoprotein changes seemed to stop increasing, or even decreased slightly after the FMP, whereas in the lower weight groups the increases continued after the FMP, but were somewhat blunted (**Fig. 7**).[46]

Among midlife women in the MBHMS, similar analyses were performed in relation to bone loss surrounding the FMP, and again, a blunting of menopause associated bone resorption was observed in the obese versus nonobese women.[47] Among both obese and nonobese women, bone loss accelerated in the 4 to 5 years around the FMP.[47] However, in obese women, bone loss subsided to baseline rates after the FMP, whereas nonobese women continued to experience a somewhat greater rate of bone loss 6 to 8 years after the FMP.[47]

Summary

Mirroring the blunted gonadotropin changes observed in obese women as they traverse the menopause, obese women also display blunted menopause-associated lipid/lipoprotein and bone changes. Whether these obesity-related modifications are directly explained by the relative elevation in estradiol in obese postmenopausal women remains unclear. In contrast with the consistency of lipid/lipoprotein and bone findings with blunted gonadotropin responses across the menopause, data suggest that obese women have an exacerbated menopausal symptom response, experiencing greater numbers of hot flashes, as well as more bothersome hot flashes, likely owing to the insulating effects of adipose tissue, although this effect may be weaker later in the menopause transition because of the blunted estradiol decrease in obese women.

CONCLUSION

Although data are limited, current information suggests there are substantial effects of obesity and adiposity on the magnitude of hormone changes experienced during the transition, as well as on the risks of chronic disease resulting from the menopause transition. The ability to partition these effects into those resulting from overall adiposity versus specific fat depots or the metabolic environment generated with excess adiposity awaits additional data. The high prevalence of obesity among women across the lifespan and the particular vulnerability of menopausal women to chronic diseases underscore the importance of further study into the potentially circular relationship between adipose tissue and menopause-associated hormone changes.

REFERENCES

1. Flegal KM, Carroll MD, Ogden CL, et al. Prevalence and trends in obesity among US adults, 1999–2008. JAMA 2010;303:235–41.
2. Santoro N, Lasley B, McConnell D, et al. Body size and ethnicity are associated with menstrual cycle alterations in women in the early menopausal transition: The Study of Women's Health across the Nation (SWAN) Daily Hormone Study. J Clin Endocrinol Metab 2004;89:2622–31.
3. Rowland AS, Baird DD, Long S, et al. Influence of medical conditions and lifestyle factors on the menstrual cycle. Epidemiology 2002;13:668–74.
4. Grenman S, Ronnemaa T, Irjala K, et al. Sex steroid, gonadotropin, cortisol, and prolactin levels in healthy, massively obese women: correlation with abdominal fat cell size and effect of weight reduction. J Clin Endocrinol Metab 1986;63:1257–61.

5. Jain A, Polotsky AJ, Rochester D, et al. Pulsatile luteinizing hormone amplitude and progesterone metabolite excretion are reduced in obese women. J Clin Endocrinol Metab 2007;92:2468–73.

6. Rochester D, Jain A, Polotsky AJ, et al. Partial recovery of luteal function after bariatric surgery in obese women. Fertil Steril 2009;92:1410–5.

7. Willett W, Stampfer MJ, Bain C, et al. Cigarette smoking, relative weight, and menopause. Am J Epidemiol 1983;117:651–8.

8. Nagata C, Takatsuka N, Inaba S, et al. Association of diet and other lifestyle with onset of menopause in Japanese women. Maturitas 1998;29:105–13.

9. Sherman B, Wallace R, Bean J, et al. Relationship of body weight to menarcheal and menopausal age: implications for breast cancer risk. J Clin Endocrinol Metab 1981; 52:488–93.

10. Palmer JR, Rosenberg L, Wise LA, et al. Onset of natural menopause in African American women. Am J Public Health 2003;93:299–306.

11. Dorjgochoo T, Kallianpur A, Gao YT, et al. Dietary and lifestyle predictors of age at natural menopause and reproductive span in the Shanghai Women's Health Study. Menopause 2008;15:924–33.

12. Bromberger JT, Matthews KA, Kuller LH, et al. Prospective study of the determinants of age at menopause. Am J Epidemiol 1997;145:124–33.

13. Gold EB, Bromberger J, Crawford S, et al. Factors associated with age at natural menopause in a multiethnic sample of midlife women. Am J Epidemiol 2001;153: 865–74.

14. Amigoni S, Morelli P, Chatenoud L, et al. Cross-sectional study of determinants of menopausal age and hormone replacement therapy use in Italian women. Climacteric 2000;3:25–32.

15. Kato I, Toniolo P, Akhmedkhanov A, et al. Prospective study of factors influencing the onset of natural menopause. J Clin Epidemiol 1998;51:1271–6.

16. Santoro N, Brockwell S, Johnston J, et al. Helping midlife women predict the onset of the final menses: SWAN, the Study of Women's Health Across the Nation. Menopause 2007;14:415–24.

17. Sammel MD, Freeman EW, Liu Z, et al. Factors that influence entry into stages of the menopausal transition. Menopause 2009;16:1218–27.

18. Freeman EW, Sammel MD, Gracia CR, et al. Follicular phase hormone levels and menstrual bleeding status in the approach to menopause. Fertil Steril 2005;83: 383–92.

19. Gracia CR, Freeman EW, Sammel MD, et al. The relationship between obesity and race on inhibin B during the menopause transition. Menopause 2005;12:559–66.

20. Freeman EW, Sammel MD, Lin H, et al. Obesity and reproductive hormone levels in the transition to menopause. Menopause 2010;17:718–26.

21. Randolph JF Jr, Sowers M, Bondarenko IV, et al. Change in estradiol and follicle-stimulating hormone across the early menopausal transition: effects of ethnicity and age. J Clin Endocrinol Metab 2004;89:1555–61.

22. Randolph JF Jr, Zheng H, Sowers MR, et al. Change in follicle-stimulating hormone and estradiol across the menopausal transition: effect of age at the final menstrual period. J Clin Endocrinol Metab 2011;96:746–54.

23. Sowers MR, Zheng H, McConnell D, et al. Estradiol rates of change in relation to the final menstrual period in a population-based cohort of women. J Clin Endocrinol Metab 2008;93:3847–52.

24. Sowers M, Randolph JF Jr, Zheng H, et al. Genetic polymorphisms and obesity influence estradiol decline during the menopause. Clin Endocrinol (Oxf) 2011;74: 618–23.

25. Su HI, Sammel MD, Freeman EW, et al. Body size affects measures of ovarian reserve in late reproductive age women. Menopause 2008;15:857–61.
26. Guthrie JR, Dennerstein L, Dudley EC. Weight gain and the menopause: a 5-year prospective study. Climacteric 1999;2:205–11.
27. Davies KM, Heaney RP, Recker RR, et al. Hormones, weight change and menopause. Int J Obes Relat Metab Disord 2001;25:874–9.
28. Wing RR, Matthews KA, Kuller LH, et al. Weight gain at the time of menopause. Arch Intern Med 1991;151:97–102.
29. Crawford SL, Casey VA, Avis NE, et al. A longitudinal study of weight and the menopause transition: results from the Massachusetts Women's Health Study. Menopause 2000;7:96–104.
30. Bjorkelund C, Lissner L, Andersson S, et al. Reproductive history in relation to relative weight and fat distribution. Int J Obes Relat Metab Disord 1996;20:213–19.
31. Sowers M, Zheng H, Tomey K, et al. Changes in body composition in women over six years at midlife: ovarian and chronological aging. J Clin Endocrinol Metab 2007;92: 895–901.
32. Donato GB, Fuchs SC, Oppermann K, et al. Association between menopause status and central adiposity measured at different cutoffs of waist circumference and waist-to-hip ratio. Menopause 2006;13:280–5.
33. Toth MJ, Tchernof A, Sites CK, et al. Menopause-related changes in body fat distribution. Ann N Y Acad Sci 2000;904:502–6.
34. Pasquali R, Casimirri F, Pascal G, et al. Influence of menopause on blood cholesterol levels in women: the role of body composition, fat distribution and hormonal milieu. Virgilio Menopause Health Group. J Intern Med 1997;241:195–203.
35. Lovejoy JC, Champagne CM, de Jonge L, et al. Increased visceral fat and decreased energy expenditure during the menopausal transition. Int J Obes (Lond) 2008;32: 949–58.
36. Janssen I, Powell LH, Crawford S, et al. Menopause and the metabolic syndrome: the Study of Women's Health Across the Nation. Arch Intern Med 2008;168:1568–75.
37. Sutton-Tyrrell K, Zhao X, Santoro N, et al. Reproductive hormones and obesity: 9 years of observation from the Study of Women's Health Across the Nation. Am J Epidemiol 2010;171:1203–13.
38. Janssen I, Powell LH, Kazlauskaite R, et al. Testosterone and visceral fat in midlife women: the Study of Women's Health Across the Nation (SWAN) fat patterning study. Obesity (Silver Spring) 2010;18:604–10.
39. Guthrie JR, Dennerstein L, Taffe JR, et al. Central abdominal fat and endogenous hormones during the menopausal transition. Fertil Steril 2003;79:1335–40.
40. Thurston RC, Sowers MR, Chang Y, et al. Adiposity and reporting of vasomotor symptoms among midlife women: the study of women's health across the nation. Am J Epidemiol 2008;167:78–85.
41. Thurston RC, Sowers MR, Sutton-Tyrrell K, et al. Abdominal adiposity and hot flashes among midlife women. Menopause 2008;15:429–34.
42. Thurston RC, Sowers MR, Sternfeld B, et al. Gains in body fat and vasomotor symptom reporting over the menopausal transition: the study of women's health across the nation. Am J Epidemiol 2009;170:766–74.
43. Ford K, Sowers M, Crutchfield M, et al. A longitudinal study of the predictors of prevalence and severity of symptoms commonly associated with menopause. Menopause 2005;12:308–17.
44. Whiteman MK, Staropoli CA, Benedict JC, et al. Risk factors for hot flashes in midlife women. J Womens Health (Larchmt) 2003;12:459–72.

45. Derby CA, Crawford SL, Pasternak RC, et al. Lipid changes during the menopause transition in relation to age and weight: the Study of Women's Health Across the Nation. Am J Epidemiol 2009;169:1352–61.
46. Matthews KA, Crawford SL, Chae CU, et al. Are changes in cardiovascular disease risk factors in midlife women due to chronological aging or to the menopausal transition? J Am Coll Cardiol 2009;54:2366–73.
47. Sowers MR, Zheng H, Jannausch ML, et al. Amount of bone loss in relation to time around the FMP and follicle-stimulating hormone staging of the transmenopause. J Clin Endocrinol Metab 2010;95:2155–62.

Reproductive Hormones and the Menopause Transition

Nanette Santoro, MD[a]*, John F. Randolph Jr, MD[b]

KEYWORDS

- Menopause • Menopause transition • Inhibin
- Anti-Mullerian hormone • Luteinizing hormone
- Follicle-stimulating hormone • Estrogen • Progesterone

Women undergo progressive follicle loss throughout life.[1] Although the majority of follicles in an individual woman's ovaries are lost in fetal life,[2] there is progressive, exponential loss of oocytes through a woman's reproductive life span. Most mathematical models of oocyte loss indicate an exponential process, and an acceleration of follicle loss as women enter the menopausal transition (MT),[3,4] indicating that a woman loses follicles at the fastest rates when she is the most reproductively aged. Moreover, there is evidence that the structural and functional quality of oocytes deteriorates with reproductive aging.[5]

In addition to changes in follicle numbers, which is the main driver of the MT, follicle dynamics also shift with the process of menopause.[6,7] The cardinal hormonal changes recognized to occur in concert with the menstrual cycle irregularity that herald entry into the MT also serve to accelerate the follicular growth process and may make it less effective. Finally, alterations in central neural processes that reliably produce an ovulatory LH surge in midreproductive life seem to become less reliable, and lead to further cycle dysfunction.[8]

This review describes the hormonal changes that accompany the process of follicle loss and menopause. We shall draw primarily, when possible, from large-sample epidemiologic studies, especially the Study of Women's Health Across the Nation (SWAN).[9] SWAN is a multiethnic, longitudinal cohort study of 3300 US women from

Funded by AG-12535 and NR-04061.
Dr Nanette Santoro is a consultant to Menogenix.
[a] Department of Obstetrics and Gynecology, University of Colorado School of Medicine, 12631 East 17th Avenue, Mail Stop B-198, AO1-Room 4010, Aurora, CO 80045, USA
[b] Department of Obstetrics and Gynecology, Division of Reproductive Endocrinology, University of Michigan, L4100 Women's Medical Hospital, 1500 East Medical Center Drive, Ann Arbor, MI 48109-0276, USA
* Corresponding author.
E-mail address: Nanette.Santoro@ucdenver.edu

Obstet Gynecol Clin N Am 38 (2011) 455–466
doi:10.1016/j.ogc.2011.05.004
0889-8545/11/$ – see front matter © 2011 Elsevier Inc. All rights reserved.

7 national sites enrolled when they were between the ages of 40 and 52. Women were followed annually in SWAN, which is now in its 14th follow-up year. Thus, most of the SWAN participants have undergone menopause and their data constitute the most representative community-based sample available to date. SWAN's Daily Hormone Study will also be discussed, because it is the most comprehensive study of menstrual cycles in midlife US women that has ever been collected.

STAGING THE MT

The MT is preceded by approximately 35 years of regular, predictable menstrual cycles. During this time, women have a well-defined intermenstrual interval of 25 to 35 days. These cycles consist of a 14-day luteal phase, and a follicular phase of at least 10 to 11 days. Before the appearance of a break in this characteristic menstrual rhythm, the oocyte supply has been dwindling, but has not yet reached a critical level. Nonetheless, although no signs are detectable to a woman, some subtle hormonal changes are happening in this midreproductive interval. Follicle-stimulating hormone (FSH), critical for the terminal stages of follicle growth, rises, albeit slowly, throughout the reproductive years.[10] In addition to this change, a woman's follicle cohort size shrinks, even though she continues to reliably ovulate every month.

The MT has been broken into 2 stages: Early and late. The initiation of the transition is when a previously regularly cycling woman experiences a skipped menstrual cycle, or notes a variation of her intermenstrual interval more than 6 days.[11] She remains in the early transition until she experiences more than 60 days' amenorrhea, at which time she transitions into the "late" MT. The late MT, characterized by prolonged amenorrhea, is accompanied by less frequent cycling, and ends with the final menstrual period (FMP). The FMP is only defined once 1 year of amenorrhea has been experienced. Each of these menstrual cycle milestones is accompanied by hormonal alterations that help the clinician to determine a woman's progress through the MT.

Methods for Evaluating Reproductive Aging and Predicting Ovarian Function

FSH
A monotropic rise in FSH is considered the endocrinologic hallmark of the MT. FSH elevations seem to be intermittent as the follicle supply dwindles, but it is an accurate reflection of a woman's ability to conceive. As such, it is more of an indicator of egg quantity than of egg quality in the early transition. FSH rises are more sustained over time in the late MT and the rise is most precipitous in the years bracketing the FMP.[12] Early follicular phase FSH, taken between cycle days 2 and 5, is the most sensitive and convenient time in the cycle to perform this measurement.

Estradiol
Along with the monotropic FSH rise characteristic of the MT, estradiol (E2) can also be elevated in the early follicular phase of the cycle, especially in the early MT.[13,14] This seems to be a reflection of the accelerated folliculogenesis and shortening of the follicular phase that occur in the early MT. Early follicular E2 levels are the last biomarker of the transition to irrevocably change, with a rapid decline beginning 2 years before the FMP and reaching stability 2 years afterward.[15]

Inhibin B
The inhibins are peptides of the transforming growth factor-β superfamily that are produced by the granulosa cells of ovarian follicles in their terminal stages of development. They consist of a common α subunit, with specificity conferred by the

β subunit. Inhibin B is produced by the granulosa cells of the growing follicle cohort and reflects both the health of the individual follicles and their overall numbers.[10] Inhibin A is a product of the dominant follicle and the corpus luteum. The shrinkage of the follicle cohort that accompanies aging is detectable by a reduction in inhibin B. Thus, early follicular phase inhibin B measurement has been proposed as way to measure ovarian reserve directly.[16,17] Inhibin B is among the earliest harbingers of the MT. Thus, loss of the follicle cohort seems to be the initiating step into the hormonal changes that ensue with the onset of the MT.

Anti-mullerian hormone or mullerian-inhibiting substance

Anti-Mullerian hormone (AMH)/Mullerian-inhibiting substance (MIS) are also transforming growth factor-β superfamily peptides, and are produced by granulosa cells. However, they are not just produced by follicles in their terminal stages of growth, but also by primary, secondary, and early antral follicles and therefore reflect more completely the follicle cohort. Circulating concentrations of AMH/MIS decline throughout reproductive life and theoretically constitute the earliest and most effective way to measure a woman's progress toward menopause. Although some studies indicate that AMH/MIS holds promise as a predictor of time to menopause, the current sensitivity of the measurement method is such that estimates of time to the FMP cannot be accomplished within a time frame less than 4 years.[18] It is hoped that the eventual development of a sufficiently sensitive assay for AMH/MIS will become a "menopause test."

Evaluations of annual serum hormones across the transition

A primary directive of the request for applications that led to the SWAN study was to "characterize the endocrinology/physiology of the perimenopause," including the assessment and discovery of biomarkers of ovarian aging. Prior longitudinal studies by McKinlay[19] and Burger[20] had begun to describe the patterns of change in serum FSH and E2 across the MT, establishing them as candidate markers of ovarian function over time that tracked both ovarian secretion (E2) and central regulation of that secretion (FSH). Both were included as annual measures in the longitudinal design of SWAN, and mandated a standardized collection protocol anchored to a reproducible timeframe in the menstrual cycle owing to significant variation in levels across the cycle. The early follicular phase was deemed the most reproducible and biologically comparable as women lost menstrual cyclicity through the MT, recognizing that changes in other menstrual cycle phases would not be evaluable with this sampling scheme. Longitudinal analyses of the accrued annual serum hormone levels included variables for day of cycle and loss of cyclicity to control for cycle variability.

An initial longitudinal analysis of FSH and E2 through 5 years of follow-up[21] noted that serum E2 concentrations decreased and FSH concentrations increased significantly with age, with more rapid change at older ages. As the study matured, and more women had undergone natural FMPs, it became possible to analyze these data anchored to the most widely utilized biomarker of ovarian aging, the FMP.[22,23] Utilizing analyses that describe change over time, previously able to decompose the MT into "epochs" of FSH and E2 change around the FMP in a parallel study of somewhat younger women,[23] the FSH pattern across the menopause transition began with an increase about 6 years before the FMP, accelerated 2 years before the FMP, decelerated beginning 0.20 years before the FMP, and attained stable levels 2 years after the FMP, independent of age at the FMP, race/ethnicity, or smoking status. The mean E2 concentration did not change until 2 years before the FMP when it began decreasing, achieving maximal rate of change at the FMP, and then

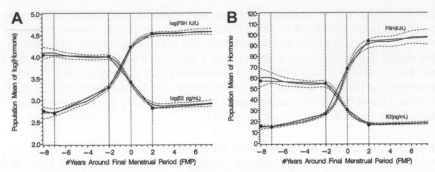

Fig. 1. Rates of change in FSH and E2 shown anchored to the FMP. (*A*) Log-transformed values. (*B*) Back-transformed values. (*From* Randolph JF Jr., Zheng H, Sowers MR, et al. Change in follicle-stimulating hormone and estradiol across the menopausal transition: effect of age at the final menstrual period. J Clin Endocrinol Metab 2011;96:746; with permission.[22])

decelerating to achieve stability 2 years after the FMP. The timespans and overall patterns of change in serum FSH and E2 across the MT were not related to age at FMP (**Fig. 1**).

In contrast with the maintenance of E2 levels until 2 years before the FMP, inhibin B and AMH concentrations fall to become undetectable by available assays 4 to 5 years before cessation of bleeding,[18] consistent with a decrease in both the size of the primordial follicle pool and the cohort of follicles recruited from that pool for each menstrual cycle. The fall in inhibin B mirrors the rise in FSH, supporting the primary role of the inhibins in the negative feedback regulation of FSH secretion.

Taken together, the dynamics of the early MT seem to be based on follicle attrition and a loss of the follicle cohort, rather than complete follicle failure. The reduction in follicle cohort size seems to be the earliest event in the transition, as evidenced by a detectable drop in inhibin B.[24] Thus, although there are still responsive follicles available, inhibin restraint of FSH secretion is lost. The resulting FSH rise leads to faster and possibly dysregulated folliculogenesis, and the menstrual cycle may grow shorter. Occasionally, the cohort size is insufficient to develop an ovulatory follicle, and the cycle is skipped, but there is no period of amenorrhea longer than 60 days (ie, 2 skipped cycles). By the late MT, follicle numbers become critically low and follicle competency (either owing to abnormal regulation or to anatomic or functional inferiority of follicles that grow later in reproductive life) is reduced such that anovulatory cycles become more common and cycles in which folliculogenesis cannot even be initiated become more common. Women then undergo a period of time of "prolonged amenorrhea" of 2 to 11 months' duration. Eventually, at a follicle complement of approximately 1000,[4] the FMP is attained and hypergonadotropic amenorrhea becomes permanent. Although the definition of the FMP as fully defined after 12 months' amenorrhea and the process is widely believed to be irreversible, it is age related and not an absolute boundary. Women over age 45 who experience 12 months' amenorrhea have a 10% probability of having a subsequent menstrual episode.[25]

MENSTRUAL CYCLE HORMONE CHANGES ACROSS THE MT

Although numerous worldwide studies have reported findings on annual or semiannual changes in serum hormones across the MT,[12,26,27] which are usually measured in the early follicular phase of the cycle, day-to-day hormone levels across a menstrual cycle have been less well characterized.

The first studies of menstrual cycle dynamics across the MT were performed by Metcalf, from New Zealand. To characterize hormone patterns over time, these investigators developed methods suitable for the collection and analysis of daily, urinary samples for gonadotropins and sex steroids. In a series of small sample size, in both cross sectional and longitudinal studies,[28-32] the Metcalf group provided the framework that has informed much current research. By examining cycles longitudinally, they observed that the proportion of ovulatory cycles decreased as women approached the FMP. Once the FMP was attained, variable estrogen excretion was observed for the first year thereafter, but no further progesterone excretion was measurable. These observations have been confirmed by subsequent investigators.

Others have since added pertinent findings by examining larger sample sizes and uncovering novel relationships. In the SWAN Daily Hormone Study, 990 women were invited to complete a daily urine collection for an entire menstrual cycle or up to 50 days if menses did not occur, and to repeat the collection annually until the FMP. Of the original 990, 848 women (86%) had interpretable data available for analysis in the baseline collection.[33] Over a 3-year follow-up period, several findings became evident from this large sample. First, a previously unappreciated relationship between hormones and body mass index (BMI) became evident in this large sample size. With increasing BMI, LH, FSH, estrogen, and progesterone metabolites all were observed to decrease significantly. Over time, progesterone metabolite excretion was reduced, both by age and by year on study. Moreover, Chinese and Japanese-American women demonstrated lower estrogen metabolite excretion compared to the other ethnic groups in SWAN (**Fig. 2**).

In the Biodemographic Models of Reproductive Aging project, samples of 17 to 134 women per reproductive stage group were assessed with 6-month, daily collections of urine.[34] These data confirmed prior, smaller studies[14] indicating an increase in estrogen exposure and increased potential for unopposed estrogen exposure as women traverse the menopause. Others have examined the hormone patterns during a menstrual cycle be performing tri-weekly serum sampling.[35] To explain some of the erratic estrogen levels observed in perimenopausal women, these investigators coined the phrase "luteal out-of-phase" cycles to describe a specific pattern of irregular cycling. In these cycles, the secondary, luteal rise of estrogen is maintained and even exaggerated, and leads to a subsequent cycle in which progesterone production is deficient. The investigators attributed this pattern to sustained FSH elevation, which "drove" estrogen production in the subsequent cycle and likely caused folliculogenesis at an inappropriately early time (ie, the preceding luteal phase).

Androgens and the Transition

The ovary, the periphery (particularly adipose tissue), and the adrenal gland are the sources of androgen production in women. A detailed picture of the patterns of androgen secretion and their correlates is covered in another article and therefore is not developed in detail in this review.

Briefly, the contributions of the ovary, periphery, and adrenal gland change over the course of the MT. As the ovarian contribution of testosterone declines with menopause, concurrent decreases in sex hormone-binding globulin, the principal, high-affinity serum carrier protein for both testosterone and E2, offsets the drop in testosterone, resulting in an overall increase in free androgen index (a measure of androgens that takes into account sex hormone-binding globulin) in many women.[36] The decrease in sex hormone-binding globulin that accompanies the MT is due to the dual influence of declining E2 levels, a function of progress to menopause, and

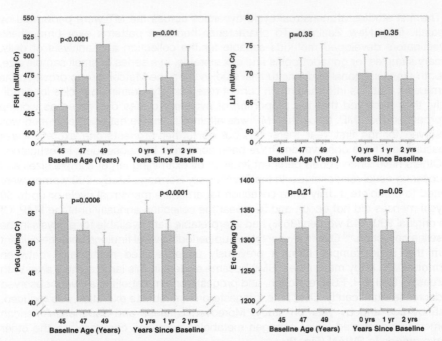

Fig. 2. Adjusted mean whole-cycle urinary reproductive hormones (with confidence intervals) by age and elapsed years since baseline (ovulatory cycles only). Note the prominent rise in FSH and decrease in pregnanediol glucuronide with both age and years on study. A more modest rise in LH is observed, and E1c does not decline with age. (*Reprinted* Santoro N, Crawford SL, Lasley WL, et al. Factors related to declining luteal function in women during the menopausal transition. J Clin Endocrinol Metab 2008;93:1711; with permission.)

increased age-related insulin resistance. Adiposity also seems to contribute, via increased peripheral conversion of androstenedione via enhanced 17-β-hydroxysteroid dehydrogenase type V.[37] Thus, women who acquire obesity in midlife or who experience substantial weight gain are likely to experience relative hyperandrogenemia. The relative androgen excess, defined as the molar ration of testosterone to E2, was observed to increase by 10.1% per year in women in the SWAN study, and its increase correlated with the development of the metabolic syndrome over time.[38]

Adrenal androgens follow a different time course from ovarian androgens, with a general decline beginning in young adulthood and continuing through the MT. Dehydroepiandrosterone sulfate (DHEAS) is the most commonly measured adrenal androgen in most studies of the MT. The decline in DHEAS was found to be reversed in most women during the late MT,[39] with 85% demonstrating an increase in the late transition.[40] Circulating DHEAS varies with ethnicity; Chinese women have the highest levels, and is significantly related to BMI. Women with higher DHEAS reported greater overall quality of life, physical functioning, and fewer depressive symptoms.[41]

Relationships between Cycle Characteristics and Patterns to Bleeding, Sleep, Symptoms, and Other Correlates of Health in Midlife Women

Menstrual cycle hormone patterns have been related to several other symptoms, signs, and risk factors in a series of studies performed in SWAN. The patterns of menstrual bleeding have been related to urinary hormone excretion patterns.[42] For the most part, changes in cycle timing (unusually long or short cycles) were associated with a failure of ovulation. Short or long durations of menstrual bleeding were also associated with anovulation. However, the relative self-reported heaviness of menstrual bleeding was more likely to be associated with leiomyomata and obesity. These findings suggest that unusually heavy menstrual bleeding typically does not have a hormonal basis, and such patterns, especially when they are persistent, should be investigated for an underlying anatomic, gynecologic cause.

Women who collected daily urine samples in the SWAN study also completed a daily diary in which they reported mood, sexual interest, and sleep quality. Women recorded whether or not they had had trouble sleeping during the previous night. Overall, a 29% increase in the odds of reporting trouble sleeping was observed as women progressed from regular cycling into the early transition.[43] Sleep quality was worst at the beginning and at the end of the menstrual cycle. The occurrence of vasomotor symptoms was also observed across the transition within a menstrual cycle.

Lipid profiles and inflammatory markers in women with varying cycle lengths in SWAN, when controlled for body size, showed no difference except for triglycerides, which increased with increasing cycle length.[44] Lower mean cycle estrone conjugates and pregnanediol glucuronide were associated with higher triglycerides, insulin levels, and inflammatory markers. In longitudinal SWAN studies, total cholesterol, low-density lipoprotein (LDL) cholesterol, lipoprotein (a), and triglycerides increased significantly in the late perimenopause/early postmenopause and with falling E2 and rising FSH independent of age, whereas HDL peaked in the late perimenopause.[45] However, when referenced to an observed FMP, only total cholesterol, LDL cholesterol, and apolipoprotein B increased with menopause; all other lipid, inflammatory, and glycemic markers changed with chronologic age.[45]

Factors, Including BMI and Race/Ethnicity, That Influence Hormones and Patterns of Hormones

Initial cross-sectional analyses of baseline annual serum hormone levels demonstrated variation in all hormones by body size, positively for testosterone and negatively for all others.[46] Ethnic variation in hormones was noted but was highly confounded by body size, and only FSH correlated with menopausal stage (**Fig. 3**).

The longitudinal analyses in SWAN of FSH and E2 noted similar patterns in the decline of E2 and the increase in FSH with age across ethnic groups, but the levels of these hormones differed by race/ethnicity.[21] The ethnic differences in E2 and FSH were independent of menopausal status, whereas the effect of BMI on serum E2 and FSH levels varied by menopausal status. Obesity markedly attenuated the FSH rise and delayed the initial increase,[21] whereas obesity, smoking behavior, and being Chinese or Japanese were associated with some variation in E2 levels, but not the pattern of E2 change. Thus, timespans and overall patterns of change in serum FSH and E2 across the MT were not related to age at FMP or smoking, whereas timespans but not overall patterns were related to obesity and race/ethnicity (**Fig. 4**).

CLINICAL IMPLICATIONS

With the maturation of SWAN and the transition to postmenopause by the vast majority of participants, both observed and obscured by hormone use or surgery, it has become possible to disentangle many of the coincident effects of both ovarian and chronologic aging on the health of women at midlife. Moreover, the complex patterns of change throughout the MT in both the cyclic and longitudinal hormone profiles are now in sharper focus and will help to direct clinical care as well as guide

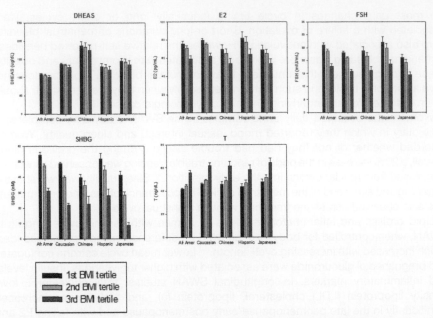

Fig. 3. Baseline serum hormones in the SWAN study sample. Each of the ethnic groups in SWAN are shown as clusters of bars; within each cluster, individual bars show BMI tertiles. (*From* Randolph JF Jr., Sowers M, Gold EB, et al. Reproductive hormones in the early menopausal transition: relationship to ethnicity, body size, and menopausal status. J Clin Endocrinol Metab 2003;88:1516.[46])

future research. It is important to note that they describe a variable pattern of change from regular, predictable menses to the absence of cyclicity with the end of bleeding.

The management of perimenopausal abnormal uterine bleeding is informed by the evidence that variation in reproductive hormones and progressively more frequent anovulatory cycles contribute primarily to cycle length changes but not hypermenorrhea. Heavy bleeding in nonobese women requires anatomic evaluation, whereas "normal" but irregular bleeding can be managed hormonally once endometrial pathology has been ruled out. Heavier but normally cyclic bleeding in the early MT is usually transient and may not require any intervention unless sustained.

Not surprisingly, frequently reported symptoms such as vasomotor symptoms, sleep complaints, and mood changes are experienced more perimenstrually, in the early and late phases of the cycle, and commonly occur well before the increasing variability in cycle length of the late MT. This confirms the practice of cyclic therapy for specific symptoms in the later luteal phase into the onset of menses when women prefer intermittent rather than continuous treatment.

There seems to be a clear menopausal effect on cardiovascular risk factors, most prominently on total cholesterol, LDL cholesterol, and apolipoprotein B, but most such factors are more related to chronologic aging. Together with the menopausal effect on body composition,[47] this suggests that strategies to limit such an increase in cholesterol and fat mass, either by lifestyle modification or medications, would be most effective if initiated during the early MT before they had taken place rather than waiting for a confirmed FMP. Whether such interventions can ultimately affect the subsequent onset and development of cardiovascular disease remains to be demonstrated by prospective trials.

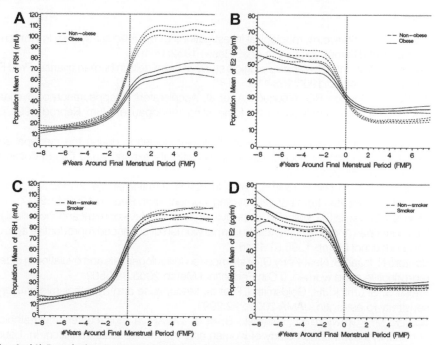

Fig. 4. (*A*) Population mean and 95% confidence intervals (CI) for mean FSH: Obese versus nonobese. (*B*) Population mean and 95% CI for mean E2: Obese versus nonobese. (*C*) Population mean and 95% CI for mean FSH: Smoker versus nonsmoker. (*D*) Population mean and 95% CI for mean E2: Smoker versus nonsmoker.

Perhaps most surprisingly, SWAN longitudinal hormone studies describe a remarkably consistent pattern of change around the FMP for women who were in their mid-to-late 40s and cycling regularly at the onset of observation. Although absolute hormone levels vary particularly by body size but also by ethnicity, and symptoms vary dramatically, the timespan of the most active hormone changes is about 4 years and centered on the FMP. This time corresponds with the most probable time of reporting symptoms, and coincides with the onset of measurable changes in bone[15] and body composition. It suggests that the late MT may be much more predictable than previously believed, and that interventions to optimize health in midlife and into old age could be reliably initiated well before the observed cessation of bleeding.

For the clinician, the current convention is that the MT has begun when a previously regularly cycling woman, regardless of age, develops increasing cycle variability such that her longest and shortest cycles differ by 1 week. Hormone changes are gradual and superimposed on progressively increasing cycle variability, and they typically last for several years. The late MT is entered when a women has an episode without bleeding for at least 60 days, indicating the progressive dysregulation of individual follicle development and frequently near the time when hormone changes accelerate about 2 years before the FMP. Bleeding ceases when follicles can no longer produce sufficient E2 to stimulate endometrial proliferation, and hormone levels stabilize again about 2 years after the FMP.

REFERENCES

1. Block E. Quantitative morphological investigations of the follicular system in women; variations at different ages. Acta Anat (Basel) 1952;14:108.
2. Baker TG. A quantitative and cytological study of germ cells in human ovaries. Proc R Soc Lond B Biol Sci 1963;158:417.
3. Faddy MJ, Gosden RG, Gougeon A, et al. Accelerated disappearance of ovarian follicles in mid-life: implications for forecasting menopause. Hum Reprod 1992;7: 1342.
4. Richardson SJ, Senikas V, Nelson JF. Follicular depletion during the menopausal transition: evidence for accelerated loss and ultimate exhaustion. J Clin Endocrinol Metab 1987;65:1231.
5. Battaglia DE, Goodwin P, Klein NA, et al. Influence of maternal age on meiotic spindle assembly in oocytes from naturally cycling women. Hum Reprod 1996;11:2217.
6. Klein NA, Battaglia DE, Miller PB, et al. Ovarian follicular development and the follicular fluid hormones and growth factors in normal women of advanced reproductive age. J Clin Endocrinol Metab 1996;81:1946.
7. Santoro N, Isaac B, Neal-Perry G, et al. Impaired folliculogenesis and ovulation in older reproductive aged women. J Clin Endocrinol Metab 2003;88:5502.
8. Weiss G, Skurnick JH, Goldsmith LT, et al. Menopause and hypothalamic-pituitary sensitivity to estrogen. JAMA 2004;292:2991.
9. Sowers MF, Crawford SL, Sternfeld B, et al. SWAN: a multi-center, multi-ethnic, community-based cohort study of women and the menopausal transition. In: Lobo RA, Kelsey J, Marcus R, editors. Menopause: biology and pathobiology. San Diego: Academic Press; 2000. p. 175.
10. Ahmed Ebbiary NA, Lenton EA, Cooke ID. Hypothalamic-pituitary ageing: progressive increase in FSH and LH concentrations throughout the reproductive life in regularly menstruating women. Clin Endocrinol (Oxf) 1994;41:199.
11. Harlow SD, Mitchell ES, Crawford S, et al. The ReSTAGE Collaboration: defining optimal bleeding criteria for onset of early menopausal transition. Fertil Steril 2008;89: 129.
12. Randolph JF Jr, Zheng H, Sowers MR, et al. Change in follicle-stimulating hormone and estradiol across the menopausal transition: effect of age at the final menstrual period. J Clin Endocrinol Metab 2011;96:746–54.
13. Santoro N, Brockwell S, Johnston J, et al. Helping midlife women predict the onset of the final menses: SWAN, the Study of Women's Health Across the Nation. Menopause 2007;14:415.
14. Santoro N, Brown JR, Adel T, et al. Characterization of reproductive hormonal dynamics in the perimenopause. J Clin Endocrinol Metab 1996;81:1495.
15. Finkelstein JS, Brockwell SE, Mehta V, et al. Bone mineral density changes during the menopause transition in a multiethnic cohort of women. J Clin Endocrinol Metab 2008;93:861.
16. Danforth DR, Arbogast LK, Mroueh J, et al. Dimeric inhibin: a direct marker of ovarian aging. Fertil Steril 1998;70:119.
17. Seifer DB, Lambert-Messerlian G, Hogan JW, et al. Day 3 serum inhibin-B is predictive of assisted reproductive technologies outcome. Fertil Steril 1997;67:110.
18. Sowers MR, Eyvazzadeh AD, McConnell D, et al. Anti-mullerian hormone and inhibin B in the definition of ovarian aging and the menopause transition. J Clin Endocrinol Metab 2008;93:3478.
19. McKinlay SM. The normal menopause transition: an overview. Maturitas 1996;23: 137.

20. Burger HG. The endocrinology of the menopause. J Steroid Biochem Mol Biol 1999;69:31.
21. Randolph JF Jr, Sowers M, Bondarenko IV, et al. Change in estradiol and follicle-stimulating hormone across the early menopausal transition: effects of ethnicity and age. J Clin Endocrinol Metab 2004;89:1555.
22. Randolph JF Jr, Zheng H, Sowers MR, et al. Change in follicle-stimulating hormone and estradiol across the menopausal transition: effect of age at the final menstrual period. J Clin Endocrinol Metab 2011;96:746.
23. Sowers MR, Zheng H, McConnell D, et al. Follicle stimulating hormone and its rate of change in defining menopause transition stages. J Clin Endocrinol Metab 2008;93: 3958.
24. Burger HG, Cahir N, Robertson DM, et al. Serum inhibins A and B fall differentially as FSH rises in perimenopausal women. Clin Endocrinol (Oxf) 1998;48:809.
25. Wallace RB, Sherman BM, Bean JA, et al. Probability of menopause with increasing duration of amenorrhea in middle-aged women. Am J Obstet Gynecol 1979;135: 1021.
26. Burger HG, Hale GE, Robertson DM, et al. A review of hormonal changes during the menopausal transition: focus on findings from the Melbourne Women's Midlife Health Project. Hum Reprod Update 2007;13:559.
27. Freeman EW, Sammel MD, Gracia CR, et al. Follicular phase hormone levels and menstrual bleeding status in the approach to menopause. Fertil Steril 2005;83:383.
28. Metcalf MG. The approach of menopause: a New Zealand study. N Z Med J 1988;101:103.
29. Metcalf MG, Donald RA, Livesey JH. Classification of menstrual cycles in pre- and perimenopausal women. J Endocrinol 1981;91:1.
30. Metcalf MG, Donald RA, Livesey JH. Pituitary-ovarian function before, during and after the menopause: a longitudinal study. Clin Endocrinol (Oxf) 1982;17:489.
31. Metcalf MG, Donald RA, Livesey JH. Pituitary-ovarian function in normal women during the menopausal transition. Clin Endocrinol (Oxf) 1981;14:245.
32. Metcalf MG, Livesey JH. Gonadotrophin excretion in fertile women: effect of age and the onset of the menopausal transition. J Endocrinol 1985;105:357.
33. Santoro N, Lasley B, McConnell D, et al. Body size and ethnicity are associated with menstrual cycle alterations in women in the early menopausal transition: The Study of Women's Health across the Nation (SWAN) Daily Hormone Study. J Clin Endocrinol Metab 2004;89:2622.
34. O'Connor KA, Ferrell RJ, Brindle E, et al. Total and unopposed estrogen exposure across stages of the transition to menopause. Cancer Epidemiol Biomarkers Prev 2009;18:828.
35. Hale GE, Hughes CL, Burger HG, et al. Atypical estradiol secretion and ovulation patterns caused by luteal out-of-phase (LOOP) events underlying irregular ovulatory menstrual cycles in the menopausal transition. Menopause 2009;16:50.
36. Burger HG, Dudley EC, Cui J, et al. A prospective longitudinal study of serum testosterone, dehydroepiandrosterone sulfate, and sex hormone-binding globulin levels through the menopause transition. J Clin Endocrinol Metab 2000;85:2832.
37. Quinkler M, Sinha B, Tomlinson JW, et al. Androgen generation in adipose tissue in women with simple obesity--a site-specific role for 17beta-hydroxysteroid dehydro-genase type 5. J Endocrinol 2004;183:331.
38. Torrens JI, Sutton-Tyrrell K, Zhao X, et al. Relative androgen excess during the menopausal transition predicts incident metabolic syndrome in midlife women: study of Women's Health Across the Nation. Menopause 2009;16:257.

39. Lasley BL, Santoro N, Randolf JF, et al. The relationship of circulating dehydroepi-androsterone, testosterone, and estradiol to stages of the menopausal transition and ethnicity. J Clin Endocrinol Metab 2002;87:3760.
40. Crawford S, Santoro N, Laughlin GA, et al. Circulating dehydroepiandrosterone sulfate concentrations during the menopausal transition. J Clin Endocrinol Metab 2009;94:2945.
41. Santoro N, Torrens J, Crawford S, et al. Correlates of circulating androgens in mid-life women: the study of women's health across the nation. J Clin Endocrinol Metab 2005;90:4836.
42. Van Voorhis BJ, Santoro N, Harlow S, et al. The relationship of bleeding patterns to daily reproductive hormones in women approaching menopause. Obstet Gynecol 2008;112:101.
43. Kravitz HM, Janssen I, Santoro N, et al. Relationship of day-to-day reproductive hormone levels to sleep in midlife women. Arch Intern Med 2005;165:2370.
44. Matthews KA, Santoro N, Lasley B, et al. Relation of cardiovascular risk factors in women approaching menopause to menstrual cycle characteristics and reproductive hormones in the follicular and luteal phases. J Clin Endocrinol Metab 2006;91:1789.
45. Matthews KA, Crawford SL, Chae CU, et al. Are changes in cardiovascular disease risk factors in midlife women due to chronological aging or to the menopausal transition? J Am Coll Cardiol 2009;54:2366.
46. Randolph JF Jr, Sowers M, Gold EB, et al. Reproductive hormones in the early menopausal transition: relationship to ethnicity, body size, and menopausal status. J Clin Endocrinol Metab 2003;88:1516.
47. Sowers M, Zheng H, Tomey K, et al. Changes in body composition in women over six years at midlife: ovarian and chronological aging. J Clin Endocrinol Metab 2007;92: 895.

Adrenal Androgens and the Menopausal Transition

Bill L. Lasley, PhD[a],*, Sybil Crawford, PhD[b],
Daniel S. McConnell, PhD[c]

KEYWORDS

- Menopausal transition • Androgens • Adrenal

Until recently, the prevailing dogma was that adrenal weak androgen production in both men and women declined after the third decade of life. In the last 10 years, this concept has changed after the analysis of the longitudinal data collected in the Study of Women's Health Across the Nation (SWAN).[1] Failure to adequately attribute phenotype, symptoms and health trajectories to the observed longitudinal changes in circulating estradiol (E2) and progesterone have led to investigations that focus on adrenal contributions to circulating sex steroids. Emerging data show that there are more ethnic and individual endocrine differences in mid-aged women in circulating adrenal steroids than in either E2 or cyclic hormone profiles, particularly during the early perimenopause.[1,2] Thus, adrenal steroid production may play a greater role in the occurrence of symptoms and the potential for healthier aging than previously recognized.

A distinct rise in circulating dehydroepiandrosterone sulfate (DHEAS) has been detected in most women during the menopausal transition (MT). This rise was detected, however, only when the annual serum levels of DHEAS were aligned according to ovarian status, defined using the World Health Organization criteria[3] (**Fig. 1**). The expected, age-related, gradual decline is observed when the same data are plotted by chronological age in premenopausal women.[2] A similar rise in DHEAS had been observed earlier in older female laboratory macaques, but has not been reported in any non-primate animal model. In women, it seems clear that most, if not all, of the DHEAS rise is attributable to the adrenal and not the ovary, because a similar rise is observed in intact and ovariectomized women.[4] Together, these observations not only underscore the importance of longitudinal investigations such as SWAN, but also explain why this specific physiologic trait went unnoticed for decades. It also highlights the value of the nonhuman primate animal model for

[a] Center for Population Health and the Environment, University of California at Davis, Davis, CA 95616, USA
[b] Department of Medicine, Division of Preventive and Behavioral Medicine, University of Massachusetts, Worcester, MA 01655, USA
[c] Department of Epidemiology, The University of Michigan, Ann Arbor, MI 48109-0404, USA
* Corresponding author.
E-mail address: bllasley@ucdavis.edu

Obstet Gynecol Clin N Am 38 (2011) 467–475
doi:10.1016/j.ogc.2011.06.001
0889-8545/11/$ – see front matter © 2011 Elsevier Inc. All rights reserved.

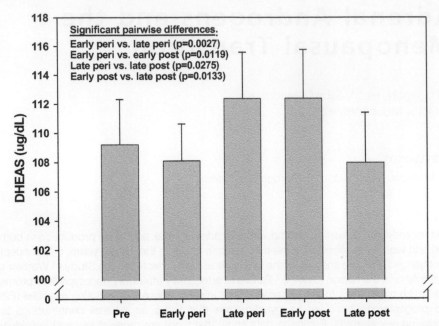

Fig. 1. Adjusted mean DHEAS (95% confidence interval) by menopause status from SWAN visits 00–09 (15,930 observations from 2,886 women). (*Reproduced from* Crawford S, Santoro N, Laughlin GA, Sowers MF, et al. Circulating Dehydroepiandrosterone Sulfate Concentrations during the Menopausal Transition. J Clin Endocrinol Metab 2009;94:2945–51. Copyright 2009, The Endocrine Society.)

human reproductive endocrinology, because this steroidogenic pathway is not found in rodent adrenals and, therefore, would not otherwise have been investigated.

Whereas the circulating levels of DHEAS in middle-aged women differ significantly between ethnicities at the beginning of the MT, the subsequent rise in DHEAS during the MT is similar, in both in the percentage of women that express it as well as the similarity in relative increase and trajectory in all 5 ethnicities studied in SWAN (**Fig. 2**).The pattern of adrenal weak androgen production that emerges when the DHEAS data are aligned by ovarian status suggests several possibilities regarding control of adrenal androgen secretion in older women. First, the ethnic differences in the circulating concentration of DHEAS in adult women indicate an ethnic-specific predisposition for the regulation of the delta-5 adrenal steroidogenic pathway (**Fig. 3**) in premenopausal women.[2] The between-ethnic similarities of the DHEAS trajectories, however, indicate a common physiologic controlling mechanism during the MT. The time course of the rise of DHEAS, which is limited to the MT and early postmenopause, suggests that changes in ovarian function are part of the controlling mechanism(s). Although the finding of an increase in circulating DHEAS demonstrates a gender divergence that seems to be intimately linked to the MT, by itself it does not necessarily indicate a physiologically important event.

A great deal of attention has been focused on the delta-4 steroidogenic pathway that produces cortisol, androstenedione (Adione), and testosterone (T; see **Fig. 3**). There are some relatively weak associations of these circulating steroids to sexual motivation, mood, and the development of metabolic syndrome over the course of SWAN.[5,6] By comparison, the longitudinal studies of SWAN have suggested that the

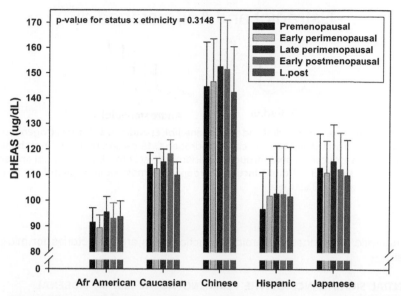

Fig. 2. Adjusted mean DHEAS (95% confidence interval) by menopause status within ethnicity from SWAN visits 00–09 (15,930 observations from 2,886 women). (*Reproduced from* Crawford S, Santoro N, Laughlin GA, Sowers MF, et al. Circulating Dehydroepiandrosterone Sulfate Concentrations during the Menopausal Transition. J Clin Endocrinol Metab 2009;94: 2945–51. Copyright 2009, The Endocrine Society.)

delta-5 steroidogenic pathway that produces dehydroepiandrosterone (DHEA), its sulfated conjugate DHEAS and androstenediol (Adiol) may play a larger role in women's healthy aging. Specifically, 2 reports[1,2] show that these 2 parallel adrenal steroidogenic pathways are controlled separately with gender-specific and ovarian

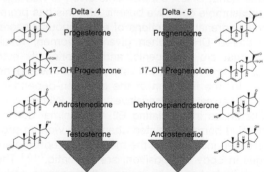

The two primary steroidogenic pathways

Fig. 3. The two primary adrenal steroidogenic pathways. The delta four pathway on the left has been considered to be the critical pathway giving rise to the mineralocorticoids and glucocorticoids as well as androstenedione and testosterone which can be aromatized peripherally to estrogen and estradiol, respectively. The delta five pathway on the right has been considered important mainly for the production of dehydroepiandrosterone and dehydroepiandrosterone sulfate which can be prohormones for peripheral conversion to more bioactive steroids. Androstenediol, because it is now recognized to occur in reatively high concentrations is now be considered to be important during the menopausal transition.

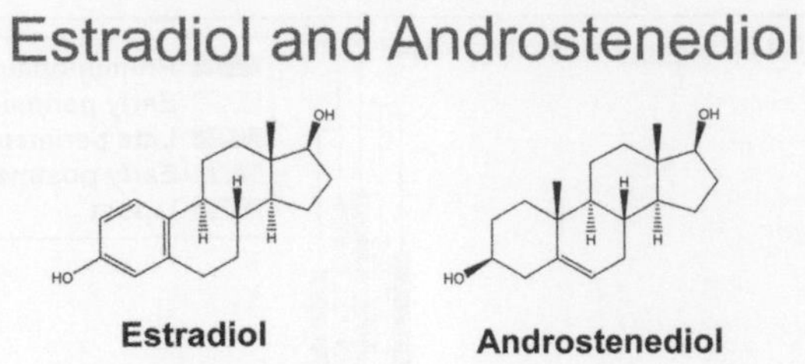

Estradiol and Androstenediol

Estradiol   **Androstenediol**

Fig. 4. Basic structures of estradiol and androstenediol. Estradiol is a classic estrogen receptor ligand while androstenediol has the classic androgen C-19 carbon structural backbone and the ability to transducer a signal through the androgen receptor. Both estradiol and androstenediol have similar 3–17 diol functional groups that most likely explain how this C-19 steroid can act as a C-18 estrogen.

stage-specific differences in steroid production rates and trajectories for mid-aged women.

POTENTIAL SIGNIFICANCE OF THE PERIMENOPAUSAL RISE IN ADRENAL ANDROGENS

It would be an oversimplification to conclude that the previous endocrine conundrums relating to the MT will now be explained by a new and more focused investigation of adrenal function, but these new data have provided insights. First, it has been long-speculated that DHEA provides the substrate for the many P450 c17 enzymes that can convert this relatively inert compound to more biologically active compounds (such as Adiol) and, with the help of 3- β-hydroxysteroid dehydrogenase-isomerase, to Adione and T (**Fig. 3**).[7,8] These products of peripheral metabolism could provide additional sex steroid activity after the loss of essential ovarian hormones at menopause. This concept is indirectly supported by the observation women with higher circulating DHEA sustain cognitive and executive function loss as they traverse the MT.[9] On the other hand, DHEA supplements given to mid-aged women do not provide significant measurable cognitive benefit, and this has promoted the need to investigate the ovarian–adrenal interactions of endogenously secreted hormones.[10] Exogenously administered DHEA, when given to women, results in circulating conversion products that are androgenic, and not primarily estrogenic.[11] These findings suggest that exogenously administered DHEA would not be directly or indirectly responsible for the retention of the estrogen-dependent integrity of the neural substrate and other estrogen-sensitive tissues. Within-woman changes and between-woman differences in circulating E2 are minimal during the early MT,[12] whereas nonreproductive hormone-related changes in women progressing through the MT, such as increased incidence of the metabolic syndrome and cardiovascular disease, and changes in body composition, are dramatic.[13,14] These observations make it difficult to attribute between-woman differences in early perimenopausal symptoms and intermediate health outcomes to changes in circulating E2. This has led to the notion that these changes are attributable to an attendant factor, presently unidentified, that would be responsible. We find it biologically plausible that adrenal androgen dynamics during the MT are at least in part an explanatory factor.

There is now evidence that Adiol, which has inherent androgenic and estrogenic bioactivities and is secreted in parallel with DHEAS and DHEA during the MT (**Fig. 4**), may be such an explanatory factor. A unique aspect of Adiol as an important, perhaps

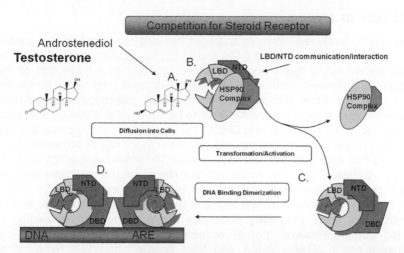

NTD: N-terminal domain, LBD: Ligand Binding Domain, DBD: DNA Binding Domain
ARE: Androgen response element, HSP90: Heat Shock Protein 90

Adapted from M. Danielsen "Nuclear receptor resource"

Fig. 5. Mechanism of steroid-steroid receptor interaction shown for testosterone and androsenediol. Both structures, as C-19 steroids, can compete for the androgen receptor (A). While androstenediol has a lower binding affinity than that of testosterone, it can bind to the receptor if its concentrations are high enough. In mid-aged women androstenediol is found in concentrations that are many fold higher than testosterone at which, it can bind to the ligand binding domain (LBD) (B). Regardless of which structure binds, the steroid-receptor complex then uncouples from the heat shock protein (HSP) to form a monimer with the ligand binding domain (LBD) exposed (C). Two of these monimers combine to form the dimer (D), that can then dock at the DNA androgen binding element (ARE) to initiate gene expression if the correct cofactors are also present. A similar process is true for the estrogen receptors.

critical, endocrine component in mid-aged women lies in its ability to transduce signals through both the androgen and estrogen receptors.[15–19] Thus, high circulating concentrations of Adiol could affect the net balance of androgens and estrogens in the body, depending on the abundance or lack of abundance of specific steroid hormone receptors in target tissues. This concept is complex because, as a weaker ligand, the ability of Adiol to transduce signals through any of these receptors depends also on the concentration of other higher affinity ligands such as T or E2 (**Fig. 5**).

The observation that there is an overall age-related decline in DHEAS, but a gender-specific rise around the time of menopause in women suggests that the delta-5 steroid biosynthetic pathway in most women is influenced by subtle changes in ovarian function as women enter the MT. Evidence in support of ovarian control of adrenal androgen production is the observation that the gender- and menopause-related rise in DHEAS in women returns to a progressive decline after menopause.[2] Taken together, the existing information indicates that the subtle changes in ovarian function that accompany the MT (a loss of inhibin B, no obvious change in estrogen dynamics, and a slight rise in follicle-stimulating hormone) trigger a transient increase in adrenal δ-5 steroid production that continues to and past the final menstrual period.

POTENTIAL ROLE OF ADIOL

Adiol, although structurally resembling an androgen, has long been recognized as a weak estrogen with a potency of 0.01% to 0.1% that of E2. Its circulating concentration in premenopausal women is less than 1 nmol/L—or about 2 to 3 times that of the average circulating concentration of E2. Because of its lower binding affinity for the estrogen receptor or other nuclear proteins that may transduce an estrogenic signal,[15] this concentration is too low for Adiol to be effective as either an androgen or estrogen.[16] However, the increase in DHEAS that starts in the early perimenopause and continues into the early postmenopause, results in much higher circulating Adiol concentrations that approach 3 to 4 nmol/L—about 100 times the average concentration of E2. At these higher circulating concentrations, protein synthesis and cell proliferation have been demonstrated in human, estrogen-sensitive cells in vitro,[18] and have been shown to elicit an estrogenic response in vivo in immature female rats.[19] Thus, Adiol could potentially contribute to circulating estrogen action in middle-aged women. However, not all women share the robust early and late perimenopausal rise in DHEAS, DHEA, and Adiol; approximately 15% remain at or near premenopausal levels. This wide range of circulating Adiol (<1–4 nmol/L), therefore, has the potential to explain the wide range of estrogen-related phenotypes and symptoms that are observed in perimenopausal women—data that have been difficult to reconcile with the relatively narrow range of circulating E2 levels during this same time period.

Virtually all menopausal hormone therapies are based on the assumption that the intervention requires the correction of low circulating estrogen concentration despite the fact that the direct measurement of low circulating E2 before the menopause is seldom used to justify this approach. In fact, the literature is not clear about the question of whether symptomatic women produce less estrogen in the early phases of the MT, with some reports indicating that estrogen production is not decreased in some women.[20–22] Clinical evidence, such as changes in estrogen-sensitive tissues, verifies that lower estrogenization is the foundation of most menopausal symptoms and is consistent with the effectiveness of E2 in ameliorating these changes. However, estrogen receptor ligands other than E2 may contribute to the clinical picture of estrogen deficiency and its attendant symptoms. The fact that there is investigative interest in such potential ligands is acknowledged in the number of failed DHEA trials that have been conducted. Furthermore, the benefits of current estrogen-based therapies seem unlikely to be totally physiologic for menopausal women, because they must be balanced against recognized risks of endometrial hyperplasia and cardiovascular diseases. In fairness to the prevailing clinical approach in applying menopausal hormone therapies to women without substantiating low estrogen production, the day-to-day fluctuations of estrogen production in women with intact ovaries defies any practical attempt to quantify either estrogen production or circulating concentrations. However, urinary hormone excretion patterns seem to indicate that there is not a general decline in estrogen production before menopause in most intact women.[22] The effectiveness of estrogen replacement to reverse menopause-related changes in middle-aged women does not necessarily support either a decrease in ovarian estrogen production or a decline in circulating E2. Although these phenomena may be contributors in the causal pathway, they have not been shown to be singularly responsible. A clear understanding of the processes and mechanism(s) that lead to the menopause and its attendant symptoms is currently limited and there is a growing body of evidence that suggests that adrenal androgens may play an important role in the estrogen/androgen balance during the MT.

TESTOSTERONE

Circulating levels of T during the MT are well established in the literature and T is clearly the principal bioactive androgen in middle-aged women.[23] Most reports are consistent in concluding that, for reproductive-aged. women approximately half of the bioactive androgens come from the ovary and half from the adrenal gland. There is less certainty regarding the ovarian contribution just before and after the final menstrual period. Most reports indicate that the postmenopausal ovary continues to secrete androgens up to and after menopause,[23,24] although a recent report using highly sensitive methods to measure circulating steroid levels indicate the ovarian contribution is less than previously accepted.[25] Although both T and Adione gradually decline with age, both of these steroids increase concomitant with the ovarian stage-specific increase in adrenal DHEAS.[2] This recent finding supports the more general, age-related decline in ovarian androgen production, but also indicates an increase in adrenal derived androgens during the MT for most women.

The Free Androgen Index (FAI) tends to be a better predictor of many health outcomes, especially cardiovascular ones, compared to T. Body mass index, waist-hip ratio, waist circumference, and the metabolic syndrome are more strongly correlated with the FAI than T.[5,6,26] Predictors of obesity included an increase in FAI and a decrease in sex hormone-binding globulin (SHBG).[26] Because the FAI has SHBG in the denominator, and SHBG is a good predictor of cardiovascular-related outcomes, these trends make good sense. The observation that free T correlates better with hyperandrogenic conditions during the MT suggests 1 of 2 possibilities. The first is that SHBG is decreased when T is elevated, a finding that is consistent with the trend of decreasing SHBG across the MT. A second possibility is more intriguing and also consistent with observations, namely that increased SHBG ligands in the form of Adione and Adiol reduces available binding sites for T, and amplify this effect.

In 2 sets of longitudinal analyses, Lasley and colleagues[2,4] found that DHEAS is negatively related to body mass index, and Sowers and colleagues[27] found that DHEAS is positively related to plasminogen activator inhibitor type 1, tissue plasminogen activator, and fibrinogen. Baseline analyses by Santoro and colleagues[5] did not find much of an association of DHEAS with body mass index, waist-hip ratio, or waist circumference. DHEAS was positively associated with better physical functioning, better self-reported health, less depression measured by the Center for Epidemiologic Studies Depression scale, and less metabolic syndrome. DHEAS was not significantly related to self-reported overall quality of life or sexual desire or arousal.

Based on the close association of circulating Adiol with circulating DHEAS during the MT, we would expect that effects of Adiol on symptoms and health outcomes would also be associated with DHEAS. However, there are few longitudinal studies in which DHEAS concentrations have been analyzed across the MT. Until such analyses are reported, no conclusion can be made. The rise in adrenal androgens before and immediately after menopause is quite variable and some women, perhaps 15%, reveal no increase in adrenal androgens.[2] Thus, a majority of women will exhibit up to a doubling of T and Adione as well as a possible 5-fold increase in Adiol as they traverse menopause. Although this rise in T represents the major androgenic contribution, the complementary contributions of Adione and Adione to total androgenicity should not be ignored. Clearly, additional investigations are required before the importance of the contribution of weak adrenal androgens to health outcomes will be completely defined. The current understanding that the adrenal participates in the estrogen:androgen balance provides more latitude in explaining androgen-related issues during the MT.

SUMMARY

The menopause-associated rise in circulating follicle-stimulating hormone,[12] the increase in the metabolic syndrome,[6,26] and other menopausal symptoms[5,22] begin to occur during the early perimenopause. However, the first significant decline in circulating E2 measured on days 3 to 7 of the menstrual cycle does not occur until 2 years before menopause—during the late perimenopause—and continues for 2 to 3 years beyond the final menstrual period. This sustained, narrow range of circulating E2 concentrations occurs at the same time that mean DHEAS, DHEA, and Adiol are increasing at their greatest rate.[2] Furthermore, the between-women differences in DHEAS, DHEA, and Adiol are the greatest of any hormone at that time.[1] More important, the 5-fold higher circulating concentrations of Adiol in individual women, compared with the concomitantly decreasing levels of circulating E2, may compensate for the lower estrogenic bioactivity of Adiol compared to E2. This relationship indicates that women with higher circulating E2 would have little benefit from even the highest concentrations of Adiol. In fact, it could be argued that the weaker ligand (Adiol) would attenuate to some degree the biological effects of E2. However, the higher concentration of Adiol in the presence of low circulating E2 could contribute significantly to the total circulating estrogen ligand pool in women during the MT, and may have clinical significance.

REFERENCES

1. Lasley BL, Santoro N, Gold EB, et al. The relationship of circulating DHEAS, testosterone and estradiol to stages of the menopausal transition and ethnicity. J Clin Endocrinol Metab 2002;87:3760–7.
2. Crawford S, Santoro N, Laughlin GA, et al. Circulating dehydroepiandrosterone sulfate concentrations during the menopausal transition. J Clin Endocrinol Metab 2009;94:2945–51.
3. World Health Organization Scientific Group. Research on Menopause in the 1990s (WHO Technical Report Series no. 866; 4). Geneva (Switzerland): World Health Organization; 1996.
4. Lasley B. Crawford S, Laughlin G, et al. Circulating dehydroepiandrosterone levels in women with bilateral salpingo-oophorectomy during the menopausal transition. Menopause 2011;18:494–8.
5. Santoro N, Torrens J, Crawford S, et al. Correlates of circulating androgens in mid-life women: the Study of Women's Health Across the Nation. J Clin Endocrinol Metab 2005;90:4836–45.
6. Torrens JI, Sutton-Tyrrell K, Zhao X, et al. Relative androgen excess during the menopausal transition predicts incident metabolic syndrome in midlife women: study of Women's Health Across the Nation. Menopause 2009;16:257–64.
7. Labrie F, Cusan L, Gomez JL, et al. Changes in serum DHEA and eleven of its metabolites during 12-month percutaneous administration of DHEA. J Steroid Biochem Mol Biol 2008;110:1–9.
8. Labrie F, Archer D, Bouchard C, et al. Intravaginal dehydroepiandrosterone (Prasterone), a physiological and highly efficient treatment of vaginal atrophy. Menopause 2009;16:907–14.
9. Davis SR, Shah SM, McKenzie DP, et al. Dehydroepiandrosterone sulfate levels are associated with more favorable cognitive function in women. J Clin Endocrinol Metab 2008;93:801–8.
10. Mamas L, Mamas E. Premature ovarian failure and dehydroepiandrosterone. Fertil Steril 2009;91:644–6.

11. Bird CE, Murphy J, Boroomand K, et al. Dehydroepiandrosterone: kinetics of metabolism in normal men and women. J Clin Endocrinol Metab 1978;47:818–22.

12. Randolph JF Jr, Sowers M, Gold EB, et al. Reproductive hormones in the early menopausal transition: relationship to ethnicity, body size, and menopausal status. J Clin Endocrinol Metab 2003;88:1516–22.

13. Janssen I, Powell LH, Crawford S, et al. Menopause and the metabolic syndrome: the Study of Women's Health Across the Nation. Arch Intern Med 2008;168:1568–75.

14. Sutton-Tyrrell K, Wildman RP, Matthews KA, et al. Sex hormone binding globulin and the free androgen index are related to cardiovascular risk factors in multiethnic premenopausal and perimenopausal women enrolled in the Study of Women's Health Across the Nation (SWAN). Circulation 2005;111:1242–9.

15. Poortman J, Prenen JAC, Schwarz F, et al. Interaction of delta-5-androstene-3-beta,17-beta-diol with estradiol and dihydrotestosterone receptors in human myometrial and mammary cancer tissue. J Clin Endocrinol Metab 1975;40:373–9.

16. Traish AM, Huang Y-H, Min K, et al. Binding characteristics of 3-H-delta-5-androstene-3-beta, 17-beta-diol to a nuclear protein in the rabbit vagina. Steroids 2004; 69:71–8.

17. Adams JB, Martyn P, Lee FT, et al. Metabolism of 17 beta-estradiol and the adrenal-derived estrogen 5-androstene-3 beta,17 beta-diol (hermaphrodiol) in human mammary cell lines. Ann NY Acad Sci 1990;595:93–105.

18. Poulan R, Labrie F. Stimulation of cell growth by C-19 steroids of adrenal origin in the ZR-75-1 human breast cancer cell line. Cancer Res 1985;46:4933–7.

19. Seymour-Munn K, Adams JB. Estrogenic effects of 5-androstene-3beta, 17beta diol at physiological concentrations and its possible implications in the etiology of breast cancer. Endocrinol 1981;112:486–91.

20. Santoro NS, Brown JB, Adel T, et al. Characterization of reproductive hormone dynamics in the perimenopause. J Clin Endocrinol Metab 1996;81:1495–501.

21. Santoro N, Lasley B, McConnell D, et al. Body size and ethnicity are associated with menstrual cycle alterations in women in the early menopausal transition: the Study of Women Across the Nation (SWAN) daily hormone study. J Clin Endocrinol Metab 2004;89:2622–31.

22. Skurnick JH, Weiss G, Goldsmith LT, et al. Longitudinal changes in hypothalamic and ovarian function in the perimenopausal women with anovulatory cycles: relationship with vasomotor symptoms. Fertil Steril 2009;91:1127–34.

23. Chen J, Sowers MR, Moran FM, et al. Circulating bioactive androgens in midlife women. J Clin Endocrinol Metab 2006;91:4387–94.

24. Longcope C, Franz C, Morello C, et al. Steroid and gonadotropin levels in women during the peri-menopausal years. Maturitas 1986;8:189–96.

25. Labrie F, Martel C, Balser J. Wide distribution of the serum dehydroepiandrosterone and sex steroid levels in postmenopausal women: role of the ovary? Menopause 2011;18:30–43.

26. Janssen I, Powell LH, Crawford S, et al. Menopause and the metabolic syndrome: the Study of Women's Health Across the Nation. Arch Intern Med 2008;168:1568–75.

27. Sowers MFR, Jannausch M, Randolph JF, et al. Androgens are associated with hemostatic and inflammatory factors among women at the mid-life. J Clin Endocrinol Metab 2005;90:6064–71.

The Menopausal Transition and Cardiovascular Risk

Claudia U. Chae, MD, MPH[a],*, Carol A. Derby, PhD[b]

KEYWORDS

- Lipids • Blood pressure • Diabetes • Metabolic syndrome
- Menopause • Perimenopause

Cardiovascular disease is the leading cause of death in women in developed countries, causing more than 400,000 deaths per year.[1] For women at the age of 40, their remaining lifetime risk is 1 in 3 for coronary heart disease (CHD), and 1 in 2 for all cardiovascular diseases.[1] The incidence rates of cardiovascular disease in women typically lag approximately 10 years behind that of men until midlife, with a marked increase in incidence rates seen after menopause.[1] In addition, the risk of cardiovascular disease is more than doubled among women who undergo bilateral oophorectomy compared with premenopausal women.[2] Therefore, it has long been postulated that estrogen is cardioprotective, and that the alteration in reproductive hormonal balance related to menopause contributes to the risk of cardiovascular disease in women. Because more than one third of life is spent in the postmenopausal state owing to increasing life expectancy, understanding the influence of menopause on future risks of cardiovascular disease is of critical importance and may also enhance our ability to identify targets for more effective preventive measures.

Because menopause, aging, and increased risk of cardiovascular disease occur concurrently, it is methodologically challenging but critical to separate out the influence of chronologic aging from that of menopause.[3] Much of the prior available data regarding menopause and cardiovascular disease risk have focused on differences in risk factors and disease rates in the premenopausal versus postmenopausal periods. Longitudinal data regarding perimenopause or the menopausal transition itself are limited but fortunately exceptions exist—including the Study of Women's Health Across the Nation (SWAN),[4] the Healthy Women Study,[5] the Melbourne Midlife Health Project,[6] the Fels Longitudinal Study,[7] and the Taiwan Chin-Shan Community

Dr Derby receives research support from Bristol Meyers Squibb.
Supported by Grant No. 2U01AG012535-16 (C.A.D.) and 5 UO1 AG12531-17 (C.U.C.) from the National Institutes of Health.
[a] Department of Medicine, Harvard Medical School, Cardiology Division, Massachusetts General Hospital, 55 Fruit Street, Boston, MA 02114 USA
[b] Department of Neurology and Department of Epidemiology and Population Health, Albert Einstein College of Medicine, 1165 Morris Park Avenue, Rousso-336, Bronx, NY 10461 USA
* Corresponding author.
E-mail address: cchae@partners.org

Cardiovascular Cohort.[8] These studies provide needed insights into the relationship between ovarian aging and cardiovascular risk in women. Regardless of the relative contributions of ovarian versus chronologic aging, the perimenopause represents a critical time period in the lifespan of women when focusing on modifiable risk factors could reduce the subsequent development of cardiovascular disease.

LIPIDS

Perhaps the strongest evidence linking menopause with adverse changes in cardiovascular risk is that suggesting proatherogenic changes in the lipid profile.[9] However, the effect of menopause on the lipoprotein profile is particularly difficult to assess, given the strong correlations of both menopause and lipids with chronologic age. From a clinical perspective, the disentangling of menopause effects from chronologic aging is important, particularly the identification of the timing of any adverse changes, in order to direct prevention efforts to reduce dyslipidemia.

The Chin-Shan Community Cardiovascular Cohort examined menopause status and levels of total cholesterol, low-density lipoprotein (LDL) cholesterol, high-density lipoprotein (HDL) cholesterol, and triglyceride levels among 401 Chinese women evaluated in 1990 and 1991 and again in 1994 and 1995.[10] Women were categorized as premenopausal at both assessments, postmenopausal at both assessments, or as having transitioned from premenopause to postmenopause during follow-up. After adjustment for age and body mass index(BMI), total cholesterol was the only lipid for which changes over time differed significantly across menopause status groups. The greatest increase in total cholesterol was among women in the group who transitioned from premenopause to postmenopause. This study assessed women at only 2 points in time. The group that transitioned from premenopause to postmenopause were not subdivided between early and late perimenopause, and the postmenopausal group included women at variable times after the final menstrual period. Thus, it was not possible to precisely adjust for age differences between the menopause status groups, and the timing of lipid changes in relation to specific stages of the menopause transition was not evaluated.

Zhou and colleagues[11] prospectively assessed menopausal status based on bleeding patterns in a cohort of 593 women aged 35 to 64 years in Beijing, China, who were followed for 4 years. Lipid levels were assessed prospectively according to concurrent menopausal status. The greatest difference in lipid levels occurred between early and late perimenopause, with total cholesterol and triglyceride levels peaking in late perimenopause. However, overall there were no differences in lipid levels for premenopausal versus postmenopausal observations, and among postmenopausal women lipids were not associated with time since menopause. This study was limited in its ability to assess the timing of lipid changes, because few women transitioned completely through menopause during the relatively short follow-up period and, similar to the Chin-Shan study,[10] a number of women were already postmenopausal at baseline.

The Fels Longitudinal Study ascertained serial measures of both lipid levels and menopausal status over a much longer follow-up period, between 1976 and 2002, for 143 women aged 40 to 60 years.[12] They reported a positive association between the menopausal transition and LDL cholesterol levels, such that mean levels were significantly lower during premenopausal observations compared with observations made in perimenopause and postmenopause. This suggests that a major increase in LDL may occur around the time of menopause; however, because the perimenopause and postmenopause observations were combined in the analyses and the sample size was small, this study does not provide information regarding the timing of lipid changes relative to the transition from late perimenopause to late postmenopause. Furthermore, results of this analysis may be confounded by the inclusion of women with either surgical or natural menopause.

The Melbourne Women's Midlife Health project prospectively described changes in cardiovascular risk factors among 150 healthy, initially premenopausal women as they traversed the menopause transition.[13] In this study, the only lipid level that demonstrated a significant change in relation to menopause was HDL cholesterol, which increased in the year preceding the final menstrual period and then declined to premenopausal levels thereafter. Changes in the other lipids were explained by age or concomitant changes in other risk factors. This report was limited by very small sample size and limited follow-up time. The women included in this analysis were a subset of a larger cohort, who were the first to complete the transition to postmenopause. Given that age at menopause is associated with smoking status and a number or demographic factors,[14] there is the potential for selection bias to affect the study results.

The SWAN study is the largest prospective study to date to assess changes in risk factors in relation to stages of the menopause transition in a multi-ethnic cohort of women who were initially premenopausal or early perimenopausal. Analyses based on the first 7 years of follow-up in SWAN[15] showed that changes in lipids during the early stages of the menopause transition were minimal, with total cholesterol, LDL cholesterol, and triglycerides peaking during late perimenopause and early postmenopause. Changes were independent of age and covariates including ethnicity, weight, smoking status, alcohol use, diet, and physical activity. Similar to the report from the Melbourne study,[13] HDL levels also peaked during late perimenopause and early postmenopause, but these changes seemed to be transient, with HDL cholesterol leveling off thereafter. Subsequent analyses based on ten years of follow-up in the SWAN cohort have shown that increases in total cholesterol and LDL occurred specifically within a 1-year interval of the final menstrual period, and were independent of age, ethnicity or baseline weight.[16] This analysis was the first to present changes in lipids in relation to the natural menopause anchored specifically to the timing of the final menstrual period.

Results from the SWAN study are consistent with an earlier report from the Healthy Women Study, which compared changes in lipids for 2 periods: The transition from premenopause to 1 year postmenopause, and the period from the first to the fifth postmenopausal years.[17] They reported that the largest increases in LDL and triglycerides occurred during the transition from premenopause to the first year postmenopause. In contrast to the SWAN findings, HDL levels decreased during this period.

There is some evidence that in addition to the concentration of the lipoproteins, their composition may change during the menopausal transition. In SWAN, apolipoprotein-B levels peaked during the year surrounding the final menstrual period.[16] Apolipoprotein-B may be a stronger predictor of cardiovascular disease risk than the LDL cholesterol level.[18] Furthermore, analyses of the SWAN cohort suggest the composition of HDL particles may shift during the menopause transition. In a subset of the SWAN cohort, although the expected inverse association of HDL with measures of subclinical vascular disease was observed among premenopausal and early perimenopausal women, the association was attenuated or reversed among late perimenopausal and postmenopausal women.[19] Preliminary cross-sectional analyses in a small subset of women suggest this attenuation of the protective effect of total HDL levels may be due to a shift in the later phases of the menopause transition toward higher HDL particle concentration, and to smaller average HDL particle size.[19] Small HDL particles may not be as cardioprotective as larger particles.[20] Further work is required to establish whether changes in the size and concentration of lipid particles during the menopausal transition are related to increases in cardiovascular risk.

In summary, the available data from prospective studies that have followed women through the menopausal transition suggest that adverse changes in the lipid profile occur within the period between early perimenopause and very early postmenopause. Thus, the optimal time for lifestyle modification and preventive interventions may be before the menopausal transition, and the available evidence underscores the need to monitor lipid levels in premenopausal and early perimenopausal women. Prospective data from the Healthy Women Study show that premenopausal levels of lipids predict the extent of subclinical vascular disease 14 to 20 years later as measured by coronary artery and aortic calcium assessed with electron beam tomography.[21,22] An earlier report from this same cohort also demonstrated that premenopausal levels of blood pressure, LDL cholesterol, HDL cholesterol, triglycerides, and BMI predict intima media thickness and carotid plaque measured from 5 to 8 years after menopause.[17] Furthermore, favorable premenopausal levels of cardiovascular risk factors, particularly not smoking and favorable lipid levels, have been shown to be protective for the development of subclinical atherosclerosis in the postmenopausal years.[21] The feasibility of preventing adverse lipid changes during the menopausal transition has been demonstrated by a randomized trial of more than 500 women, in which a lifestyle intervention that included diet and exercise was able to blunt increases in LDL cholesterol during the transition from perimenopause to postmenopause.[23]

BLOOD PRESSURE

The relationship between endogenous estrogens and blood pressure is complex and may be mediated by multiple mechanisms, both genomic and non-genomic,[24] including hormonal influences on vascular tone and remodeling, the renin–angiotensin system, and oxidative stress.[25] Premenopausal women have lower blood pressures than age-matched men, with an increase in blood pressure seen in the first decade after menopause.[26] Early onset of menopause and duration of the postmenopausal period are associated with higher blood pressures,[27] and women with hypoestrogenemic states are at increased risk of developing hypertension.[28,29] Approximately 75% of postmenopausal women in the United States are hypertensive.[30]

It remains challenging to discern the specific effects of menopause-related hormonal changes on blood pressure given the coexistence of multiple other risk factors for hypertension, including age, obesity, arterial stiffening, and changes in insulin resistance, in this age group. Cross-sectional studies have provided conflicting data regarding the association between menopausal status and blood pressure and whether differences are accounted for by age, BMI, or other confounders.[31,32] Because of the limitations of cross-sectional studies, longitudinal studies have provided more reliable data regarding the independent influence of the menopausal transition on blood pressure.

In longitudinal data from SWAN, based on 10 years of follow-up,[16] changes in cardiovascular risk factors were examined in relation to the timing of the final menstrual period. These data demonstrated that changes in systolic and diastolic blood pressures through the menopausal transition were related to chronologic aging and that there was no influence of the final menstrual period on blood pressure. These data are consistent with other data from SWAN that failed to find any relationship between hormonal changes during the menopausal transition and blood pressure.[33]

The lack of measurable effect of the menopausal transition itself on blood pressure in SWAN is similar to the findings from the Melbourne Women's Midlife Health Project, in which changes in diastolic blood pressure were related to age, BMI, and changes in other risk factors.[13] In the Chin-Shan Community Cardiovascular Cohort Study,[10] changes in systolic and diastolic blood pressures were not related to the menopausal transition; in fact, there was a trend toward a greater increase in systolic blood pressure among women who remained premenopausal compared with those who transitioned during the follow-up period, whereas diastolic blood pressure was unaffected by menopause, age, or BMI. In the Healthy Women Study,[17] observed increases in blood pressure were greater during postmenopause than during perimenopause. Premenopausal systolic blood pressure was a predictor of subsequent carotid intimal medial thickness and plaque; when changes in risk factors between the premenopausal and the first year postmenopausal examinations were analyzed, only change in pulse pressure was related to both intima media thickness and plaque.

Although there does not seem to be a strong relationship between the menopausal transition itself and subsequent hypertension, the increase in hypertension in midlife and thereafter among women emphasizes the importance of monitoring blood pressure closely in these age groups and treating hypertension aggressively to reduce the future risk of cardiovascular disease.[34,35] In SWAN, among the 1255 women who were perimenopausal at baseline and not taking antihypertensive medication, 57.7% had normal blood pressure, 31.6% were prehypertensive and therefore at high risk of developing hypertension, and 10.7% were hypertensive.[36] An additional 205 perimenopausal women in SWAN were being treated with antihypertensive medications, of whom 58.5% met Seventh Report of the Joint National Committee on Prevention, Detection, Evaluation, and Treatment of High Blood Pressure criteria for having blood pressures at or below treatment goal.[36] When examined by ethnicity, prevalence rates of hypertension in the premenopausal and perimenopausal women in SWAN were 2-fold higher among Hispanic women and nearly 3-fold higher among African-American women compared with Caucasian women, with suboptimal rates of treatment and control.[37] Unfortunately, these rates are similar to nationally representative samples of women.[26] Therefore, greater attention to lifestyle modification and primary prevention measures to control blood pressure, as well as the diagnosis and effective treatment of hypertension in perimenopausal and postmenopausal women, are needed.

GLUCOSE, INSULIN, AND THE METABOLIC SYNDROME

Data from cohort studies that have followed women through the menopause transition do not support a strong influence of the menopause transition on glucose or insulin levels, or on the risk of developing type 2 diabetes. In the Melbourne Midlife Health project, there was no difference in changes in fasting glucose or insulin levels for women who transitioned from premenopause or early perimenopause to postmenopause, and those who remained premenopausal or early perimenopausal over 5 years of follow-up.[38] Although increases in insulin were also independent of age, they were positively associated with increases in BMI.[38] Similarly, analyses based on 10 years of follow-up in the SWAN cohort found no association between the final menstrual period and insulin or glucose levels.[16] Data from the Healthy Women Study suggest that changes in glucose may occur during the 5 years after menopause rather than during the perimenopausal period.[17] This may be because of postmenopausal increases in the proportion of body fat during the postmenopausal period.[17]

Longitudinal data suggest that the menopausal transition may be associated with the metabolic syndrome, a collection of metabolic risk factors, including impaired glucose metabolism, hypertension, dyslipidemia, and abdominal obesity, that is associated with increased risk of cardiovascular disease and type 2 diabetes.[39] Given the lack of evidence for menopause-related effects on insulin or glucose levels, it is likely that increases in the metabolic syndrome during the transition are attributable to changes in these other components. In the SWAN cohort, the incidence of the metabolic syndrome increased from 6 years prior until 6 years after the final menstrual period, independent of age and other cardiovascular risk levels.[40] The risk of developing metabolic syndrome was not related to changes in either estradiol or total testosterone, but increases in bioavailable testosterone or SHBG were similarly associated with excess risk. Additional analyses in this cohort have demonstrated that the development of relative androgen excess, defined as change over time in the ratio of testosterone to estradiol, was associated with increased risk of incident metabolic syndrome.[41] Taken together, these studies suggest that the interplay of testosterone and estradiol, rather than the absolute levels of either, may underlie the observed increases in metabolic syndrome risk during menopause. These results are in agreement with results from a recent, large meta-analysis suggesting that lower SHBG is associated with the metabolic syndrome, and that women with the metabolic syndrome have higher levels of total and free testosterone.[42] An adverse effect of androgens on insulin resistance has been proposed as a potential mechanism, although further studies are required to assess this hypothesis.[41,43]

SUBCLINICAL ATHEROSCLEROSIS

Estrogen exerts direct effects on the arterial wall, which may impact both vascular tone and the development of atherosclerosis.[44–47] Estrogen has been shown to have vasodilatory effects, which may be related to effects on calcium channels, potentiation of endothelium-dependent vasodilation, or upregulation of prostacyclin synthesis.[44,45,48–50] Estrogen may inhibit atherosclerosis by impeding smooth muscle cell proliferation, inhibiting deposition of LDL cholesterol in the vascular wall, or by inhibiting platelet aggregation and stress-induced endothelial injury.[44,45,48,51]

Menopausal influences on vascular structure and function have been suggested by studies of gender differences in age-related change in vascular reactivity. Among adult men, endothelial dysfunction increases gradually with age, whereas among women endothelial dysfunction accelerates around the age of menopause.[52–55] Longitudinal data regarding the relation of the stages of the menopause transition to the development of subclinical vascular disease are sparse. An ancillary study in the SWAN cohort, SWAN Heart,[56] is currently assessing the relationship of the menopausal transition to the natural history of subclinical atherosclerosis. In this study, late perimenopause and decreased estradiol levels were associated with larger adventitial diameter of the common carotid artery, after adjustment for age and multivariable adjustment for concurrent risk factor status.[57]

Data from SWAN Heart have also suggested that symptoms of hot flashes during the menopausal transition may be a marker for adverse vascular changes.[56,58] In the SWAN Heart cohort, the presence of hot flashes is associated with endothelial dysfunction with decreased flow-mediated dilation, and with higher levels of aortic calcification[56] and intima media thickness of the common carotid artery.[58] Given the evidence for the protective effects of estrogen on the vascular wall, and correlations of low estradiol concentrations with hot flashes, low estradiol concentrations in perimenopausal women have been proposed as a mechanism by which hot flashes are linked to indices of subclinical vascular disease. Alternatively, because hot flashes occur at a time of adverse changes in established cardiovascular risk factors, shared risk factors may also explain the observed association.[56] Further studies are required to elucidate the mechanisms by which hot flashes during the menopause transition may be linked to adverse vascular changes.

CLINICAL CONSIDERATIONS

Although much remains to be learned about the relationship between the menopausal transition and cardiovascular risk in women, the menopausal transition represents both a biologically and clinically relevant time point to address risk factor modification in women. For example, based on findings from SWAN and other studies, the lipid and apolipoprotein changes associated with perimenopause seem to be independent of chronologic age and may be proatherogenic. Additional study is needed to further examine these changes and their association with cardiovascular outcomes, and to determine which aspects of these changes are most important in determining future risk, including particle composition. Nevertheless, the finding of a critical time period, the year immediately around the FMP, as the time of the most adverse changes in lipid profiles,[16] underscores the need to monitor women's lipid profiles as they approach menopause and the importance of instituting proven lifestyle measures and drug therapy when needed to reduce risk. Although the available data do not clearly demonstrate associations between the menopausal transition and other non-lipid cardiovascular risk factors that are independent of chronologic aging, additional studies are needed.

It remains to be seen whether menopausal status or measurable biologic or hormonal changes related to the transition provide independent and incremental value to the risk estimates provided by traditional risk factors. However, this concept merits further study given the limitations of existing risk stratification models in women. For example, the Framingham Risk Score classifies most women as low risk for CHD despite differences in risk factor burden, because of the importance of age in its 10-year risk equation. Unless a woman is over 70 years of age, it is uncommon that she will score high enough by the Framingham Risk Score to be considered for pharmacologic therapy, such as lipid-lowering medications.[59] Furthermore, women are also more likely to experience non-CHD cardiovascular events such as stroke or heart failure. An updated Framingham Risk Score for general cardiovascular disease, including CHD, angina, stroke, peripheral vascular disease, and heart failure, has been developed to address these issues.[60]

Another ongoing controversy involves the potential role of hormone therapy in the perimenopausal period.[61,62] The Women's Health Initiative (WHI) trials demonstrated an overall increased risk of cardiovascular disease events in healthy postmenopausal women with a uterus (aged 50–79 years; mean age, 63.2; mean follow-up, 5.2 years) randomized to oral conjugated equine estrogen (CEE) 0.625 mg/d and medroxyprogesterone acetate 2.5 mg/d,[63] and no overall effect on coronary risk in women without a uterus (aged 50–79 years; mean age, 63.6; mean follow-up, 7.1 years) randomized to oral CEE 0.625 mg/d compared with placebo.[64] However, the "timing hypothesis" proposes that younger women without preexisting atherosclerosis could benefit from hormone therapy, as suggested by animal models[65] and epidemiologic data.[66] This question remains unresolved. Subsequent analyses of WHI trial data have suggested that women who initiated hormone therapy closer to the menopause tended to have reduced CHD risk, but this difference was not significant.[67] A meta-analysis pooling data from 23 hormone therapy trials, including WHI, showed a similar trend.[68] Additional analyses of WHI data, which included both the clinical trial and observational study data, examined the effect of hormone therapy soon after the menopause on multiple health outcomes, and found that the overall benefit/risk balance was unfavorable for combined CEE/medroxyprogesterone acetate therapy and neutral for CEE alone.[69] Most recently, extended follow-up of the estrogen-alone component of WHI (10.7 years) found that CHD-related outcomes were more favorable for younger women (age 50–59) treated with CEE compared with older women; a similar pattern was seen when time since menopause was examined, rather than age.[70] An ongoing trial, the Kronos Early Estrogen Replacement Study, is examining the effect of hormone therapy (oral CEE 0.45 mg/d or 50 μg transdermal estradiol, in combination with cyclic oral micronized progesterone 200 mg for 12 days each month) in preventing progression of carotid intima medial thickness and coronary calcification in women aged 42 to 58 years who are within 36 months of their final menstrual period.[71] Additional information is needed regarding the effects of hormone therapy initiated during the perimenopausal period on the risk of cardiovascular disease and other health outcomes, and whether effects differ based on the type, dose, and mode of hormone therapy or based on the characteristics of the women themselves.

Nevertheless, based on the data available thus far, we may conclude that the menopausal transition represents a time of substantial adverse changes in cardiovascular risk factors for women, related to both chronologic and ovarian aging. Given these relationships, the tracking of premenopausal and perimenopausal risk factor burden with future risk of vascular disease,[17] as well as the significant increase in cardiovascular disease that occurs after menopause, women and their health care providers should be vigilant about risk factor monitoring in the premenopausal and perimenopausal years. Lifestyle modification and therapeutic interventions should be implemented before the menopausal transition to counter these adverse risk factor changes and reduce women's future risk of cardiovascular disease.

REFERENCES

1. Roger VL, Go AS, Lloyd-Jones DM, et al. Heart disease and stroke statistics—2011 update: a report from the American Heart Association. Circulation 2011;123:e18–e209.
2. Atsma F, Bartelink ML, Grobbee DE, et al. Postmenopausal status and early menopause as independent risk factors for cardiovascular disease: a meta-analysis. Menopause 2006;13:265–79.
3. Bittner V. Menopause, age, and cardiovascular risk: a complex relationship. J Am Coll Cardiol 2009;54:2374–5.
4. Sowers MF, Crawford S, Sternfeld B, et al. Design, survey sampling and recruitment methods of SWAN: a multi-center, multi-ethnic, community-based cohort study of women and the menopausal transition. In: Lobos R, Marcus R, Kelsey JL, editors. Menopause. New York (NY): Academic Press; 2000. p. 175–88.
5. Matthews KA, Kelsey SF, Meilahn EN, et al. Educational attainment and behavioral and biologic risk factors for coronary heart disease in middle-aged women. Am J Epidemiol 1989;129:1132–44.
6. Dennerstein L, Smith AMA, Morse C, et al. Menopausal symptoms in Australian women. Med J Aust 1994;159:232–6.
7. Roche AF. Growth, maturation, and body composition: the Fels Longitudinal Study, 1929–1991. Cambridge (UK): Cambridge University Press; 1991.
8. Lee Y, Lin RS, Sung FC, et al. Chin-Shan Community Cardiovascular Cohort in Taiwan-baseline data and five-year follow-up morbidity and mortality. J Clin Epidemiol 2000;53:838–46.
9. Derby CA. Cardiovascular pathophysiology. In: Lobos R, Marcus R, Kelsey JL, editors. Menopause, New York (NY): Academic Press; 2000. p. 229–43.
10. Torng PL, Su TC, Sung FC, et al. Effects of menopause on intraindividual changes in serum lipids, blood pressure, and body weight—the Chin-Shan Community Cardiovascular Cohort Study. Atherosclerosis 2002;161:409–15.

11. Zhou JL, Lin SQ, Shen Y, et al. Serum lipid profile changes during the menopausal transition in Chinese women: a community-based cohort study. Menopause 2010; 17:997–1003.
12. Schubert CM, Rogers NL, Remsberg KE, et al. Lipids, lipoproteins, lifestyle, adiposity and fat-free mass during middle age: The Fels Longitudinal Study. Int J Obes (Lond) 2006;30:251–60.
13. Do KA, Green A, Guthrie JR, et al. Longitudinal study of risk factors for coronary heart disease across the menopausal transition. Am J Epidemiol 2000;151:584–93.
14. Gold EB, Bromberger J, Crawford S, et al. Factors associated with age at natural menopause in a multiethnic sample of midlife women. Am J Epidemiol 2001;153: 865–74.
15. Derby CA, Crawford SL, Pasternak RC, et al. Lipid changes during the menopause transition in relation to age and weight: the Study of Women's Health Across the Nation. Am J Epidemiol 2009;169:1352–61.
16. Matthews KA, Crawford SL, Chae CU, et al. Are changes in cardiovascular disease risk factors in midlife women due to chronological aging or to the menopausal transition? J Am Coll Cardiol 2009;54:2366–73.
17. Matthews KA, Kuller LH, Sutton-Tyrrell K, et al. Changes in cardiovascular risk factors during the perimenopause and postmenopause and carotid artery atherosclerosis in healthy women. Stroke 2001;32:1104–11.
18. Andrikoula M, McDowell IF. The contribution of ApoB and ApoA1 measurements to cardiovascular risk assessment. Diabetes Obes Metab 2008;10:271–8.
19. Woodard GA, Brooks MM, Barinas-Mitchell E, et al. Lipids, menopause, and early atherosclerosis in Study of Women's Health Across the Nation Heart women. Menopause Nov 19, 2010. [Epub ahead of print].
20. Mora S, Otvos JD, Rifai N, et al. Lipoprotein particle profiles by nuclear magnetic resonance compared with standard lipids and apolipoproteins in predicting incident cardiovascular disease in women. Circulation 2009;119:931–9.
21. Matthews KA, Kuller LH, Chang Y, et al. Premenopausal risk factors for coronary and aortic calcification: a 20-year follow-up in the Healthy Women Study. Prev Med 2007;45:302–8.
22. Kuller LH, Matthews KA, Sutton-Tyrrell K, et al. Coronary and aortic calcification among women 8 years after menopause and their premenopausal risk factors: the Healthy Women Study. Arterioscler Thromb Vasc Biol 1999;19:2189–98.
23. Kuller LH, Simkin-Silverman LR, Wing RR, et al. Women's Healthy Lifestyle Project: a randomized clinical trial: results at 54 months. Circulation 2001;103:32–7.
24. Mendelsohn ME, Karas RH. The protective effects of estrogen on the cardiovascular system. N Engl J Med 1999;340:1801–11.
25. Barton M, Meyer MR. Postmenopausal hypertension: mechanisms and therapy. Hypertension 2009;54:11–8.
26. Burt VL, Whelton P, Roccella EJ, et al. Prevalence of hypertension in the US adult population. Results from the Third National Health and Nutrition Examination Survey, 1988–1991. Hypertension 1995;25:305–13.
27. Izumi Y, Matsumoto K, Ozawa Y, et al. Effect of age at menopause on blood pressure in postmenopausal women. Am J Hypertens 2007;20:1045–50.
28. Shaw LJ, Bairey Merz CN, Azziz R, et al. Postmenopausal women with a history of irregular menses and elevated androgen measurements at high risk for worsening cardiovascular event-free survival: results from the National Institutes of Health—National Heart, Lung, and Blood Institute sponsored Women's Ischemia Syndrome Evaluation. J Clin Endocrinol Metab 2008;93:1276–84.

29. Mercuro G, Zoncu S, Saiu F, et al. Menopause induced by oophorectomy reveals a role of ovarian estrogen on the maintenance of pressure homeostasis. Maturitas 2004;47:131–8.

30. Ong KL, Cheung BM, Man YB, et al. Prevalence, awareness, treatment, and control of hypertension among United States adults 1999–2004. Hypertension 2007;49:69–75.

31. Portaluppi F, Pansini F, Manfredini R, et al. Relative influence of menopausal status, age, and body mass index on blood pressure. Hypertension 1997;29:976–9.

32. Zanchetti A, Facchetti R, Cesana GC, et al. Menopause-related blood pressure increase and its relationship to age and body mass index: the SIMONA epidemiological study. J Hypertens 2005;23:2269–76.

33. Sutton-Tyrrell K, Wildman RP, Matthews KA, et al. Sex-hormone-binding globulin and the free androgen index are related to cardiovascular risk factors in multiethnic premenopausal and perimenopausal women enrolled in the Study of Women Across the Nation (SWAN). Circulation 2005;111:1242–9.

34. Collins P, Rosano G, Casey C, et al. Management of cardiovascular risk in the peri-menopausal woman: a consensus statement of European cardiologists and gynaecologists. Eur Heart J 2007;28:2028–40.

35. Chobanian AV, Bakris GL, Black HR, et al. Seventh report of the Joint National Committee on Prevention, Detection, Evaluation, and Treatment of High Blood Pressure. Hypertension 2003;42:1206–52.

36. Derby CA, FitzGerald G, Lasser NL, et al. Application of national screening criteria for blood pressure and cholesterol to perimenopausal women: prevalence of hypertension and hypercholesterolemia in the Study of Women's Health Across the Nation. Prev Cardiol 2006;9:150–9.

37. Lloyd-Jones DM, Sutton-Tyrrell K, Patel AS, et al. Ethnic variation in hypertension among premenopausal and perimenopausal women: Study of Women's Health Across the Nation. Hypertension 2005;46:689–95.

38. Guthrie JR, Ball M, Dudley EC, et al. Impaired fasting glycaemia in middle-aged women: a prospective study. Int J Obes Relat Metab Disord 2001;25:646–51.

39. Grundy SM. Metabolic syndrome: a multiplex cardiovascular risk factor. J Clin Endocrinol Metab 2007;92:399–404.

40. Janssen I, Powell LH, Crawford S, et al. Menopause and the metabolic syndrome: the Study of Women's Health Across the Nation. Arch Intern Med 2008;168:1568–75.

41. Torrens JI, Sutton-Tyrrell K, Zhao X, et al. Relative androgen excess during the menopausal transition predicts incident metabolic syndrome in midlife women: Study of Women's Health Across the Nation. Menopause 2009;16:257–64.

42. Brand JS, van der Tweel I, Grobbee DE, et al. Testosterone, sex hormone-binding globulin and the metabolic syndrome: a systematic review and meta-analysis of observational studies. Int J Epidemiol 2011;40:189–207.

43. Polotsky HN, Polotsky AJ. Metabolic implications of menopause. Semin Reprod Med 2010;28:426–34.

44. Rosano GM, Chierchia SL, Leonardo F, et al. Cardioprotective effects of ovarian hormones. Eur Heart J 1996;17(Suppl D):15–9.

45. Samaan SA, Crawford MH. Estrogen and cardiovascular function after menopause. J Am Coll Cardiol 1995;26:1403–10.

46. Kublickiene K, Luksha L. Gender and the endothelium. Pharmacol Rep 2008;60: 49–60.

47. Mendelsohn ME. Protective effects of estrogen on the cardiovascular system. Am J Cardiol 2002;89:12E–17E.

48. Gupta S, Rymer J. Hormone replacement therapy and cardiovascular disease. Int J Gynaecol Obstet 1996;52:119–25.
49. Collins P, Rosano GM, Jiang C, et al. Cardiovascular protection by oestrogen—a calcium antagonist effect? Lancet 1993;341:1264–5.
50. Glasser SP, Selwyn AP, Ganz P. Atherosclerosis: risk factors and the vascular endothelium. Am Heart J 1996;131:379–84.
51. Wild RA. Estrogen: effects on the cardiovascular tree. Obstet Gynecol 1996;87:27S–35S.
52. Celermajer DS, Sorensen KE, Bull C, et al. Endothelium-dependent dilation in the systemic arteries of asymptomatic subjects relates to coronary risk factors and their interaction. J Am Coll Cardiol 1994;24:1468–74.
53. Celermajer DS, Sorensen KE, Spiegelhalter DJ, et al. Aging is associated with endothelial dysfunction in healthy men years before the age-related decline in women. J Am Coll Cardiol 1994;24:471–6.
54. Taddei S, Virdis A, Ghiadoni L, et al. Menopause is associated with endothelial dysfunction in women. Hypertension 1996;28:576–82.
55. Jensen-Urstad K, Johansson J. Gender difference in age-related changes in vascular function. J Intern Med 2001;250:29–36.
56. Thurston RC, Sutton-Tyrrell K, Everson-Rose SA, et al. Hot flashes and subclinical cardiovascular disease: findings from the Study of Women's Health Across the Nation Heart Study. Circulation 2008;118:1234–40.
57. Wildman RP, Colvin AB, Powell LH, et al. Associations of endogenous sex hormones with the vasculature in menopausal women: the Study of Women's Health Across the Nation (SWAN). Menopause 2008;15:414–21.
58. Thurston RC, Sutton-Tyrrell K, Everson-Rose SA, et al. Hot flashes and carotid intima media thickness among midlife women. Menopause Jan 14, 2011. [Epub ahead of print].
59. Sibley C, Blumenthal RS, Merz CN, et al. Limitations of current cardiovascular disease risk assessment strategies in women. J Womens Health (Larchmt) 2006;15:54–6.
60. D'Agostino RBS, Vasan RS, Pencina MJ, et al. General cardiovascular risk profile for use in primary care: the Framingham Heart Study. Circulation 2008;117:743–53.
61. Barrett-Connor E. Hormones and heart disease in women: the timing hypothesis. Am J Epidemiol 2007;166:506–10.
62. Manson JE, Bassuk SS. Invited commentary: Hormone therapy and risk of coronary heart disease-why renew the focus on the early years of menopause? Am J Epidemiol 2007;166:511–7.
63. Rossouw JE, Anderson GL, Prentice RL, et al. Risks and benefits of estrogen plus progestin in healthy postmenopausal women: principal results from the Women's Health Initiative randomized controlled trial. JAMA 2002;288:321–33.
64. Anderson GL, Limacher M, Assaf AR, et al. Effects of conjugated equine estrogen in postmenopausal women with hysterectomy: the Women's Health Initiative randomized controlled trial. JAMA 2004;291:1701–12.
65. Mikkola TS, Clarkson TB. Estrogen replacement therapy, atherosclerosis, and vascular function. Cardiovasc Res 2002;53:605–19.
66. Grodstein F, Manson JE, Stampfer MJ. Hormone therapy and coronary heart disease: the role of time since menopause and age at hormone initiation. J Womens Health (Larchmt) 2006;15:35–44.
67. Rossouw JE, Prentice RL, Manson JE, et al. Postmenopausal hormone therapy and risk of cardiovascular disease by age and years since menopause. JAMA 2007;297:1465–77.

68. Salpeter SR, Walsh JM, Greyber E, et al. Brief report: Coronary heart disease events associated with hormone therapy in younger and older women. A meta-analysis. J Gen Intern Med 2006;21:363–6.

69. Prentice RL, Manson JE, Langer RD, et al. Benefits and risks of postmenopausal hormone therapy when it is initiated soon after menopause. Am J Epidemiol 2009; 170:12–23.

70. LaCroix AZ, Chlebowski RT, Manson JE, et al. Health outcomes after stopping conjugated equine estrogens among postmenopausal women with prior hysterectomy: a randomized controlled trial. JAMA 2011;305:1305–14.

71. Miller VM, Black DM, Brinton EA, et al. Using basic science to design a clinical trial: baseline characteristics of women enrolled in the Kronos Early Estrogen Prevention Study (KEEPS). J Cardiovasc Transl Res 2009;2:228–39.

Vasomotor Symptoms and Menopause: Findings from the Study of Women's Health across the Nation

Rebecca C. Thurston, PhD[a,b,*], Hadine Joffe, MD, MSc[c]

KEYWORDS

- Hot flashes • Hot flushes • Vasomotor symptoms
- Menopause • Climacteric symptoms
- Menopausal symptoms

The Study of Women's Health across the Nation (SWAN) is among the largest and most ethnically diverse longitudinal studies of the menopausal transition. SWAN enrolled 3302 midlife women across 5 racial/ethnic groups, and has followed these women for more than 10 years. During this time, a wealth of information about SWAN participants was collected annually, including information about vasomotor and other menopause-related symptoms, health behaviors, social and psychological functioning, as well as a range of physiologic indices. Thus, SWAN, with its longitudinal design, multiethnic sample, and biopsychosocial perspective, has allowed unique insights into vasomotor symptoms (VMS), serving to advance the field of midlife women's health. Herein we have summarized some of the insights gained from SWAN about this common and often troublesome midlife symptom. Specifically, we review the epidemiology and physiology of VMS, risk factors for VMS, and associated quality of life and health conditions. We emphasize findings from SWAN given the wealth of information gained from this unique cohort study.

In addition to the SWAN funding described in the overview, this work was also supported by NIH grants AG029216 (Thurston) and NH082922 (Joffe).

Hadine Joffe has received research support from Bayer HealthCare Pharmaceuticals (co-PI), Forest Laboratories (co-I), GlaxoSmithKline (co-I), and served as an advisor/consultant to Sunovion.

[a] Department of Psychiatry, University of Pittsburgh School of Medicine, 3811 O'Hara Street, Pittsburgh, PA 15213, USA

[b] Department of Epidemiology, University of Pittsburgh Graduate School of Public Health, 130 DeSoto Street, Pittsburgh, PA 15261, USA

[c] Department of Psychiatry, Center for Women's Mental Health, Massachusetts General Hospital, Harvard Medical School, 185 Cambridge Street, Suite 2000, Boston, MA 02114, USA

* Corresponding author. Department of Psychiatry, University of Pittsburgh School of Medicine, 3811 O'Hara Street, Pittsburgh, PA 15213.

E-mail address: thurstonrc@upmc.edu

DEFINITION AND EPIDEMIOLOGY OF VMS

VMS, or hot flashes and night sweats, are often considered the cardinal symptoms of menopause. VMS are episodes of profuse heat accompanied by sweating and flushing, experienced predominantly around the head, neck, chest, and upper back. VMS are experienced by the majority of women during the menopausal transition. In SWAN, 60% to 80% of women experience VMS at some point during the menopausal transition, with prevalence rates varying by racial/ethnic group.[1] Research from SWAN indicates that the occurrence and frequency of VMS peak in the late perimenopause and early postmenopausal years,[1] or the several years surrounding the final menstrual period. However, research from a range of studies has shown that a sizable minority of women report VMS earlier in midlife, before the onset of menstrual cycle changes,[2] and well into their 60s and 70s, decades after the menopause transition.[3,4] Given the prevalence and duration of VMS among midlife women, it is critical to understand the underlying biology of this symptom, the extent to which VMS may impair quality of life, and whether VMS may serve as a marker for other important health conditions.

PHYSIOLOGY OF VMS
Reproductive Hormones

The physiology of hot flashes is not fully understood, and likely represents an interplay between multiple central and peripheral physiologic systems. Reproductive hormones likely play an integral role, as evidenced by the onset of VMS occurring in the context of the dramatic reproductive hormone changes of the menopausal transition and by the therapeutic role of exogenous estrogen in their treatment. SWAN analyses show that levels of endogenous hormones are associated with VMS. On an annual basis, SWAN participants (n = 3302) reported on their experience of VMS over the prior 2 weeks and provided a blood sample for measurement of estradiol (E2), follicle-stimulating hormone (FSH), testosterone, dehydroepiandrosterone sulfate, and sex hormone–binding globulin. Considered separately, higher FSH and lower E2 levels were associated with a greater likelihood of reporting VMS (over 5 years), whereas only higher FSH levels were associated with VMS when both hormones were considered.[5]

A subset of SWAN women (n = 742) also participated in the SWAN Daily Hormone Study, which involved annual urine collection over a complete menstrual cycle (or a comparable period of time for women without menstrual cycles) for assessment of urinary FSH, luteinizing hormone, the progesterone metabolite pregnanediol glucuronide, and estrone conjugates. Women also completed a daily VMS diary during this time. In this analysis, findings were similar to those in the full cohort among women who had evidence of impaired ovulatory activity, with higher FSH and lower estrone conjugate levels associated with a greater likelihood of reporting VMS.[6] This pattern was not observed among women who seemed to be ovulatory, among whom the only hormone associated with VMS was higher pregnanediol glucuronide levels. Taken together, these findings indicate that lower estrogen and higher FSH levels are associated with VMS reporting, particularly for women with anovulatory cycles. However, although all perimenopausal women experience these hormonal changes, not all women have VMS. Therefore, other physiologic systems beyond the reproductive axis must be at play.

Thermoregulation

Leading models characterize VMS, at least in part, as thermoregulatory heat dissipation events. There is some evidence of a narrowing of the thermoneutral zone in symptomatic postmenopausal women, or the zone in which core body temperature is maintained without triggering thermoregulatory homeostatic mechanisms such as sweating or shivering.[7] Therefore, for symptomatic women, small fluctuations in core body temperature can exceed this zone and trigger heat dissipation mechanisms such as sweating and peripheral vasodilation (a hot flash). Research indicating that E2 administration reduces VMS and widens the thermoneutral zone adds support to this model.[8] Although there are some empirical data to support this model, more research is needed. Other systems implicated in the etiology of hot flashes include central serotonergic, noradrenergic, opioid, adrenal, and autonomic systems, as well as vascular processes, but little evidence is available to clearly elucidate their role in the genesis of hot flashes.[9-13]

Genetics

SWAN and other studies have sought to characterize associations between genetic polymorphisms and VMS. To date, estrogen receptor polymorphisms and selected single nucleotide polymorphisms of genes involved in the biosynthesis and metabolism of different estrogens (E2, estrone, estriol) have been explored. Variants in genes that encode for estrogen receptor-α and in enzymes involved in synthesis of and conversion between more and less potent estrogens have been found to predict the likelihood of VMS in the different racial/ethnic groups studied in SWAN (n = 1538).[14,15] Although there have been some inconsistencies between findings, similar results have been seen in other studies investigating single nucleotide polymorphisms involved in synthesis and metabolism of estrogens,[16-19] as well as estrogen receptor-α.[20] In general, these associations persist after adjusting for other important contributory factors, including reproductive hormone levels. Given the established variability between race/ethnic groups in genetic polymorphisms, SWAN results provide an important contribution to our understanding of gene/VMS associations because of the inclusion of large numbers of women from different racial/ethnic minority groups. Taken together, these results suggest that the link between VMS and genetic polymorphisms may be due to polymorphisms that alter sex steroid hormone activity. However, it is not known whether these genetic determinants exert their effects centrally in the brain or peripherally on the autonomic nervous system, vasculature, or other systems potentially involved in the genesis of VMS.

RISK FACTORS FOR VMS
Race/Ethnicity

VMS show pronounced racial/ethnic variations. Of the 5 racial/ethnic groups studied in SWAN, African-American women were most likely to report VMS. African American women were also more likely to describe their VMS as bothersome, even after controlling for their increased rate of reporting VMS relative to Caucasian women. Caucasian and Hispanic women in SWAN are broadly similar in their rates of reporting VMS. However, pronounced variation across different ethnic groups of Hispanic women has been noted in SWAN, with the highest rates of VMS reported among Central American women and lowest rates among Cuban women.[21] Chinese and Japanese women in SWAN are least likely to report VMS, with Japanese women least likely to report VMS or to describe them as bothersome.[1,22]

The reasons for these racial/ethnic differences are likely varied and not fully understood. Although key factors associated with VMS show pronounced racial/ethnic variation, including body mass index (BMI), E2 levels, smoking, hormone use, and socioeconomic position, racial/ethnic differences in VMS in SWAN persist after controlling for these factors.[1] Others have suggested that the low level of VMS among Asian versus Caucasian women is due to Asian women's relatively high soy intake. However, in SWAN, this does not seem to be the case,[1,23] consistent with findings from randomized, controlled trials, which have produced mixed or inconclusive results regarding the use of soy or isoflavones for the management of VMS.[24-26] Moreover, experiencing and reporting of any physical symptom, including VMS, is complex and influenced by a range of perceptual and reporting processes. Cultural variations in how women experience, interpret, label, and report VMS may also play a role in observed racial/ethnic differences in VMS.[27]

Obesity

A key risk factor for VMS is obesity. For many years, obesity was thought to be protective against VMS because androgens are aromatized into estrogens in body fat.[28] Women with more adipose tissue would thereby be expected to have a lower risk of VMS. One important finding from SWAN and other large, observational studies is that obesity may be a risk factor, rather than a protective characteristic, for VMS during the perimenopause and early postmenopause. For example, in SWAN (n = 3302) women with no or infrequent VMS had an average BMI of 28 kg/m², whereas those with more frequent VMS (having VMS at on ≥days in the past 2 weeks) had an average BMI of 31 kg/m².[1] This association between VMS and higher BMI persisted after controlling for related risk factors. Findings of positive associations between BMI and VMS are more consistent with a thermoregulatory model of VMS, in which adipose tissue acts as an insulator, preventing the heat dissipating action of VMS, thereby increasing their occurrence or severity. However, the mechanisms responsible for links between obesity and VMS are not understood, and may include other physiologic mechanisms, including a possible role of other endocrine functions of adipose tissue.[29] Moreover, the positive associations between obesity and VMS may be most applicable to women earlier in the menopausal transition (eg, in the perimenopause or early postmenopause).[30-34]

The analytic approaches used to examine the association between obesity and VMS primarily use calculated BMI, which encompasses both lean and fat mass, and therefore cannot discern the relative contributions of fat and lean mass as predictors of VMS. Because the contribution of adipose tissue to risk for VMS may result from its thermoregulatory properties or its endocrine products, understanding specifically how adiposity is related to VMS is important. SWAN analyses have examined the association of adiposity to VMS using 3 different approaches. The first of these investigations examined adiposity as measured by bioelectrical impedance analysis (n = 1776), which yields measures of both fat and lean mass. A higher total percentage of body fat, but not lean mass, was related to an increased likelihood of VMS after controlling for confounding factors such as reproductive hormones, smoking, race/ethnicity, education and negative affect.[35] A second analysis from SWAN utilized computed tomography measures of abdominal adiposity (n = 461). Computed tomography yields measures of total abdominal adiposity, including subcutaneous adiposity, or the adipose tissue between the skin and the abdominal muscle wall, and visceral adiposity, or the adipose tissue behind the abdominal muscle wall and in the peritoneal space around the organs. Notably, subcutaneous fat is particularly insulating.[36] Results indicated that higher abdominal adiposity, and particularly subcutaneous adiposity, was associated with an increased likelihood of reporting hot flashes.[37] These associations were not accounted for by confounding factors or reproductive hormones (E2 and FSH). Finally, a third analysis from SWAN utilized measures of bioelectrical impedance analysis over a 4-year period, thereby allowing examination of change in adiposity over time in relation to VMS (n = 1659). This analysis is particularly relevant given that weight gain is common during midlife.[38] Findings indicated that, relative to women who maintained stable body fat, gains in body fat from one year to the next were associated with an increased likelihood of reporting VMS at the subsequent visit.[39] These associations were independent of confounding factors and changes in reproductive hormones. Taken together, these findings indicate that among perimenopausal and early postmenopausal women, adiposity was associated with an increased likelihood of having VMS, a finding consistent with both a thermoregulatory model of VMS and also an endocrine model of adiposity and VMS.

Health Behaviors

The potential role of health behaviors in VMS has been of particular interest. One of the most consistently observed health behaviors associated with VMS is smoking. In SWAN, over the course of 6 years of follow-up, current smokers had a more than 60% increased likelihood of reporting VMS relative to nonsmokers,[1] adjusted for confounding factors such as education, BMI, menopausal status, and race/ethnicity. In fact, SWAN results show that both active smoking and passive smoke exposure are associated with a greater likelihood of VMS.[23] It has been hypothesized that the association between smoking and VMS is due to the anti-estrogenic effects of cigarette smoking.[40] However, challenging this explanation is evidence from SWAN indicating that differences in endogenous E2 levels did not account for the association between smoking and VMS.[23]

Other notable health behaviors, such as dietary factors and physical activity, have shown much weaker associations with VMS. In SWAN, dietary factors such as total kilocalorie, fat, fiber, caffeine, alcohol intake, or specific vitamin intake have not been associated with VMS, after accounting for confounding factors such as education, smoking, and BMI.[1,23] Although initial reports showed a beneficial effect of the isoflavone, genistein, in relation to VMS,[23] this association was not observed in later longitudinal analyses.[1] Another health behavior of particular interest is physical activity.[41] Physical activity has also not been consistently associated with VMS in SWAN and other studies, after adjustment for confounding factors.[1,41] It is notable that physical activity may have dual roles in relation to VMS, positively impacting factors such as mood and body weight, which may improve VMS, but also acutely raising core body temperature, which could theoretically increase the occurrence of VMS. Together, these SWAN investigations suggest that smoking is the health behavior most clearly related to VMS, with diet and physical activity showing much weaker or inconsistent associations with VMS.

Negative Affect

Negative mood (affect) has consistently been associated with VMS across investigations. In SWAN (n = 3302), higher levels of anxiety, depressive symptoms, and perceived stress at study entry have been associated with an increased likelihood of VMS occurring over the subsequent 6 years.[1] In fact, the psychological factor most consistently associated with hot flashes is anxiety, an association that has been observed in SWAN and other studies.[42] In addition to an increase in the occurrence and frequency of VMS, women with greater negative affect tend to rate their VMS as more bothersome, even after accounting for the higher frequency of their VMS. The relationships between negative affect and VMS are not fully understood, and may involve a complex interplay between physiologic and psychological factors. It is well-established that negative affect can influence symptom reporting, with a tendency toward elevated symptom reporting in the context of negative affect.[43] For example, women with a greater sensitivity to physical symptoms in general may be more likely to subsequently report VMS.[1] Research with physiologic hot flash monitors has confirmed the importance of negative affect in the reporting of hot flashes, showing a greater likelihood that hot flashes are reported when they are not detected physiologically.[44,45] However, the relationship between negative affect and VMS is bidirectional, because VMS also influence mood.

Other Social and Demographic Factors

Multiple other social and psychological factors have been associated with an increased likelihood of VMS. Child abuse and neglect are prevalent in the SWAN population and are associated with a range of poor physical and mental health outcomes. VMS are no exception. Women who endorsed a history of child abuse or neglect (38% of the sample assessed) were more likely to report VMS during the menopausal transition even after controlling for multiple factors, including negative affect, sociodemographic factors, and health behaviors.[46] Another important sociodemographic risk factor for VMS is low socioeconomic position. Women who are in lower socioeconomic positions, including women with lower educational attainment, lower income, or who endorse difficulty paying for basics are more likely to report VMS relative to their higher socioeconomic position counterparts.[1] The reasons for the association between socioeconomic position and VMS, an association observed across studies, are not well understood. Lower socioeconomic position is associated with smoking, higher BMI, higher perceived stress, and higher negative affect,[47,48] and is concentrated among certain minority racial/ethnic groups.[49] However, in SWAN, the association between low socioeconomic position and VMS could not be accounted for by any of these potentially confounding factors. It is notable that the influence of low socioeconomic position or early exposures such as child abuse on health is likely the result of multiple social, psychological, and physiologic processes operating over a life course, presenting a challenge to explaining these associations with any set of assessments administered at midlife.[47,50]

ASSOCIATED QUALITY-OF-LIFE SYMPTOMS

SWAN has investigated the association between VMS and key quality-of-life outcomes that may be influenced by the presence of VMS. These include sleep, mood, and cognitive function. Because each of these symptom domains is covered separately in other sections of this special edition, we briefly discuss available SWAN data that address specifically the association between VMS and these common symptoms affecting quality of life. In SWAN analyses, VMS have been strongly associated with reduced health-related quality-of-life, although menopause stage itself was not associated with health-related quality-of-life.[51,52] The negative association between VMS and health-related quality-of-life is strongest among those with more frequent VMS.[51]

Sleep

SWAN results have shown strong associations between VMS and perceived sleep disturbance in cross-sectional analyses,[53] longitudinal studies that follow women annually across the menopausal transition,[54] and in daily diary studies that capture a more detailed pattern of the close association between reported VMS and sleep problems.[55] VMS have been associated with all aspects of perceived sleep disturbance that contribute to poor sleep continuity and quality, including falling asleep, staying asleep, and early morning awakening.[54] In all analyses, VMS reporting stands out as a consistent factor that contributes to reporting of poor sleep after controlling for other important predictive factors. These data are consistent with numerous other studies that have similarly described a strong association between reported VMS and perceived sleep disturbance. The SWAN Sleep Study has collected extensive data that address the association between VMS and objectively measured sleep using polysomnography. Results of ongoing analyses bearing on the association between VMS and health-related quality-of-life–measured sleep are eagerly awaited given the more controversial extant literature on the association between VMS and objectively measured sleep parameters.

Mood

VMS and mood seem to be related in numerous and potentially complex ways. Initial evidence for links between VMS and depression comes from studies such as SWAN showing that high levels of depressive symptoms[56–58] as well as clinically significant depression[59–61] are most common during the perimenopause and early postmenopause, when VMS are most prevalent. SWAN and other studies have also found that perimenopausal women with VMS are more likely to develop depression after the onset of VMS than are perimenopausal women without VMS,[56,59–64] although these links may be due to other factors associated with having a depressive episode, such as a prior history of anxiety disorder and stressful life events.[59]

Studies have shown that VMS can both precede and follow, as well as occur concurrently with, depression,[65] indicating that the link between VMS and depression may be explained by a number of different causal pathways. When depression co-occurs with or follows VMS, VMS may result in mood disturbance because VMS can impair sleep, which is an important risk factor for depression. Alternatively, VMS may be an initial symptomatic manifestation of perturbations in neural systems that also underlie depression. Indirect evidence suggests that the serotonergic and noradrenergic systems, neurotransmitter systems commonly linked with depression, may be involved in the etiology of VMS,[10–13,66] raising the possibility that central nervous system processes contribute to both VMS and depression vulnerability.

However, many women with VMS do not experience depression. The observation that VMS occur in the absence of depression and that depression occurs in midlife women without VMS indicates that neither condition is required for the other symptom to manifest. Further investigation is warranted to understand the causal relationship between these 2 common midlife symptoms.

Cognitive Function

SWAN analyses (n = 2362) have shown that there is a transient decrement in cognitive performance during the perimenopause, which is characterized by a diminished ability to learn that subsequently resolves as women become postmenopausal.[67] Additional SWAN analyses (n = 1903) have indicated that this transient decrement is not explained by VMS.[68] These data are consistent with some,[69] but not all,[70] other smaller studies that similarly found an absence of an association between VMS and verbal memory performance when VMS are measured by self-report. In contrast, studies measuring VMS objectively show an inverse correlation between VMS and cognitive performance,[71] suggesting that physiologic changes underlying VMS may be linked directly and centrally with cognitive function.

EMERGING LINKS BETWEEN VMS AND DISEASE OUTCOMES

VMS have traditionally been conceptualized as an important quality-of-life issue during the menopausal transition, and they have generally not been assumed to have specific implications for physical health. However, emerging research from SWAN and other studies has begun to call this assumption into question.

Cardiovascular Risk

Initial work from several large trials of hormone therapy, including the Women's Health Initiative and the Heart and Estrogen Replacement Study suggested links between VMS and cardiovascular disease (CVD) risk. In both studies, the elevated coronary heart disease event risk associated with hormone therapy use were highest among women reporting moderate to severe VMS at the study entry, and in the Women's Health Initiative, the older women with VMS.[72,73] We have added to these initial observations in SWAN, exploring potential links between VMS and CVD. Much of this research has been conducted in the context of the SWAN Heart Study (n = 588), an ancillary study to SWAN that collected data on several measures of subclinical CVD, including brachial artery flow mediated dilation, a marker of endothelial dysfunction; coronary artery and aortic calcification, measures of calcified plaques in these arterial beds; and carotid intima media thickness (IMT), a well-established marker of atherosclerosis. These subclinical CVD measures are useful to understand risk for CVD among disease-free individuals, as all 3 measures have been prospectively associated with elevated cardiovascular event rates among individuals without clinical CVD.[74–76] Findings indicated that women reporting hot flashes, and in the case of IMT, more frequent hot flashes, had poorer endothelial function, greater aortic calcification, and greater IMT compared with their counterparts without hot flashes.[77,78] These associations persisted after controlling for confounding demographic and other known cardiovascular risk factors as well as E2 levels. Findings for night sweats were similar to those for hot flashes, but somewhat attenuated. Notably, associations between hot flashes and IMT were most pronounced for women who were overweight or obese, as well as for women who experienced hot flashes across multiple annual visits, suggesting that hot flashes may be most informative with respect to CVD risk when they are persistent and when they occur in individuals with other CVD risk factors, such as obesity. The precise reasons for and nature of the association between VMS and CVD risk require further investigation and explication. However, one interpretation of these findings is that hot flashes may be a symptomatic manifestation of underlying adverse changes in a woman's vasculature.

Bone Health

Emerging research from SWAN and other studies has linked VMS and bone mineral density and bone turnover. In the first of these SWAN analyses (n = 2213), women reporting VMS had lower bone mineral density.[79] This association was observed across women of all menopausal stages in the sample, but particularly among the postmenopausal women. The associations between VMS and bone mineral density varied by specific bone site studies, most apparent at the lumbar spine and hip among postmenopausal women, and at the femoral neck among women earlier in the menopausal transition. In a second set of SWAN analyses (n = 2283), the occurrence of VMS was further examined in relation to a highly sensitive marker of bone turnover, urinary N-telopeptide. In these analyses, perimenopausal and postmenopausal women with VMS had higher bone turnover (higher urinary N-telopeptide levels) than their counterparts without VMS.[80] In both analyses of bone density and bone turnover, associations largely persisted after controlling for potential confounders, although E2 and FSH levels accounted for some, but not all, of these associations. Potential reasons for associations between VMS and bone health require further investigation, including an exploration of the potential contribution of the hypothalamic–pituitary–adrenal axis and the sympathetic nervous system.[79] However, these results suggest that VMS may be an important indicator of some aspect of declining

ovarian function that is not captured by menstrual cycle changes or annual reproductive hormone levels.

SUMMARY

SWAN has yielded unique insights about VMS, the cardinal symptom of menopause.
We have learned that VMS are experienced by most midlife women, but show
pronounced racial/ethnic differences that cannot be explained by other known VMS
risk factors. Key risk factors for VMS include low education, smoking, and negative
affect. Obesity, previously thought to be protective against VMS, is actually a risk
factor for VMS among perimenopausal and early postmenopausal women. Further,
VMS are associated with poorer quality of life, negative mood, and sleep problems
during midlife. The association between VMS and mood is complex, bidirectional, and
possibly explained by multiple pathways, including sleep and neural mechanisms.
Finally, emerging information from SWAN indicates that VMS may be linked to certain
adverse physical health outcomes, including subclinical CVD and lower bone density.
Thus, SWAN has been a rich source of information about this common and often
troublesome midlife symptom. Ongoing findings from SWAN will continue to yield
important information about VMS in the years to come.

REFERENCES

1. Gold E, Colvin A, Avis N, et al. Longitudinal analysis of vasomotor symptoms and
   race/ethnicity across the menopausal transition: Study of Women's Health Across the
   Nation (SWAN). Am J Public Health 2006;96:1226–35.
2. Freeman EW, Grisso JA, Berlin J, et al. Symptom reports from a cohort of African
   American and white women in the late reproductive years. Menopause 2001;8:
   33–42.
3. Barnabei VM, Cochrane BB, Aragaki AK, et al. Menopausal symptoms and treatment-
   related effects of estrogen and progestin in the Women's Health Initiative. Obstet
   Gynecol 2005;105:1063–73.
4. Barnabei VM, Grady D, Stovall DW, et al. Menopausal symptoms in older women and
   the effects of treatment with hormone therapy. Obstet Gynecol 2002;100:1209–18.
5. Randolph JF Jr, Sowers M, Bondarenko I, et al. The relationship of longitudinal change
   in reproductive hormones and vasomotor symptoms during the menopausal transition. J Clin Endocrinol Metab 2005;90:6106–12.
6. Gold EB, Lasley B, Crawford SL, et al. Relation of daily urinary hormone patterns to
   vasomotor symptoms in a racially/ethnically diverse sample of midlife women: study of
   women's health across the nation. Reprod Sci 2007;14:786–97.
7. Freedman RR, Krell W. Reduced thermoregulatory null zone in postmenopausal
   women with hot flashes. Am J Obstet Gynecol 1999;181:66–70.
8. Freedman RR, Blacker CM. Estrogen raises the sweating threshold in postmenopausal women with hot flashes. Fertil Steril 2002;77:487–90.
9. Thurston R, Christie I, Matthews K. Hot flashes and cardiac vagal control: a link to
   cardiovascular risk? Menopause 2010;17:456–61.
10. Woods NF, Mitchell ES, Smith-Dijulio K. Cortisol levels during the menopausal
    transition and early postmenopause: observations from the Seattle Midlife Women's
    Health Study. Menopause 2009;16:708–18.
11. Freedman RR, Woodward S. Elevated a2-adrenergic responsiveness in menopausal
    hot flushes: pharmacologic and biochemical studies. In: Lomax P, Schonbaum E,
    editors. Thermoregulation: the pathophysiological basis of clinical disorders. Basel:
    Krager; 1992:6–9.

12. Casper RF, Yen SS. Neuroendocrinology of menopausal flushes: an hypothesis of flush mechanism. Clin Endocrinol (Oxf) 1985;22:293–312.
13. Sturdee DW. The menopausal hot flush—anything new? Maturitas 2008;60:42–9.
14. Crandall CJ, Crawford SL, Gold EB. Vasomotor symptom prevalence is associated with polymorphisms in sex steroid-metabolizing enzymes and receptors. Am J Med 2006;119(9 Suppl 1):S52–60.
15. Sowers MR, Wilson AL, Karvonen-Gutierrez CA, et al. Sex steroid hormone pathway genes and health-related measures in women of 4 races/ethnicities: the Study of Women's Health Across the Nation (SWAN). Am J Med 2006;119(9 Suppl 1):S103–10.
16. Rebbeck TR, Su HI, Sammel MD, et al. Effect of hormone metabolism genotypes on steroid hormone levels and menopausal symptoms in a prospective population-based cohort of women experiencing the menopausal transition. Menopause 2010; 17:1026–34.
17. Schilling C, Gallicchio L, Miller SR, et al. Genetic polymorphisms, hormone levels, and hot flashes in midlife women. Maturitas 2007;57:120–31.
18. Woods NF, Mitchell ES, Tao Y, et al. Polymorphisms in the estrogen synthesis and metabolism pathways and symptoms during the menopausal transition: observations from the Seattle Midlife Women's Health Study. Menopause 2006;13:902–10.
19. Visvanathan K, Gallicchio L, Schilling C, et al. Cytochrome gene polymorphisms, serum estrogens, and hot flushes in midlife women. Obstet Gynecol 2005;106: 1372–81.
20. Malacara JM, Perez-Luque EL, Martinez-Garza S, et al. The relationship of estrogen receptor-alpha polymorphism with symptoms and other characteristics in post-menopausal women. Maturitas 2004;49:163–9.
21. Green R, Polotsky AJ, Wildman RP, et al. Menopausal symptoms within a Hispanic cohort: SWAN, the Study of Women's Health Across the Nation. Climacteric 2010; 13:376–84.
22. Thurston RC, Bromberger JT, Joffe H, et al. Beyond frequency: who is most bothered by vasomotor symptoms? Menopause 2008;15:841–7.
23. Gold EB, Block G, Crawford S, et al. Lifestyle and demographic factors in relation to vasomotor symptoms: baseline results from the Study of Women's Health Across the Nation. Am J Epidemiol 2004;159:1189–99.
24. Nelson HD, Vesco KK, Haney E, et al. Nonhormonal therapies for menopausal hot flashes: systematic review and meta-analysis. JAMA 2006;295:2057–71.
25. Bolanos R, Del Castillo A, Francia J. Soy isoflavones versus placebo in the treatment of climacteric vasomotor symptoms: systematic review and meta-analysis. Menopause 2010;17:660–6.
26. Lethaby AE, Brown J, Marjoribanks J, et al. Phytoestrogens for vasomotor menopausal symptoms. Cochrane Database Syst Rev 2007;4:CD001395.
27. Crawford SL. The roles of biologic and nonbiologic factors in cultural differences in vasomotor symptoms measured by surveys. Menopause 2007;14:725–33.
28. Ryan K, Berkowitz R, Barbieri R, et al. Kistner's gynecology and women's health. 7th edition. St. Louis: Mosby, Inc; 1999.
29. Alexander C, Cochran CJ, Gallicchio L, et al. Serum leptin levels, hormone levels, and hot flashes in midlife women. Fertil Steril 2010;94:1037–43.
30. Whiteman MK, Staropoli CA, Langenberg PW, et al. Smoking, body mass, and hot flashes in midlife women. Obstet Gynecol 2003;101:264–72.
31. den Tonkelaar I, Seidell JC, van Noord PA. Obesity and fat distribution in relation to hot flashes in Dutch women from the DOM-project. Maturitas 1996;23:301–5.

32. Gold EB, Sternfeld B, Kelsey JL, et al. Relation of demographic and lifestyle factors to symptoms in a multi-racial/ethnic population of women 40–55 years of age. Am J Epidemiol 2000;152:463–73.

33. Hyde Riley E, Inui TS, Kleinman K, et al. Differential association of modifiable health behaviors with hot flashes in perimenopausal and postmenopausal women. J Gen Intern Med 2004;19:740–6.

34. Sabia S, Fournier A, Mesrine S, et al. Risk factors for onset of menopausal symptoms: results from a large cohort study. Maturitas 2008;60:108–21.

35. Thurston RC, Sowers MR, Chang Y, et al. Adiposity and reporting of vasomotor symptoms among midlife women: the study of women's health across the nation. Am J Epidemiol 2008;167:78–85.

36. Anderson GS. Human morphology and temperature regulation. Int J Biometeorol 1999;43:99–109.

37. Thurston RC, Sowers MR, Sutton-Tyrrell K, et al. Abdominal adiposity and hot flashes among midlife women. Menopause 2008;15:429–34.

38. Sternfeld B, Wang H, Quesenberry CP Jr, et al. Physical activity and changes in weight and waist circumference in midlife women: findings from the Study of Women's Health Across the Nation. Am J Epidemiol 2004;160:912–22.

39. Thurston RC, Sowers MR, Sternfeld B, et al. Gains in body fat and vasomotor symptom reporting over the menopausal transition: the study of women's health across the nation. Am J Epidemiol 2009;170:766–74.

40. Michnovicz JJ, Hershcopf RJ, Naganuma H, et al. Increased 2-hydroxylation of estradiol as a possible mechanism for the anti-estrogenic effect of cigarette smoking. N Engl J Med 1986;315:1305–9.

41. Greendale GA, Gold EB. Lifestyle factors: are they related to vasomotor symptoms and do they modify the effectiveness or side effects of hormone therapy? Am J Med 2005;118(Suppl 12B):148–54.

42. Freeman EW, Sammel MD, Lin H, et al. The role of anxiety and hormonal changes in menopausal hot flashes. Menopause 2005;12:258–66.

43. Pennebaker J. The psychology of physical symptoms. New York: Springer-Verlag; 1982.

44. Thurston R, Matthews K, Hernandez J, et al. Improving the performance of physiologic hot flash measures with support vector machines. Psychophysiology 2009;46:285–92.

45. Thurston RC, Blumenthal JA, Babyak MA, et al. Emotional antecedents of hot flashes during daily life. Psychosom Med 2005;67:137–46.

46. Thurston RC, Bromberger J, Chang Y, et al. Childhood abuse or neglect is associated with increased vasomotor symptom reporting among midlife women. Menopause 2008;15:16–22.

47. Adler NE, Boyce WT, Chesney MA, et al. Socioeconomic inequalities in health. No easy solution. JAMA 1993;269:3140–5.

48. Thurston RC, Kubzansky LD, Kawachi I, et al. Do depression and anxiety mediate the link between educational attainment and CHD? Psychosom Med 2006;68:25–32.

49. Williams DR, Collins C. US socioeconomic and racial differences in health: patterns and explanations. Annu Rev Sociol 1995;21:349–86.

50. Link BG, Phelan J. Social conditions as fundamental causes of disease. J Health Soc Behav 1995;Spec No:80–94.

51. Avis NE, Colvin A, Bromberger JT, et al. Change in health-related quality of life over the menopausal transition in a multiethnic cohort of middle-aged women: Study of Women's Health Across the Nation. Menopause 2009;16:860–9.

52. Avis NE, Ory M, Matthews KA, et al. Health-related quality of life in a multiethnic sample of middle-aged women: Study of Women's Health Across the Nation (SWAN). Med Care 2003;41:1262–76.

53. Kravitz HM, Ganz PA, Bromberger J, et al. Sleep difficulty in women at midlife: a community survey of sleep and the menopausal transition. Menopause 2003;10: 19–28.

54. Kravitz HM, Zhao X, Bromberger JT, et al. Sleep disturbance during the menopausal transition in a multi-ethnic community sample of women. Sleep 2008;31:979–90.

55. Kravitz HM, Janssen I, Santoro N, et al. Relationship of day-to-day reproductive hormone levels to sleep in midlife women. Arch Intern Med 2005;165:2370–6.

56. Bromberger JT, Assmann SF, Avis NE, et al. Persistent mood symptoms in a multiethnic community cohort of pre- and perimenopausal women. Am J Epidemiol 2003;158:347–56.

57. Bromberger JT, Harlow S, Avis N, et al. Racial/ethnic differences in the prevalence of depressive symptoms among middle-aged women: The Study of Women's Health Across the Nation (SWAN). Am J Public Health 2004;94:1378–85.

58. Bromberger JT, Matthews KA, Schott LL, et al. Depressive symptoms during the menopausal transition: The Study of Women's Health Across the Nation (SWAN). J Affect Disord 2007;103:267–72.

59. Bromberger JT, Kravitz HM, Matthews K, et al. Predictors of first lifetime episodes of major depression in midlife women. Psychol Med 2009;39:55–64.

60. Cohen LS, Soares CN, Vitonis AF, et al. Risk for new onset of depression during the menopausal transition: the Harvard study of moods and cycles. Arch General Psychiatry 2006;63:385–90.

61. Freeman EW, Sammel MD, Lin H, et al. Associations of hormones and menopausal status with depressed mood in women with no history of depression. Arch Gen Psychiatry 2006;63:375–82.

62. Bromberger JT, Meyer PM, Kravitz HM, et al. Psychologic distress and natural menopause: a multiethnic community study. Am J Public Health 2001;91:1435–42.

63. Bromberger JT, Schott LL, Kravitz HM, et al. Longitudinal change in reproductive hormones and depressive symptoms across the menopausal transition: results from the Study of Women's Health Across the Nation (SWAN). Arch Gen Psychiatry 2010;67:598–607.

64. Joffe H, Hall JE, Soares CN, et al. Vasomotor symptoms are associated with depression in perimenopausal women seeking primary care. Menopause 2002; 9:392–8.

65. Freeman EW, Sammel MD, Lin H. Temporal associations of hot flashes and depression in the transition to menopause. Menopause 2009;16:728–34.

66. Deecher DC, Dorries K. Understanding the pathophysiology of vasomotor symptoms (hot flushes and night sweats) that occur in perimenopause, menopause, and post-menopause life stages. Arch Women's Mental Health 2007;10:247–57.

67. Greendale GA, Huang MH, Wight RG, et al. Effects of the menopause transition and hormone use on cognitive performance in midlife women. Neurology 2009;72:1850–7.

68. Greendale GA, Wight RG, Huang MH, et al. Menopause-associated symptoms and cognitive performance: results from the study of women's health across the nation. Am J Epidemiol 2010;171:1214–24.

69. LeBlanc ES, Neiss MB, Carello PE, et al. Hot flashes and estrogen therapy do not influence cognition in early menopausal women. Menopause 2007;14:191–202.

70. Joffe H, Hall JE, Gruber S, et al. Estrogen therapy selectively enhances prefrontal cognitive processes: a randomized, double-blind, placebo-controlled study with functional magnetic resonance imaging in perimenopausal and recently postmenopausal women. Menopause 2006;13:411–22.

71. Maki PM, Drogos LL, Rubin LH, et al. Objective hot flashes are negatively related to verbal memory performance in midlife women. Menopause 2008;15:848–56.
72. Rossouw JE, Prentice RL, Manson JE, et al. Postmenopausal hormone therapy and risk of cardiovascular disease by age and years since menopause. JAMA 2007;297: 1465–77.
73. Huang AJ, Sawaya GF, Vittinghoff E, et al. Hot flushes, coronary heart disease, and hormone therapy in postmenopausal women. Menopause 2009;16:639–43.
74. Yeboah J, Crouse JR, Hsu FC, et al. Brachial flow-mediated dilation predicts incident cardiovascular events in older adults: the Cardiovascular Health Study. Circulation 2007;115:2390–7.
75. Iribarren C, Sidney S, Sternfeld B, et al. Calcification of the aortic arch: risk factors and association with coronary heart disease, stroke, and peripheral vascular disease. JAMA 2000;283:2810–5.
76. Rumberger JA, Brundage BH, Rader DJ, et al. Electron beam computed tomographic coronary calcium scanning: a review and guidelines for use in asymptomatic persons. Mayo Clin Proc 1999;74:243–52.
77. Thurston RC, Sutton-Tyrrell K, Everson-Rose S, et al. Hot flashes and carotid intima media thickness among midlife women. Menopause 2011;18(4):352–8.
78. Thurston RC, Sutton-Tyrrell K, Everson-Rose SA, et al. Hot flashes and subclinical cardiovascular disease: Findings from the Study of Women's Health Across the Nation Heart Study. Circulation 2008;118:1234–40.
79. Crandall CJ, Zheng Y, Crawford SL, et al. Presence of vasomotor symptoms is associated with lower bone mineral density: a longitudinal analysis. Menopause 2009;16:239–46.
80. Crandall CJ, Tseng CH, Crawford SL, et al. Association of menopausal vasomotor symptoms with increased bone turnover during the menopausal transition. J Bone Miner Res 2011;26:840–9.

Bone and the Perimenopause

Joan C. Lo, MD[a,b,*], Sherri-Ann M. Burnett-Bowie, MD, MPH[c,d], Joel S. Finkelstein, MD[c,d]

KEYWORDS

- Osteoporosis • Perimenopause • Menopause • Bone
- Fractures

The loss of ovarian function during the menopausal transition has a profound impact on female skeletal health. Currently, it is estimated that 1 in every 2 Caucasian women will experience an osteoporotic fracture during her lifetime,[1] contributing to considerable morbidity and an enormous economic burden within the aging female population. However, most studies have been conducted in postmenopausal women, with fewer investigations focusing specifically on perimenopausal bone health. The Study of Women's Health Across the Nation (SWAN) is the largest prospective cohort to date where changes in bone mineral density (BMD) and bone turnover have been examined in relation to ovarian aging among women followed across the menopausal transition.[2,3] As defined by bleeding pattern in SWAN, early perimenopause is characterized by increasing menstrual irregularity but less than 3 months of amenorrhea, late perimenopause by amenorrhea lasting greater than 3 months but less than 1 year, and postmenopause by the absence of menstrual bleeding for 12 consecutive months or more.[3,4] A recent, multistudy collaboration has further recommended that the early menopause transition be defined by a persistent, 7-day or greater difference in consecutive cycle lengths and the late menopause transition by at least 60 days of amenorrhea.[5,6] A serum follicle-stimulating hormone (FSH) level of 40 IU/L or greater has also been found to be an independent marker of the transition that may facilitate predicting the time to the final menstrual period.[6,7]

Conducted in a large multiethnic population of more than 2000 women across 5 clinical centers in the United States, the SWAN bone study has contributed greatly to

Disclosures: Drs Lo and Burnett-Bowie have received research funding from Amgen, Inc.
a Division of Research, Kaiser Permanente Northern California, 2000 Broadway, Oakland, CA 94612, USA
b Department of Medicine, University of California San Francisco, San Francisco, CA, USA
c Department of Medicine, Endocrine Unit, Thier 1051, Harvard Medical School, 50 Blossom Street, Boston, MA 02114, USA
d Massachusetts General Hospital, Boston, MA 02114, USA
* Corresponding author. Division of Research, Kaiser Permanente Northern California, 2000 Broadway, Oakland, CA 94612.
E-mail address: Joan.C.Lo@kp.org

our understanding of both early and late changes in bone metabolism during perimenopause, associated clinical and race/ethnic differences, and the implication of these findings for optimization of postmenopausal bone health. This review focuses on bone loss during the menopausal transition, changes surrounding the final menstrual period, and the role of endogenous hormones and ethnic variation in predicting BMD and bone loss. Specific findings from SWAN and other studies, data on perimenopausal fractures, fracture risk, and implications for clinical management are also discussed.

BONE LOSS DURING THE MENOPAUSAL TRANSITION
Changes in BMD

Although there is a large body of literature examining BMD among postmenopausal women, and a moderate body of literature examining BMD among premenopausal women, fewer studies have monitored BMD serially in a cohort of women who were initially premenopausal and continued monitoring BMD until women experienced their final menstrual period.[8–11] Some of these earlier studies reported that BMD remained stable in premenopausal women, whereas others found that BMD begins to decline well before the final menstrual period.[3,12–17] However, many of the early studies lacked clear definitions of menopausal status, and prior studies often examined BMD as a function of chronologic age instead of menopause stage or time from the final menstrual period. SWAN investigators examined changes in BMD of the lumbar spine and total hip across 6 annual visits in nearly 2000 participants with carefully characterized perimenopausal stage.[3] There was little change in BMD during the premenopausal or early perimenopausal period. Bone loss accelerated dramatically during late perimenopause and continued through the early postmenopause.[3] This acceleration in bone loss during the late perimenopause (**Fig. 1**) was characterized by a 1.8% to 2.3% annual rate of bone loss in the lumbar spine and 1.0% to 1.4% in the hip.[3] Body weight was found to be an important predictor of the rate of bone loss, independent of differences in race/ethnicity. Compared with women in the highest tertile of body weight, rate of bone loss was 35% to 55% greater among women in the lowest tertile of body weight.[3]

Similar rates of accelerated bone loss have also been reported in the Melbourne Women's Midlife Health Project where an average annual rate of BMD decline of 2.5%

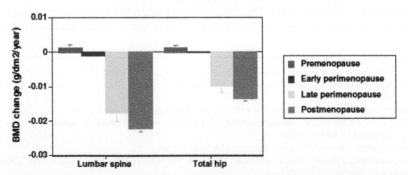

Fig. 1. Annual adjusted rates of change in BMD of the lumbar spine and total hip during the menopausal transition among 1902 SWAN participants. Error bars represent 95% confidence limits. (From Finkelstein JS, Brockwell SE, Mehta V, et al. Bone mineral density changes during the menopausal transition in a multiethnic cohort of women. J Clin Endocrinol Metab 2008;93:861–8; with permission.)

in the lumbar spine and 1.7% in the femoral neck occurred in the time surrounding the final menstrual period.[18] These findings are comparable to early data obtained in perimenopausal women residing in France, where the average annual decline in vertebral BMD was in the range of 2.35%.[19] The association of higher body mass or body mass index with slower rates of bone loss at various skeletal sites (including the forearm, hip and spine) has also been described in several studies, consistent with the known protective effect of body size and adiposity on bone loss and fracture risk.[11,17,18,20]

The Role of Endogenous Hormones

Bone loss in postmenopausal women has historically been attributed to estrogen deficiency. A detailed review of changes in ovarian and pituitary hormones during the menopausal transition is described elsewhere in this issue of *Obstetrics and Gynecology Clinics of North America* (Reproductive Hormones and Menopause). There are numerous studies in older postmenopausal women demonstrating a significant association between circulating estrogen levels, BMD and fracture risk.[21,22] However, in premenopausal and perimenopausal women, it is difficult to extrapolate a single estradiol level, even when obtained during a well-defined portion of the menstrual cycle, to an entire menstrual cycle or series of menstrual cycles. This is because estradiol levels change from day to day and vary over a range of more than 10-fold across the course of a normal menstrual cycle.[23] There is also evidence that fluctuations in estradiol may be more pronounced in the perimenopause, at least in its earlier stages.[24] Thus, in contrast with the postmenopause when estradiol levels are quite stable, perimenopausal estradiol levels might not be expected to correlate well with BMD and bone loss during the perimenopause, more because of the difficulty in assessing estrogen status rather than a lack of a true relationship. Moreover, the effect of fluctuating estradiol on BMD and bone loss is not well understood. It is possible that the periods of normal-to-high estradiol followed by periods of low estradiol that are characteristic of the perimenopause may relate differently to bone than the more stable and consistent levels seen in midreproductive-aged women.

Perimenopause is characterized by an increase in bone resorption and reduction in BMD.[25] These findings are accompanied by higher serum FSH levels, although estrogen levels may remain within the premenopausal range during the early transition.[25] In premenopausal and early perimenopausal Australian women examined across the menopausal transition, the estradiol level measured at the final time point was significantly associated with perimenopausal bone loss.[26] In a separate examination of Swedish women undergoing prospective measurement of distal radius BMD at menopause, postmenopausal serum estradiol level was also found to correlate with changes in BMD.[27]

In SWAN, significant cross-sectional associations were observed between baseline serum FSH levels and BMD, but not between baseline serum estradiol levels and BMD, in premenopausal and early perimenopausal women.[28] Baseline FSH levels and changes in FSH levels were associated with longitudinal changes during the menopausal transition,[29] whereas annual measures of serum estradiol did not predict bone loss. Estradiol concentrations below 35 pg/mL were associated with lower BMD levels during the transition, however.[29] Examination of BMD change in the context of FSH staging in the Michigan Bone Health and Metabolism Study (**Fig. 2**) showed that bone loss in the lumbar spine and femoral neck became evident when FSH increased into the range of 34 to 56 IU/L, which occurred approximately 2 years before the final menstrual period.[17] The annualized rate of bone loss in the lumbar spine increased from 1.7% in perimenopausal women with FSH levels of 34 to 56 IU/L to 3.3% during

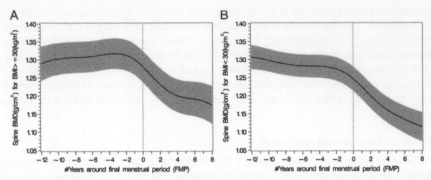

Fig. 2. The pattern of population mean lumbar spine and femoral neck BMD values in relation to the final menstrual period with 95% upper and lower confidence intervals (black solid line with shaded areas). The Michigan Bone Health and Metabolism Study. (From Sowers MR, Zheng H, Jannausch ML, et al. Amount of bone loss in relation to time around the final menstrual period and follicle-stimulating hormone staging of the transmenopause. J Clin Endocrinol Metab 2010;95:2155–62; with permission.)

the 2 years after the final menstrual period and then declined to 1.1% per year in subsequent postmenopausal years.[17]

There has also been increasing awareness of other potential hormones that may contribute to bone loss during ovarian aging.[30] For example, it has been reported that mice with null mutations in the FSH receptor gene do not manifest bone loss, despite atrophic ovaries and uterus and disordered estrous cycles, suggesting that FSH is required for bone loss to occur in states of estrogen deficiency.[31,32] However, because mice with null mutations in the FSH receptor gene have elevated testosterone levels,[33] the lack of bone loss may be due to direct effects of testosterone on bone. Other gonadal peptides, such as inhibin A, inhibin B, and activin, have also been purported to contribute to changes in BMD with ovarian aging. Both inhibin A and inhibin B suppress osteoblast and osteoclast development and they oppose the stimulatory effects of activin and bone morphogenetic proteins on bone formation.[34] Whether any of these compounds truly contributes to the regulation of bone homeostasis during the perimenopause is currently unclear. Progesterone has also been implicated in the regulation of bone mass. The decline in progesterone concentrations associated with anovulation or luteal phase deficiency[35] and the reduction in inhibin secretion evident during the perimenopause may represent an additional mechanism for bone loss independent of circulating estrogen.[30,34,36] In a subset of premenopausal and early perimenopausal SWAN women in whom urinary excretion of estrogen and progesterone metabolites was assessed daily for 1 menstrual cycle each year, no association between measures of luteal function and BMD was observed[37]; however, larger studies are needed to examine the specific impact of changes in ovulatory function on BMD in midlife women. Finally, new data have led some experts to hypothesize that other, intrinsic, age-related factors may be important in the pathogenesis of postmenopausal osteoporosis, particularly with regard to loss of trabecular bone.[30]

Changes in Bone Turnover

Bone turnover markers have been used for many years in the research setting to monitor the response to specific osteoporosis therapies.[38] Peptides made by osteoblasts, including bone-specific alkaline phosphatase, osteocalcin, and procol-lagen type I N-propeptide are often used to assess bone formation, whereas products of type I collagen degradation, including the cross-linked N-terminal and C-terminal telopeptides of type I collagen [N-telopeptide (NTX) or serum C-telopeptide] are often used to assess bone matrix degradation. In cross-sectional analyses, bone resorption markers are consistently higher in untreated postmenopausal osteoporotic women than in premenopausal women, whereas bone formation markers are more vari-able.[39–42] Higher levels of bone turnover markers have been shown in many, but not all studies,[40,43–45] to predict subsequent bone loss[40,46,47] or fracture risk[40,41,44,48] (independent of BMD changes) in postmenopausal women not receiving anti-osteoporosis treatment.

There remain, however, many gaps in knowledge that hinder the utilization of bone turnover markers in clinical practice. Few studies have measured bone turnover markers in perimenopausal women or in a racially diverse cohort of women. In a cross-sectional analysis, urinary NTX and osteocalcin were measured in 2375 SWAN participants who were either premenopausal or early perimenopausal.[49] Mean NTX and osteocalcin levels were slightly higher in the perimenopausal women compared with the premenopausal women; however, these differences were not significant. Another cross-sectional analysis of 2313 premenopausal or early perimenopausal SWAN subjects demonstrated ethnic/racial differences in osteocalcin and urinary NTX levels wherein Caucasian subjects had the highest levels of both markers, even after adjusting for anthropometric and lifestyle differences.[50] The increased bone turnover observed in Caucasian subjects may explain the lower BMD, as discussed later in this chapter, seen in these subjects as compared with women from other racial groups. Additionally, only a few studies have assessed longitudinal changes in bone turnover markers during the menopause and the published reports have been limited by small cohort size. In a 3-year study of 15 premenopausal women where 6 women became postmenopausal, bone resorption markers were unchanged before the final menses but started to increase 6 months after the final menstrual period.[51] The mean within-subject increase in bone resorption markers was 30% to 50%.[51] In an 8-year study of 104 premenopausal women, 34 women became menopausal over the observation period with significant within-individual increases in bone resorption markers.[52] Longitudinal changes in bone resorption markers in the SWAN study are currently being analyzed; given SWAN's cohort size and racial diversity, these data will add substantively to our knowledge of the effect of the menopause on bone turnover markers. Because of substantial within-individual variability of these mark-ers, lack of uniform reference standards, and challenges with interpretation, the use of bone turnover markers has been limited primarily to the research domain. However, with increasing knowledge of the hormonal and physiologic factors that affect bone turnover markers, a stronger clinical role for bone turnover measurements may become evident in the future.[38,40]

Race/Ethnic Differences

It is well known that BMD and osteoporotic fracture risk vary by race/ethnicity, with unadjusted BMD values typically lowest in Asian women, intermediate in Caucasian women, and highest in African-American women. Fracture rates follow a different pattern, however, with the highest rates in Caucasians, intermediate rates in Asians, and the lowest rates in African Americans. Some of the observed differences in BMD among race/ethnic groups could be because of differences in bone size (one of the limitations of dual energy x-ray absorptiometry, which measures areal and not 3-dimensional BMD). However, race/ethnic differences have similarly been reported in population studies utilizing quantitative computed tomography, which measures volumetric BMD[53] and adjusting BMD values in SWAN for bone size did not eliminate race/ethnic differences in BMD.[54]

The specific sampling structure of the SWAN Bone Study across 5 clinical centers, each with approximately half the participants selected based on being of non-Hispanic Caucasian race and the remaining based on African-American, Chinese, and Japanese race with annual BMD measurements during follow-up provides one of the few population-based studies able to examine race/ethnic differences in BMD and bone loss across the menopausal transition.[2] At the baseline evaluation, the racial variation in BMD (highest in African Americans followed by Caucasians and lowest in Chinese and Japanese women) was found to be largely due to differences in body weight.[54] After adjustment for weight and other confounders, there were minimal differences in lumbar spine BMD among African-American, Chinese, or Japanese women, all of whom had higher adjusted BMD compared with Caucasian women.[54] Unadjusted femoral neck BMD was highest in African Americans, intermediate in Caucasians, and lowest in Japanese and Chinese women with mean differences of 14% to 24% between African Americans and the other groups. After careful weight matching, the difference in femoral neck BMD between African Americans and the other groups was reduced to approximately 8% and the difference between Asians and Caucasians was eliminated. It is only because SWAN has large numbers of women from each of these racial/ethnic groups that weight matching and adjustment was possible, thus allowing new insights into racial/ethnic differences in BMD. Across the menopausal transition, rates of bone loss were greatest among Chinese and Japanese women, intermediate among Caucasian women, and lowest among African-American women; however, like the baseline differences in BMD, these variations were also largely accounted for by differences in body weight rather than race/ethnicity per se.[3] Taken together, SWAN has helped to reinforce the finding that Caucasian race is a risk factor for bone loss, and that adjusting for body weight is critical in the determination of peak bone mass as well as a woman's risk of bone loss during the menopausal transition.

PERIMENOPAUSAL FRACTURE RISK

Population-based studies, conducted mainly in Caucasian women, have contributed substantially to our understanding of fracture patterns across the aging lifespan. Among 10,902 middle-aged Swedish women followed for up to 11 years, the largest proportion of low-energy fractures occurred in the forearm (37%) followed by the ankle (12%), spine and proximal humerus (9% each), hands or feet (8%), and hip (8%).[55] Overall, the incidence of fracture was quite low, estimated at 5.5 per 1000 person-years for forearm fractures and approximately 3 per 1000 person-years for the proximal humerus.[55] Risk factors for incident fracture included older age, prior fracture, diabetes mellitus, and poor health status; greater body mass index was associated with an increased risk of proximal humerus and ankle fractures but lower risk of forearm fractures.[55] Among 3068 perimenopausal women aged 47 to 53 years residing in Finland, 8.5% sustained a fracture during a mean follow-up period of 3.6 years, with most fractures again occurring in the extremities (26% wrist, 16% ankle, 19% hands or feet, and 15% rib).[56] The presence of low BMD, prior fracture history, nonuse of hormone replacement therapy, and 3 or more chronic illnesses and smoking were found to be independent risk factors for perimenopausal fracture.[56] In a similarly aged cohort of 1857 women undergoing BMD screening in Scotland, the 2-year incidence of self-reported fracture was 2.4%; risk factors associated with an increased fracture risk included low spine BMD, prior fracture history, family history of hip fracture, and postmenopausal status.[57] Among 2171 women enrolled in SWAN and followed for up to 8 years, 245 reported an incident fracture.[58] The subset of women with diabetes (5%) underwent an earlier menopause transition and experienced a 2-fold increased risk of incident fracture compared with women without diabetes.[58] Fracture risk is also influenced by other predisposing conditions, including genetic factors, relevant comorbidities and exposures (eg, rheumatoid arthritis, malabsorptive syndromes, systemic glucocorticoids, aromatase inhibitors), differences in structural bone geometry, and risk of falls.[1]

CLINICAL MANAGEMENT CONSIDERATIONS
Diet and Lifestyle Factors

The dietary and lifestyle recommendations for optimal bone health and fracture prevention during the perimenopause are the same as those recommended for postmenopausal women. These include a well-balanced diet, regular exercise, smoking cessation, avoidance of excessive alcohol consumption, and fall prevention measures.[1,59] Attention should also be given to changes in weight, particularly in light of the known association of weight loss with increasing rates of bone loss and subsequent fracture risk.[60]

Calcium and Vitamin D

Maintenance of adequate calcium and vitamin D intake remain an important component of preventive bone health. Several studies have shown that calcium and vitamin D supplementation improves BMD and reduces fracture risk in late postmenopausal women.[61-65] The Women's Health Initiative trial found that calcium (500 mg twice daily) and vitamin D (400 IU/d) supplementation in healthy postmenopausal women increased hip BMD modestly, but did not reduce hip fracture risk significantly in the cohort as a whole, although fracture risk was reduced significantly in women who adhered to study treatment.[66] However, it should be noted that women in the Women's Health Initiative trial received a relatively low dose of vitamin D (400 IU) and more than half were concurrently receiving hormone replacement therapy.[67] In early postmenopausal women (within the first 5 years of their final menstrual period), calcium administration slows bone loss from sites composed largely of cortical bone, but has little effect on skeletal sites composed largely of trabecular bone.[67-70] The relationship between calcium supplementation and fracture risk in perimenopausal or early postmenopausal women is less clear.[67,70]

Even though the beneficial effects of calcium administration in perimenopausal women are not well established, most experts recommend that perimenopausal women should be counseled regarding optimal calcium intake. Currently, both the National Academy of Sciences and the National Osteoporosis Foundation recommend a total daily intake of 1200 mg elemental calcium (combining dietary and supplement sources) for women over age 50.[1,59,71] Dietary calcium sources are preferred owing to greater calcium absorption and possibly because of a lower risk of vascular disease, particularly in light of a recent meta-analysis that reported that calcium supplementation increases the risk of cardiovascular events.[72,73] Calcium supplements, when taken, should be in conjunction with meals to maximize gastrointestinal absorption. Select populations at higher risk for reduced dietary calcium intake include older individuals and those with lactose intolerance, vegetarian diet, or poor eating habits.[59,74] A list of calcium-rich foods can be found through the Office for Dietary Supplements, National Institutes of Health (available at: http://ods.od.nih.gov/factsheets/calcium/).

Vitamin D may reduce fracture risk through a number of mechanisms. Correcting vitamin D deficiency can improve calcium absorption and thereby treat secondary hyperparathyroidism and osteomalacia.[75,76] Additionally, correcting vitamin D deficiency can decrease fracture risk by improving muscle strength and reducing the risk of falls.[77] There is ongoing debate as to the minimum 25-hydroxyvitamin D level required for skeletal benefits. A meta-analysis of 7 clinical trials with 9820 subjects suggested that a daily dose of vitamin D 700 to 800 IU is required to achieve a 25-hydroxyvitamin D level of 40 ng/mL, which is associated with 26% and 23% reduction in hip and nonvertebral fracture risk, respectively.[62] However, the findings of this meta-analysis are discordant with the 2010 National Academy of Sciences recommendations that women younger and older than 50 years should consume 600 and 800 IU of vitamin D daily, respectively, and that the minimum desired 25-hydroxyvitamin D level for skeletal benefits is 20 ng/mL.[71] Even with the ongoing debate, certain populations are at increased risk for vitamin D deficiency and may require higher doses of vitamin D (1000–2000 IU/d or pharmacologic therapy). Serum 25-hydroxyvitamin D levels reflect the dietary intake of vitamin D and the synthesis of vitamin D in response to ultraviolet B exposure of the skin.[78,79] Thus, women with pigmented skin or limited sun exposure owing to use of sunscreen or occlusive clothing are at particular risk for vitamin D deficiency.[80] Dietary sources of vitamin D can be found through the Office for Dietary Supplements, National Institutes of Health (available at: http://ods.od.nih.gov/factsheets/vitaminD/).

BMD Screening in Perimenopausal Women

Dual energy x-ray absorptiometry is the most widely available and validated modality for measurement of BMD and continues to be the preferred method for assessing osteoporosis.[81] The National Osteoporosis Foundation recommends BMD testing for women in the menopausal transition if there is a specific risk factor associated with increased fracture risk (eg, prior fragility fracture or high-risk medication), but recognizes that BMD assessment may not be indicated if the results will not influence treatment decisions.[1] When BMD measurements are performed, The World Health Organization (WHO) criteria for osteoporosis apply to postmenopausal women, using the reference range for young adult Caucasian women for calculation of BMD T score.[81,82] The North American Menopause Society advises that the WHO criteria can be used for classification of perimenopausal women, but that care should be taken to interpret BMD results appropriately in this setting.[59] For premenopausal women, the International Society for Clinical Densitometry advises that race-adjusted Z score (instead of T score) be used, with a Z-score of −2.0 or lower defined as "below the expected range for age" and a Z-score above −2.0 defined as "above the expected range for age" for women before the menopause.[82]

There are currently no recommendations for osteoporosis screening in healthy perimenopausal women. The 2011 US Preventive Task Force recommends screening for osteoporosis in postmenopausal women below age 65 years if their fracture risk is equivalent to that of a 65-year-old white woman with no other risk factors.[83] This screening threshold translates to a 9.3% 10-year risk of major osteoporotic fractures calculated using the web-based WHO Fracture Risk Assessment Tool FRAX (available at: www.shef.ac.uk/frax). Using these recommendations, the majority of healthy perimenopausal women would likely not be recommended for BMD screening. Alternatively, women with low body weight comprise a higher risk subgroup where BMD testing during late perimenopause has been suggested.[3,84] As yet, there are no controlled studies examining the benefit of early detection and intervention for low BMD,[83] with the exception of specific premenopausal patient subsets (eg, breast cancer, chronic glucocorticoid therapy).

Fracture Risk Assessment

Few studies have examined the application of FRAX in perimenopausal and early postmenopausal women, most of whom have a relatively low fracture risk.[85] For the US population, early revisions to FRAX were made in 2009 based on updated US fracture incidence rates, resulting in lower rates of major osteoporotic fracture, particularly at the younger ages.[86] Other risk factors considered in FRAX include age, gender, race/ethnicity, parental history of hip fracture, other clinical risk factors, and femoral neck BMD. A recent study conducted in France, using data from 2651 perimenopausal and early postmenopausal women with dual energy x-ray absorptiometry measurements and an average follow-up of 13 years, suggested that FRAX may not improve the discriminatory value of hip BMD alone for fracture risk prediction.[87] At an individual level, FRAX is a useful clinical risk assessment tool that may also aid in patient counseling. For the US population, the National Osteoporosis Foundation has recommended cost-effective osteoporosis treatment thresholds of 3% for 10-year risk of hip fracture or 20% for 10-year risk of major osteoporotic fracture using the WHO FRAX model in women with osteopenia.[88]

Treatment Considerations

There are currently no established guidelines pertaining to the treatment and prevention of osteoporosis in perimenopausal women. For perimenopausal women who have a high fracture risk or for those in whom osteoporosis treatment is indicated, the selection of therapy should be considered individually. A detailed discussion of available osteoporosis therapies and their risks and benefits is beyond the scope of this article. Briefly, bisphosphonate drugs are considered first-line drugs for the treatment of postmenopausal osteoporosis, with evidence for reduction in risk of hip, vertebral, and nonvertebral fractures.[59] However, because the optimal duration of bisphosphonate treatment remains unknown, practitioners may weigh consideration of other antiresorptive therapies for postmenopausal women with osteoporosis who are relatively young, depending on osteoporosis disease severity. Use of antiresorptive agents in perimenopausal women carries a potential hazard of prenatal exposure. Although fertility is rare and rarely desired in this age group, noncontracepting, sexually active perimenopausal women require specific counseling before taking bisphosphonates. Raloxifene, a selective estrogen receptor modulator shown to prevent bone loss and reduce vertebral fracture risk in elderly postmenopausal women, may be an option for younger postmenopausal women with osteoporosis, although its efficacy in preventing nonvertebral and hip fractures is uncertain.[59] Because raloxifene administration may reduce BMD in premenopausal women,[89] it should not be used for the prevention of bone loss in perimenopausal women. For perimenopausal women with menopausal symptoms, treatment with estrogen plus progestin (or estrogen alone if the woman has had a hysterectomy) can be considered, although when hormone replacement therapy is assessed solely for osteoporosis indications, the risks and benefits should be weighed in conjunction with other non–estrogen-based therapies.[1,59] There are currently no recommendations with regard to estrogen therapy for prevention of postmenopausal bone loss. Once estrogen is discontinued, there does not seem to be a persisting benefit on BMD, bone loss, or fracture risk.[90–92]

In conclusion, the findings from prospective examination of BMD change across the menopausal transition demonstrate an early and accelerated rate of bone loss, particularly in the lumbar spine. Bone loss begins to accelerate 1 to 2 years before the menopause, concurrent with the prolonged amenorrhea that characterizes the late menopausal transition.[3,17] Importantly, these rates of bone loss are also influenced by body size, with greater bone loss among nonobese women and those with lower body mass, independent of race/ethnicity.[3,17] The greatest reduction in BMD occurs in the year before the final menstrual period and the first 2 years after the final menstrual period, with lower rates of loss during the ensuing 1 to 7 years.[17] Clinical management considerations during the perimenopause include maintenance of adequate dietary calcium and vitamin D intake, attention to modifiable risk factors and consideration of osteoporosis screening in high risk populations with assessment of fracture risk. The indications, benefits, and risks of pharmacologic osteoporosis therapy should be individually assessed as there are currently no established guidelines addressing the treatment and prevention of osteoporosis in perimenopausal women.

ACKNOWLEDGMENTS

The contents of this publication are solely the responsibility of the authors and do not represent the official views of the National Institutes of Health, Kaiser Permanente, the University of California, or Massachusetts General Hospital.

REFERENCES

1. Clinician's Guide to Prevention and Treatment of Osteoporosis. Washington, DC: National Osteoporosis Foundation; 2010. p. 1–36.
2. Neer RM. Bone loss across the menopausal transition. Ann N Y Acad Sci 2010;1192: 66–71.
3. Finkelstein JS, Brockwell SE, Mehta V, et al. Bone mineral density changes during the menopause transition in a multiethnic cohort of women. J Clin Endocrinol Metab 2008;93:861–8.
4. Lasley BL, Santoro N, Randolf JF, et al. The relationship of circulating dehydroepi-androsterone, testosterone, and estradiol to stages of the menopausal transition and ethnicity. J Clin Endocrinol Metab 2002;87:3760–7.
5. Harlow SD, Crawford S, Dennerstein L, et al. Recommendations from a multi-study evaluation of proposed criteria for staging reproductive aging. Climacteric 2007;10: 112–9.
6. Ferrell RJ, Sowers M. Longitudinal, epidemiologic studies of female reproductive aging. Ann N Y Acad Sci 2010;1204:188–97.
7. Randolph JF Jr, Crawford S, Dennerstein L, et al. The value of follicle-stimulating hormone concentration and clinical findings as markers of the late menopausal transition. J Clin Endocrinol Metab 2006;91:3034–40.
8. Ahlborg HG, Johnell O, Nilsson BE, et al. Bone loss in relation to menopause: a prospective study during 16 years. Bone 2001;28:327–31.
9. Falch JA, Sandvik L. Perimenopausal appendicular bone loss: a 10-year prospective study. Bone 1990;11:425–8.
10. Ravn P, Hetland ML, Overgaard K, et al. Premenopausal and postmenopausal changes in bone mineral density of the proximal femur measured by dual-energy X-ray absorptiometry. J Bone Miner Res 1994;9:1975–80.
11. Reeve J, Walton J, Russell LJ, et al. Determinants of the first decade of bone loss after menopause at spine, hip and radius. QJM 1999;92:261–73.
12. Bainbridge KE, Sowers MF, Crutchfield M, et al. Natural history of bone loss over 6 years among premenopausal and early postmenopausal women. Am J Epidemiol 2002;156:410–7.
13. Recker R, Lappe J, Davies K, et al. Characterization of perimenopausal bone loss: a prospective study. J Bone Miner Res 2000;15:1965–73.

14. Recker RR, Lappe JM, Davies KM, et al. Change in bone mass immediately before menopause. J Bone Miner Res 1992;7:857–62.
15. Sowers M, Crutchfield M, Bandekar R, et al. Bone mineral density and its change in pre-and perimenopausal white women: the Michigan Bone Health Study. J Bone Miner Res 1998;13:1134–40.
16. Slemenda C, Hui SL, Longcope C, et al. Sex steroids and bone mass. A study of changes about the time of menopause. J Clin Invest 1987;80:1261–9.
17. Sowers MR, Zheng H, Jannausch ML, et al. Amount of bone loss in relation to time around the final menstrual period and follicle-stimulating hormone staging of the transmenopause. J Clin Endocrinol Metab 2010;95:2155–62.
18. Guthrie JR, Ebeling PR, Hopper JL, et al. A prospective study of bone loss in menopausal Australian-born women. Osteoporos Int 1998;8:282–90.
19. Pouilles JM, Tremollieres F, Ribot C. The effects of menopause on longitudinal bone loss from the spine. Calcif Tissue Int 1993;52:340–3.
20. Rannevik G, Jeppsson S, Johnell O, et al. A longitudinal study of the perimenopausal transition: altered profiles of steroid and pituitary hormones, SHBG and bone mineral density. Maturitas 1995;21:103–13.
21. Cummings SR, Browner WS, Bauer D, et al. Endogenous hormones and the risk of hip and vertebral fractures among older women. Study of Osteoporotic Fractures Research Group. N Engl J Med 1998;339:733–8.
22. Greendale GA, Edelstein S, Barrett-Connor E. Endogenous sex steroids and bone mineral density in older women and men: the Rancho Bernardo Study. J Bone Miner Res 1997;12:1833–43.
23. Filicori M, Santoro N, Merriam GR, et al. Characterization of the physiological pattern of episodic gonadotropin secretion throughout the human menstrual cycle. J Clin Endocrinol Metab 1986;62:1136–44.
24. Santoro N, Brown JR, Adel T, et al. Characterization of reproductive hormonal dynamics in the perimenopause. J Clin Endocrinol Metab 1996;81:1495–501.
25. Ebeling PR, Atley LM, Guthrie JR, et al. Bone turnover markers and bone density across the menopausal transition. J Clin Endocrinol Metab 1996;81:3366–71.
26. Guthrie JR, Lehert P, Dennerstein L, et al. The relative effect of endogenous estradiol and androgens on menopausal bone loss: a longitudinal study. Osteoporos Int 2004;15:881–6.
27. Ahlborg HG, Johnell O, Turner CH, et al. Bone loss and bone size after menopause. N Engl J Med 2003;349:327–34.
28. Sowers MR, Finkelstein JS, Ettinger B, et al. The association of endogenous hormone concentrations and bone mineral density measures in pre- and perimenopausal women of four ethnic groups: SWAN. Osteoporos Int 2003;14:44–52.
29. Sowers MR, Jannausch M, McConnell D, et al. Hormone predictors of bone mineral density changes during the menopausal transition. J Clin Endocrinol Metab 2006;91: 1261–7.
30. Khosla S, Melton LJ 3rd, Riggs BL. The unitary model for estrogen deficiency and the pathogenesis of osteoporosis: is a revision needed? J Bone Miner Res 2011;26:441–51.
31. Iqbal J, Sun L, Kumar TR, et al. Follicle-stimulating hormone stimulates TNF production from immune cells to enhance osteoblast and osteoclast formation. Proc Natl Acad Sci U S A 2006;103:14925–30.
32. Sun L, Peng Y, Sharrow AC, et al. FSH directly regulates bone mass. Cell 2006;125: 247–60.

33. Abel MH, Huhtaniemi I, Pakarinen P, et al. Age-related uterine and ovarian hypertrophy in FSH receptor knockout and FSHbeta subunit knockout mice. Reproduction 2003;125:165–73.
34. Nicks KM, Fowler TW, Akel NS, et al. Bone turnover across the menopause transition: The role of gonadal inhibins. Ann N Y Acad Sci 2010;1192:153–60.
35. Santoro N, Crawford SL, Lasley WL, et al. Factors related to declining luteal function in women during the menopausal transition. J Clin Endocrinol Metab 2008;93:1711–21.
36. Seifert-Klauss V, Prior JC. Progesterone and bone: actions promoting bone health in women. J Osteoporos 2010;2010:845180.
37. Grewal J, Sowers MR, Randolph JF Jr, et al. Low bone mineral density in the early menopausal transition: role for ovulatory function. J Clin Endocrinol Metab 2006;91: 3780–5.
38. Vasikaran S, Eastell R, Bruyere O, et al. Markers of bone turnover for the prediction of fracture risk and monitoring of osteoporosis treatment: a need for international reference standards. Osteoporos Int 2011;22:391–420.
39. Akesson K, Ljunghall S, Jonsson B, et al. Assessment of biochemical markers of bone metabolism in relation to the occurrence of fracture: a retrospective and prospective population-based study of women. J Bone Miner Res 1995;10:1823–9.
40. Delmas PD, Eastell R, Garnero P, et al. The use of biochemical markers of bone turnover in osteoporosis. Committee of Scientific Advisors of the International Osteoporosis Foundation. Osteoporos Int 2000;11(Suppl 6):S2–17.
41. Garnero P, Hausherr E, Chapuy MC, et al. Markers of bone resorption predict hip fracture in elderly women: the EPIDOS Prospective Study. J Bone Miner Res 1996; 11:1531–8.
42. Garnero P, Shih WJ, Gineyts E, et al. Comparison of new biochemical markers of bone turnover in late postmenopausal osteoporotic women in response to alendronate treatment. J Clin Endocrinol Metab 1994;79:1693–700.
43. Bauer DC, Sklarin PM, Stone KL, et al. Biochemical markers of bone turnover and prediction of hip bone loss in older women: the study of osteoporotic fractures. J Bone Miner Res 1999;14:1404–10.
44. Garnero P. Markers of bone turnover for the prediction of fracture risk. Osteoporos Int 2000;11(Suppl 6):S55–65.
45. Melton LJ 3rd, Crowson CS, O'Fallon WM, et al. Relative contributions of bone density, bone turnover, and clinical risk factors to long-term fracture prediction. J Bone Miner Res 2003;18:312–8.
46. Hansen MA, Overgaard K, Riis BJ, et al. Role of peak bone mass and bone loss in postmenopausal osteoporosis: 12 year study. BMJ 1991;303:961–4.
47. Rosen CJ, Chesnut CH 3rd, Mallinak NJ. The predictive value of biochemical markers of bone turnover for bone mineral density in early postmenopausal women treated with hormone replacement or calcium supplementation. J Clin Endocrinol Metab 1997;82:1904–10.
48. Riis BJ, Hansen MA, Jensen AM, et al. Low bone mass and fast rate of bone loss at menopause: equal risk factors for future fracture: a 15-year follow-up study. Bone 1996;19:9–12.
49. Sowers MR, Greendale GA, Bondarenko I, et al. Endogenous hormones and bone turnover markers in pre- and perimenopausal women: SWAN. Osteoporos Int 2003; 14:191–7.
50. Finkelstein JS, Sowers M, Greendale GA, et al. Ethnic variation in bone turnover in pre- and early perimenopausal women: effects of anthropometric and lifestyle factors. J Clin Endocrinol Metab 2002;87:3051–6.

51. Hassager C, Colwell A, Assiri AM, et al. Effect of menopause and hormone replacement therapy on urinary excretion of pyridinium cross-links: a longitudinal and cross-sectional study. Clin Endocrinol (Oxf) 1992;37:45–50.
52. Nordin BE, JM WI, Clifton PM, et al. A longitudinal study of bone-related biochemical changes at the menopause. Clin Endocrinol (Oxf) 2004;61:123–30.
53. Ito M, Lang TF, Jergas M, et al. Spinal trabecular bone loss and fracture in American and Japanese women. Calcif Tissue Int 1997;61:123–8.
54. Finkelstein JS, Lee ML, Sowers M, et al. Ethnic variation in bone density in premenopausal and early perimenopausal women: effects of anthropometric and lifestyle factors. J Clin Endocrinol Metab 2002;87:3057–67.
55. Holmberg AH, Johnell O, Nilsson PM, et al. Risk factors for fragility fracture in middle age. A prospective population-based study of 33,000 men and women. Osteoporos Int 2006;17:1065–77.
56. Huopio J, Kroger H, Honkanen R, et al. Risk factors for perimenopausal fractures: a prospective study. Osteoporos Int 2000;11:219–27.
57. Torgerson DJ, Campbell MK, Thomas RE, et al. Prediction of perimenopausal fractures by bone mineral density and other risk factors. J Bone Miner Res 1996;11: 293–7.
58. Khalil N, Sutton-Tyrrell K, Strotmeyer ES, et al. Menopausal bone changes and incident fractures in diabetic women: a cohort study. Osteoporos Int 2011;22: 1367–76.
59. Management of osteoporosis in postmenopausal women: 2010 position statement of The North American Menopause Society. Menopause 2010;17:25–54.
60. Ensrud KE, Ewing SK, Stone KL, et al. Intentional and unintentional weight loss increase bone loss and hip fracture risk in older women. J Am Geriatr Soc 2003;51: 1740–7.
61. Avenell A, Gillespie WJ, Gillespie LD, et al. Vitamin D and vitamin D analogues for preventing fractures associated with involutional and post-menopausal osteoporosis. Cochrane Database Syst Rev 2009;2:CD000227.
62. Bischoff-Ferrari HA, Willett WC, Wong JB, et al. Fracture prevention with vitamin D supplementation: a meta-analysis of randomized controlled trials. JAMA 2005;293: 2257–64.
63. Chapuy MC, Arlot ME, Duboeuf F, et al. Vitamin D3 and calcium to prevent hip fractures in the elderly women. N Engl J Med 1992;327:1637–42.
64. Dawson-Hughes B, Harris SS, Krall EA, et al. Effect of calcium and vitamin D supplementation on bone density in men and women 65 years of age or older. N Engl J Med 1997;337:670–6.
65. Grant AM, Avenell A, Campbell MK, et al. Oral vitamin D3 and calcium for secondary prevention of low-trauma fractures in elderly people (Randomised Evaluation of Calcium Or vitamin D, RECORD): a randomised placebo-controlled trial. Lancet 2005;365:1621–8.
66. Jackson RD, LaCroix AZ, Gass M, et al. Calcium plus vitamin D supplementation and the risk of fractures. N Engl J Med 2006;354:669–83.
67. Finkelstein JS. Calcium plus vitamin D for postmenopausal women— bone appetit? N Engl J Med 2006;354:750–2.
68. Citron JT, Ettinger B, Genant HK. Spinal bone mineral loss in estrogen-replete, calcium-replete premenopausal women. Osteoporos Int 1995;5:228–33.
69. Dawson-Hughes B, Dallal GE, Krall EA, et al. A controlled trial of the effect of calcium supplementation on bone density in postmenopausal women. N Engl J Med 1990; 323:878–83.

70. Reid IR, Mason B, Horne A, et al. Randomized controlled trial of calcium in healthy older women. Am J Med 2006;119:777–85.

71. Dietary reference intakes for calcium and vitamin D. Washington, DC: Institute of Medicine of the National Academies; 2011.

72. Bolland MJ, Avenell A, Baron JA, et al. Effect of calcium supplements on risk of myocardial infarction and cardiovascular events: meta-analysis. BMJ 2010;341: c3691.

73. Bolland MJ, Barber PA, Doughty RN, et al. Vascular events in healthy older women receiving calcium supplementation: randomised controlled trial. BMJ 2008;336: 262–6.

74. Bailey RL, Dodd KW, Goldman JA, et al. Estimation of total usual calcium and vitamin D intakes in the United States. J Nutr 2010;140:817–22.

75. Chapuy MC, Schott AM, Garnero P, et al. Healthy elderly French women living at home have secondary hyperparathyroidism and high bone turnover in winter. EPIDOS Study Group. J Clin Endocrinol Metab 1996;81:1129–33.

76. Holick MF. Vitamin D deficiency. N Engl J Med 2007;357:266–81.

77. Bischoff-Ferrari HA, Dawson-Hughes B, Staehelin HB, et al. Fall prevention with supplemental and active forms of vitamin D: a meta-analysis of randomised controlled trials. BMJ 2009;339:b3692.

78. Holick MF, MacLaughlin JA, Clark MB, et al. Photosynthesis of previtamin D3 in human skin and the physiologic consequences. Science 1980;210:203–5.

79. Norman AW. Sunlight, season, skin pigmentation, vitamin D, and 25-hydroxyvitamin D: integral components of the vitamin D endocrine system. Am J Clin Nutr 1998;67: 1108–10.

80. Wortsman J, Matsuoka LY, Chen TC, et al. Decreased bioavailability of vitamin D in obesity. Am J Clin Nutr 2000;72:690–3.

81. Kanis JA, McCloskey EV, Johansson H, et al. A reference standard for the description of osteoporosis. Bone 2008;42:467–75.

82. Baim S, Binkley N, Bilezikian JP, et al. Official Positions of the International Society for Clinical Densitometry and executive summary of the 2007 ISCD Position Development Conference. J Clin Densitom 2008;11:75–91.

83. Screening for osteoporosis: U.S. preventive services task force recommendation statement. Ann Intern Med 2011;154:356–64.

84. Waugh EJ, Lam MA, Hawker GA, et al. Risk factors for low bone mass in healthy 40-60 year old women: a systematic review of the literature. Osteoporos Int 2009;20: 1–21.

85. Tremollieres F, Cochet T, Cohade C, et al. Fracture risk in early postmenopausal women assessed using FRAX. Joint Bone Spine 2010;77:345–8.

86. Ettinger B, Black DM, Dawson-Hughes B, et al. Updated fracture incidence rates for the US version of FRAX. Osteoporos Int 2010;21:25–33.

87. Tremollieres FA, Pouilles JM, Drewniak N, et al. Fracture risk prediction using BMD and clinical risk factors in early postmenopausal women: sensitivity of the WHO FRAX tool. J Bone Miner Res 2010;25:1002–9.

88. Tosteson AN, Melton LJ 3rd, Dawson-Hughes B, et al. Cost-effective osteoporosis treatment thresholds: the United States perspective. Osteoporos Int 2008;19: 437–47.

89. Eng-Wong J, Reynolds JC, Venzon D, et al. Effect of raloxifene on bone mineral density in premenopausal women at increased risk of breast cancer. J Clin Endocrinol Metab 2006;91:3941–6.

90. Cauley JA, Seeley DG, Ensrud K, et al. Estrogen replacement therapy and fractures in older women. Study of Osteoporotic Fractures Research Group. Ann Intern Med 1995;122:9–16.
91. Cauley JA, Zmuda JM, Ensrud KE, et al. Timing of estrogen replacement therapy for optimal osteoporosis prevention. J Clin Endocrinol Metab 2001;86:5700–5.
92. Schneider DL, Barrett-Connor EL, Morton DJ. Timing of postmenopausal estrogen for optimal bone mineral density. The Rancho Bernardo Study. JAMA 1997;277:543–7.

Perimenopause and Cognition

Gail A. Greendale, MD[a]*, Carol A. Derby, PhD[b],
Pauline M. Maki, PhD[c]

KEYWORDS

- Perimenopause • Menopause • Estrogen
- Follicle-stimulating hormone • Cognitive function
- Cardiovascular risk factors • Ovariectomy

Is the perimenopausal transition detrimental to cognitive function? This is an often-asked question in clinical practice, because self-reported memory problems are common during midlife.[1,2] The Seattle Midlife Women's Health Study reported that of 230 women aged 33 to 55 years who were interviewed about their perceived cognitive function, 60% noticed an unfavorable memory change "over the past few years."[1] In this cross-sectional survey, women reported problems with recall of words and numbers, disruptions in everyday behavior (eg, losing household items), difficulty concentrating, needing to use memory aids, and forgetting events (eg, appointments). Factors that were associated with perceived memory dysfunction were being a worker, job stress and multiple life roles—but not perimenopause transition stage—suggesting that the perceived memory difficulties were predominantly a function of stress and multiple burdens resulting in diminished attention and concentration. The Study of Women's Health Across the Nation (SWAN) also reported a cross-sectional association[2] between self-reported forgetfulness and being perimenopausal.[2] Forgetfulness was common in middle age: In this sample of 12,425 women aged 40 to 55 years, unadjusted for sociodemographic factors, 31% of premenopausal, 44% of early or late perimenopausal, and 42% of naturally menopausal women endorsed forgetfulness. After adjustment for race/ethnicity, age, education, economic hardship, marital status, parity, body size, health habits, and symptoms of anxiety, depression,

---

Supported by grant nos. 5 U01 AG012539-17 (G.A.G.); 2 PO1 AG03949 and 2U01AG012535-16 (C.A.D.); and 1 R01 MH083782-01A1 (P.M.M.)
Dr Derby receives research funding from Bristol-Meyers-Squibb.
[a] Division of Geriatrics, David Geffen School of Medicine at UCLA, 10945 Le Conte Avenue, Suite 2339, Los Angeles CA 90095-1687 USA
[b] Albert Einstein College of Medicine, Department of Neurology, Department of Epidemiology and Population Health, 1165 Morris Park Avenue, Rousso 336, Bronx, NY 10461 USA
[c] Center for Cognitive Medicine, University of Illinois at Chicago, College of Medicine, Department of Psychiatry and Psychology, 912 South Wood Street, Chicago IL 60612 USA
* Corresponding author.
E-mail address: ggreenda@mednet.ucla.edu.

Obstet Gynecol Clin N Am 38 (2011) 519–535
doi:10.1016/j.ogc.2011.05.007
0889-8545/11/$ – see front matter © 2011 Elsevier Inc. All rights reserved.

and poor sleep, perimenopausal women were 1.4 times more likely to report forgetfulness than premenopausal women. Thus, in the SWAN cross-sectional survey, self-reported forgetfulness did seem to be related to perimenopause independently of several relevant characteristics, including stress symptoms.

In addition to the desire to address women's clinical questions, research interest in the relation between perimenopause and cognition is fueled by preclinical evidence that estrogens have salutary neurophysiologic effects, leading researchers to postulate that a drop in estrogen (which occurs during perimenopause) would be detrimental to cognition.[3,4] For example, the hippocampus and prefrontal cortex, which serve episodic and working memory, are rich in estrogen receptors.[3] In animal and in vitro models, by genomic and non-genomic pathways, estrogens elevate levels of neurotransmitters such as serotonin and acetylcholine, promote neuronal growth and formation of synapses, act as antioxidants, and have regulatory effects on calcium homeostasis and second messenger systems.[3-7]

Beyond attempting to understand the concurrent effects of perimenopause on cognition, an emerging paradigm is endeavoring to connect biological changes that occur in other systems during the menopause transition with the risk of future cognitive dysfunction. This novel framework proposes that perimenopausal worsening of cardiovascular risk factors may result in cognitive decline and dementia in late life, and therefore conceives of the perimenopause as a potential window of opportunity for targeting modifiable cardiovascular risk factors in an effort to delay or prevent these conditions in the future.[8]

In this article, we detail the theoretical basis underlying why cognitive function may be affected by the perimenopause, review the results of longitudinal studies of measured cognitive performance during the perimenopause, and describe the potential linkages between perimenopausal cardiovascular risk and cognitive function in later life. We concentrate on data that come directly from the perimenopausal transition stage whenever possible; however, in some instances such data are not available. Therefore, we include some preclinical or clinical information based on menopausal animal models or early postmenopausal women when relevant.

MECHANISMS UNDERLYING THE RELATION BETWEEN PERIMENOPAUSE AND COGNITION
Changes in Sex Steroids May Have Indirect and Direct Neurologic Effects

When considering the mechanisms by which the perimenopause might impact cognitive function, it is important to consider both the indirect and direct effects of hormonal changes on the brain. Indirect effects are the effects of hormonal changes on brain systems associated with menopausal symptoms such as mood, sleep disturbance, and hot flashes. Direct effects are effects on neural systems subserving cognitive functions. Indirect effects are reviewed first.

The Serotonin System, Mood, and Cognition

SWAN demonstrated that objective changes in cognition across the menopausal transition were not accounted for by self-reported menopausal symptoms (hot flashes, anxiety, depression, and sleep disturbance).[9] However, the anxiety and depressive symptoms themselves were associated with small decrements in psychomotor speed, consistent with emerging evidence from basic science studies, showing that the effects of estrogen on depression and anxiety are largely mediated by estrogen receptor-β effects on serotonin and hypothalamic–pituitary–adrenal (HPA) axis function.[9-12]

Interventional research done in early postmenopausal women (mean age, 52 years) suggests that estrogen effects on serotonergic function may be a key mechanism relating mood and cognitive symptoms in the menopausal transition.[13] One open-label study randomized 19 early menopausal women to either a tryptophan depletion procedure (a reversible pharmacologic challenge that results in low levels of sero-tonin) or a sham (control) procedure before and after 8 weeks of transdermal estradiol treatment.[13] Verbal memory decreased significantly after the tryptophan depletion challenge, but estradiol treatment buffered this effect. Spatial learning did not decrease significantly as a result of tryptophan depletion; estrogen had no influence on spatial learning. In addition, estradiol enhanced mood on the day after the depletion challenge. This study provides experimental support for the beneficial effect of estrogen on serotonergic function in relation to both memory and mood. Additional support for the thesis that estrogen acts through the serotonergic system to modulate mood and cognitive performance comes from a study examining the effects of estrogen supplementation on serotonin systems and cognitive function in 10 early postmenopausal women (mean age, 54 years) who completed cognitive assessments and positron emission tomography scans before and after 10 weeks of treatment with transdermal estradiol.[14] The positron emission tomography radioligand deuteroaltan-serin was used to probe the influence of estrogen on 5-HT (2A) receptor binding. With estradiol treatment, 5-HT (2A) receptor binding significantly increased in right frontal cortex. Estradiol treatment also enhanced category fluency (a measure of executive function) and Trails A (a measure of psychomotor speed).

The Cortisol Pathway, Menopause Symptoms, and Cognition

Women often attribute cognitive problems to hot flashes, the cardinal symptom of the menopausal transition. Several investigations report no relation between performance on cognitive tests and self-reported hot flashes.[9,15,16] However, 1 small study found that moderate-to-severe objectively measured hot flashes, but not subjectively reported hot flashes, were related to declines in verbal memory.[17] In that investiga-tion, women subjectively reported only 40% of their objective hot flashes. Thus, the possibility that hot flashes contribute to the memory deficits observed in the menopausal transition remains open.

Higher cortisol levels or greater cortisol reactivity may be 1 mechanism that links hot flashes, and depressive or anxiety symptoms to perimenopausal decrements in cognitive performance. Cortisol increases after a hot flash,[18] and experimental administration of corticosteroids produces verbal memory impairment, and higher endogenous cortisol levels are associated with poorer performance on memory tasks.[19-26] Estrogen may also buffer the stress response. Young women show less cortisol responsivity to a laboratory stressor compared with men.[27] Although research on dynamic change in the HPA axis is lacking in perimenopausal women, in premenopausal women, HPA responsiveness varies across the menstrual cycle, with some studies showing greater responsiveness during the luteal versus follicular phase,[19,28] but others showing the opposite effect.[29] Seeman and colleagues[30] also found a greater HPA response to a stress challenge in postmenopausal women compared with older men.[30] Indeed, a meta-analysis of results from 34 laboratory stress studies concluded that the effect of aging on cortisol responsivity is 3 times greater in women than in men.[31]

The only published data about changes in the HPA axis during the perimenopause are from the Seattle Midlife Women's Health Study, which examined longitudinal changes in HPA activation.[32,33] An increase in overnight urinary cortisol levels during the late perimenopause was observed; cortisol levels returned to lower levels when women reached postmenopause.

Perimenopausal Changes in Sex Steroids: Direct Neurologic Effects

Estrogen fluctuations and withdrawal have myriad direct effects on the central nervous system (CNS) that have the potential to influence cognitive functions such as psychomotor speed and memory. Examples of estrogen-related CNS actions include increasing levels of neurotransmitters, enhancing neuron growth and formation of synapses, acting as antioxidants, and having regulatory effects on calcium homeostasis and second messenger systems.[3-7] A critical determinant of the effects of estrogen on the CNS and other health outcomes, including cardiovascular disease,[34,35] seems to be the timing of estrogen exposure in relation to the menopausal transition and/or age. In the case of cognitive outcomes, some evidence supports the "critical window hypothesis"—that exposure early in the menopausal transition or postmenopausal period confers cognitive benefit whereas exposure later in the menopausal transition confers neutral or detrimental effects.[36,37]

Animal Models of Menopause: Ovariectomy

Our understanding of the CNS mechanisms of estrogen action comes from basic science studies and human studies. Basic science studies in rodents and non-human primates rely on an ovariectomy (OVX) model of surgical menopause, which results in the abrupt withdrawal of estrogen (and other ovarian hormones). OVX models, therefore, do not mimic a natural menopausal transition. Additionally, OVX models do not produce levels of follicle-stimulating hormone (FSH), gonadotropin-releasing hormone, luteinizing hormone, and testosterone that are typical of the natural menopause.[38] Data from the OVX model suggest that estrogen effects on the cholinergic system are a critical factor contributing to memory declines associated with estrogen loss. Cholinergic systems play a central role in age-related changes in attention and memory function.[39]

Animal Models of Menopause: Induced Ovarian Failure

There are ongoing efforts to create and test an animal model of the natural menopause that parallels features of the human perimenopause, including a gradual reduction of estrogen and progesterone, and more typical levels of FSH, gonadotropin-releasing hormone, luteinizing hormone, and testosterone. One of these models, accelerated ovarian failure, represents a gradual loss of ovarian steroid hormones over time.[40] This effort centers on a technique developed in mice that relies upon exposure to 4-vinylcyclohexene diepoxide (VCD) to selectively destroy primordial and primary follicles. Mice exposed to VCD show hormonal features typical of the human perimenopause, including estrous acyclicity, fluctuating estrogen levels, and ultimately undetectable estrogen levels. Emerging evidence from the VCD model demonstrates the importance of considering the approach to modeling the perimenopause when evaluating the impact of the perimenopause on cognition and brain function.[40]

In the first study to compare the cognitive effects of surgical versus transitional VCD model of the menopause, Acosta and colleagues[40] compared middle-aged rats assigned to (1) sham surgery, (2) OVX surgery, (3) VCD, or (4) VCD then OVX (VCD/OVX). The inclusion of the latter group provided the opportunity to examine the effects of removal of residual ovarian output (eg, androgen) after VCD and follicular depletion. The value of the VCD model in modeling perimenopausal hormone levels was evident in the finding that the 2 groups with intact ovaries (sham and VCD) had lower luteinizing hormone and FSH levels, and higher androstenedione levels, compared with the 2 groups with no ovaries (OVX and VCD-OVX). Only the sham group exhibited high progesterone levels relative to all other groups. The behavioral effects of OVX versus VCD were evident on a measure of spatial working memory and short-term retention. Specifically, the VCD group showed more errors compared with the sham and VCD-OVX groups, whereas the OVX group was marginally different from the VCD group and did not differ from sham. Memory tests were carried out before and after pharmacologic reduction of acetylcholine (via scopolamine treatment), but the extent to which this manipulation reduced memory performance was similar across groups, suggesting no differential sensitivity to cholinergic loss in the OVX versus VCD model. The predictors of memory performance differed in the OVX versus VCD models. In OVX animals (OVX and VCD-OVX), higher FSH was associated with fewer working memory errors after scopolamine challenge. In VCD animals, higher androstenedione levels were associated with more working memory errors. These data suggest some caution in extrapolating findings concerning the impact of the perimenopause on cognitive function from models of surgical menopause to transitional models of menopause.

This research team next investigated the cognitive effects of estrogen therapy, specifically conjugated equine estrogen (CEE), in OVX and VCD animals.[41] The primary finding was that CEE had a beneficial effect on cognition in the OVX rats, but had a negative or neutral impact in the VCD rats in 3 separate cognitive tests. First, on the delay trial of a spatial and reference memory test, CEE enhanced performance in OVX animals but did not impact performance in VCD animals. Second, CEE enhanced working memory performance across increasing levels of difficulty in OVX animals, whereas CEE decreased the performance in VCD animals. Third, on a measure of long delay (8-hour) spatial memory, CEE enhanced memory retention in OVX rats, but had no benefit in VCD rats. As in the previous investigation, androstenedione levels predicted poorer cognition in the VCD animals, such that higher levels were associated with worse performance regardless of CEE treatment. These findings suggest a need for caution in extrapolating data concerning estrogen therapy and cognitive function from OVX models to a transitional VCD model.

Critical Timing: OVX Effects Differ by Age

Among OVX studies, those examining the effects of OVX on cognition and brain function in middle-aged rats are especially important in understanding the impact of hormonal changes during the menopausal transition. Two studies by Markowska and Savonenko[42,43] demonstrated the importance of considering the age of animal when examining the impact of OVX on cognition. The first study examined the impact of OVX and estrogen supplementation on cognitive performance in middle-aged female rats, beginning 1 month after OVX or sham surgery, and monthly thereafter as they aged. The most prominent effect of OVX in middle-aged female rats was accelerated aging in working memory function, but not in reference memory. The cognitive impairment emerged gradually, first occurring 4 months after OVX. Initially, the decrement was observed in tasks that placed more demands on working memory, and then was detected progressively in the easier tasks. Five months after OVX, when the animals reached old age, half of the animals received estrogen and half received vehicle. Estrogen administration improved deficits on 1 measure of working memory in old rats only when administered in a manner that mimicked estrogen fluctuations across the estrous. OVX also increased cognitive sensitivity to cholinergic withdrawal (via scopolamine) in aging rats, but estrogen was not effective in reversing those cognitive deficits in those older animals. These findings contrasted with previous demonstrations that estrogen reverses memory deficits induced by scopolamine in younger rats.[44,45] Overall, this study demonstrated that abrupt estrogen withdrawal has differing cognitive effects across a variety of cognitive measures, but does seem to accelerate cognitive aging on some measures. Additionally, the finding suggests that the beneficial effects of estrogen in reversing memory deficits induced by cholinergic withdrawal in younger animals are not evident in older animals. Thus, after abrupt hormonal decline, estrogen interacts with the cholinergic system to enhance memory in younger rats but not older rats.

A follow-up study by Savonenko and Markowska[43] directly contrasted the cognitive effects of OVX in middle-aged and older rats, and the effects of estrogen supplementation and cholinergic withdrawal in the 2 age groups.[43] The cognitive task was a T-maze active avoidance task, which depends on the integrity of the hippocampus and amygdala, as well as the cholinergic system. Results supported a critical "time window" in middle age during which estrogen supplementation conferred benefits and after which time estrogen supplementation was ineffective. Specifically, when the cholinergic system was compromised by scopolamine, middle-aged and older rats showed different sensitivities to estrogen withdrawal by OVX and estrogen supplementation. Among middle-aged rats, estrogen withdrawal did not increase sensitivity to the memory impairments that follow scopolamine challenge. In older age rats, estrogen withdrawal exacerbated the effect of scopolamine. Similarly, in middle-aged rats, estrogen supplementation decreased the extent to which scopolamine impaired performance on the T-maze. By contrast, estrogen supplementation was ineffective in protecting against scopolamine-induced memory deficits in older rats. These findings suggest that the effects of estrogen withdrawal and supplementation are evident on this particular task only when the cholinergic system was experimentally compromised by scopolamine.

Human Pharmacologic Challenge Studies Support Critical Timing

An age-related "window of opportunity" for estrogen to benefit cognition in women is supported by a cholinergic challenge trial by Dumas and colleagues.[46] A stratified sample of postmenopausal women, aged 50 to 62 years or 70 to 81 years, were randomly assigned to receive oral estradiol (2 mg/d) or placebo for 3 months. The women then completed a cholinergic challenge, which consisted of 3 conditions: (1) 2.5 mg/kg scopolamine (anti-muscarinic challenge), (2) 20 mg mecamylamine (anti-nicotinic challenge), and (3) placebo, in randomized order. In both age groups, there was a decrease in memory during the anticholinergic challenge. Estrogen at the 2 mg/d dose reversed the challenge-induced impairment on verbal memory in the younger, but not in the older, group. These findings parallel findings from the basic science literature, suggesting that estrogen ameliorates memory impairments owing to cholinergic withdrawal in young, but not older, postmenopausal women. Notably, an earlier clinical trial by this same research team demonstrated that treatment with 1 mg oral estradiol reversed scopolamine-induced declines in attention and psychomotor speed, suggesting that estrogen interacts with the cholinergic system to influence psychomotor speed and attention.[47]

Human Neuroimaging Studies: A Window to Estrogen's CNS Effects

The impact of ovarian hormone withdrawal on brain function and the importance of the cholinergic system in the context of ovarian hormone withdrawal are evident in a series of neuroimaging studies by Craig and colleagues.[48–50] In these studies, healthy premenopausal women underwent pharmacologic ovarian hormone suppression with leuprolide acetate, and given a verbal memory task. Hormone suppression produced decreased activation in the left prefrontal cortex, anterior cingulate, and medial frontal gyrus.[49] A subsequent study demonstrated that brain function returned to baseline when ovarian hormone levels returned to normal.[48] Like ovarian hormone withdrawal, scopolamine treatment reduced activation in the left inferior frontal gyrus during verbal encoding, and the combination of estrogen suppression and cholinergic suppression led to dramatic decreases in activity in this area.[50] The left inferior frontal gyrus is involved in processing of the meaning of verbal material. Together these data suggest that estrogen withdrawal might negatively affect the extent to which verbal information is meaningfully processed and estrogen supplementation might enhance the encoding of verbal information into memory by enhancing the depth of semantic processing.

Estrogen also seems to enhance hippocampal function when administered in the perimenopausal period.[51] A recent functional magnetic resonance imaging study investigated brain function in 2 groups of women, one that initiated hormone therapy beginning in the perimenopause and continuing to older age, and the other that used no menopausal hormone therapy. At the time of the neuroimaging, women were on average 60 years of age. The neuroimaging task was a delayed word list task (verbal memory) that included an encoding phase, a 15-minute delay, and a retrieval phase to parallel clinical neuropsychological measures of verbal memory. Early continued use of estrogen was associated with enhanced verbal memory and enhanced function in the hippocampus during memory retrieval, concordant with the critical timing hypothesis. Similar findings of a benefit of early estrogen treatment on hippocampal volume have been reported.[52]

Relation of Critical Timing and Health Cell Bias Theories

An alternative to the critical timing hypothesis is the "healthy cell bias" of estrogen introduced by Brinton.[53] The healthy cell bias posits that as the continuum of neurologic health progresses from healthy to unhealthy, the effects of estrogen supplementation progresses from beneficial to neutral or detrimental. In this paradigm, estrogen confers beneficial effects for neurologic function and survival if neurons are healthy at the time of estrogen exposure. Conversely, estrogen exposure negatively impacts neurologic function and survival if neurologic health is compromised. Given that cells are more likely to be healthy earlier in the perimenopausal period than later in the postmenopausal period, the healthy cell bias and the critical window hypothesis overlap. There is mounting evidence that the negative impact of hormone therapy is most evident in women whose cognitive performance is lower than expected at the time of estrogen exposure.[54,55] Also consistent with the healthy cell bias hypothesis is evidence from a randomized, clinical trial that even older women can benefit from estrogen provided that they perform at or above expected levels of performance on verbal memory tasks.[56]

HUMAN LONGITUDINAL STUDIES OF PERIMENOPAUSE AND COGNITIVE PERFORMANCE
Longitudinal Studies of Measured Cognitive Performance During Perimenopause

There are 4 published longitudinal reports on the subject of perimenopause and measured cognitive performance.[9,57–59] Three of these studies focused on the relation between the perimenopause transition and cognition and the fourth addressed the question of whether perimenopausal symptoms contribute to the subtle decrements in cognitive function observed during perimenopause.

The Kinmen Women-Health Investigation (KIWI) studied longitudinal cognitive performance in a sample of 694 Chinese residents of Kinman, Taiwan.[57] At baseline,

KIWI participants were premenopausal and averaged 46 years of age. Cognitive tests included assays of verbal memory, verbal fluency, mental flexibility, and processing speed. At an 18-month follow-up assessment, performance on all cognitive tests improved, an expected learning effect (see below for further explanation of learning effects).[60] However, women who transitioned to perimenopause during the follow-up period manifested significantly less improvement in verbal fluency than did those who did not transition.

The remaining 3 longitudinal analyses of measured cognitive performance during the menopause transition come from SWAN. SWAN is a multisite, community-based, longitudinal cohort study, ongoing at 7 clinical centers in the United States.[61] At baseline, SWAN participants were between 42 and 52 years old, premenopausal or early perimenopausal and self-identified (per protocol requisite) as African-American, Caucasian, Chinese, Japanese, or Hispanic.

At SWAN baseline, only the SWAN Chicago site assessed cognitive performance, using a test of processing speed and a test of working memory (the ability to keep information in mind and manipulate it). All 7 SWAN sites began measuring cognition at the fourth annual follow-up visit. The SWAN cohort cognitive assessment included the same 2 tests that had been used by Chicago-SWAN and added a third test of verbal memory.[62-65]

The Chicago SWAN site-specific results included information from about 800 women followed for an average of 2 years.[58] Like the KIWI study, Chicago SWAN witnessed small improvements over time in cognitive processing speed and working memory, consistent with expected learning in this age range. But, unlike KIWI, advancement to perimenopause during the observation period did not dampen the learning effect. Subsequently, a 4-year longitudinal analysis based on the entire SWAN cohort (n = 2362) found that being perimenopausal transiently reduced measured cognitive performance.[59] A learning effect was also evident in this larger study: Cognitive processing speed improved with each annual visit during premenopause, early perimenopause, and postmenopause. But during late perimenopause women did not demonstrate learning (improved cognitive processing speed) with repeated testing. Similarly, during premenopause and postmenopause, verbal memory scores got better at each follow-up, but although participants were early or late perimenopausal their verbal memory tests did not improve. Compared with the Chicago site-specific report, the SWAN cohort sample size was much larger, the follow-up time doubled, and the effects of previous and current hormone use were accounted for in the statistical models; each of these factors likely contributed to the different results.

In both KIWI and SWAN, the cognitive performance difficulties during perimenopause were subtle: They were evidenced by a lack of improvement with repeated annual testing, not a decline in scores. This underscores the relevance of the "learning effect" in studies of midlife cognitive performance. When serial cognitive tests are given to middle aged individuals, increasing scores with repeated administrations are the norm; this is termed "the learning effect." A lack improvement with successive test administrations during midlife, therefore, may be interpreted as an indicator of abnormal cognitive function.[60] KIWI and SWAN participants ranged in age from 40 to 61 years, and thus would be expected to improve with repeated tests. The lack of learning, isolated to the perimenopausal stage of the transition, argues for a transient detrimental effect of the perimenopause on cognitive performance.

Mechanistic Hypotheses

What mechanisms might account for a perimenopause-associated alteration in cognitive function? As reviewed, an estrogen-related pathway is plausible: Estrogen benefits hippocampal and prefrontal cortical function, potentially enhancing verbal memory and executive function, cognitive domains that are consistent with the results from KIWI and SWAN.[4,6,66,67] The drop in estrogen that accompanies perimenopause could, therefore, negatively impact cognitive performance.[68]

Menopause transition symptoms could also lead to poorer cognitive performance. The most recent SWAN analysis addressed the question of whether vasomotor, depressive, anxiety, or sleep disturbance symptoms, which are associated with perimenopause, are themselves related to poorer cognitive function during the transition.[9,69–77] SWAN reported that higher levels of depressive and anxiety symptoms were directly related to slightly poorer cognitive performance. However, the presence of menopause transition symptoms did not account for the cognitive decrements observed during perimenopause. Specifically, women with more depressive symptoms did worse on the test of cognitive processing speed and those with higher degrees of anxiety demonstrated less learning in the domain of verbal memory. Neither sleep disturbances nor vasomotor symptoms had a direct effect on concurrent cognitive performance and learning. These results are consistent with evidence that attention and concentration deficits accompany depressive and anxiety disorders.[78–81] But, when all 4 of these menopause transition symptoms (vasomotor, depressive, anxiety, and sleep disturbance) were added to models of menopause transition stage and cognition, the negative effect of late perimenopause on learning was unaltered, suggesting that the presence of these symptoms did not account for the perimenopause-associated learning decrement.

PERIMENOPAUSAL CARDIOVASCULAR RISK AND COGNITION

The perimenopause is associated with adverse changes in a number of cardiovascular risk factors (reviewed by Chae and Derby in this volume). A growing body of evidence links cardiovascular risk status, particularly during midlife, with cognitive decline and dementia later in life. Furthermore, women with the highest levels of vascular risk factors during perimenopause remain in the highest risk groups after menopause, resulting in protracted exposure to this potentially damaging cardiovascular risk profile.[82] Thus, the perimenopause may be a critical time in the lifespan when preventive efforts to reduce the risk of subsequent cognitive disability are warranted.

Vascular Disease and Dementia

Traditionally, Alzheimer's disease and vascular dementia, the leading causes of dementia in the elderly, have been considered distinct clinical entities. However, accumulating evidence suggests an association between vascular disease and cognitive decline and dementia regardless of subtype, with vascular pathology contributing to at least half of all dementia cases.[83–86] Furthermore, data from imaging and cliniconeuropathologic correlation studies suggest that the presence of vascular pathology exacerbates the clinical expression of Alzheimer's disease.[87–91] Vascular risk factors are associated with cognitive decline and dementia in older populations.[83,85,86,90] A summary index of vascular risk factor status, the Framingham Stroke risk profile, has been associated longitudinally with deficits in a range of cognitive functions.[92] Finally, white matter hyperintensities, markers of ischemia in the brain, have been linked to deficits in cognitive function, particularly frontal/executive functions (eg, planning, strategy use, and task switching).[93-97]

Midlife Risk Factors and Cognition

Given that the natural history of both Alzheimer's disease and vascular disease span decades, the impact of vascular risk factors on cognitive decline and dementia may be cumulative over the lifespan.[84] Just as subclinical vascular disease begins decades before clinically overt cardiovascular disease, the neurodegenerative changes that underlie dementia begin many years before clinical diagnosis. There is accumulating evidence linking risk factor status during middle age with cognitive decline and dementia in older age.[8] A retrospective cohort study of participants in the Kaiser Permanente medical care plan demonstrated that presence of diabetes, hypertension, high cholesterol, or smoking measured at approximately age 40 each predicted the diagnosis of dementia 20 to 30 years later. The presence of all 4 of these risk factors during midlife doubled the risk of developing dementia in later life.[98]

Cardiovascular risk factors ascertained in midlife predict risk of cognitive decline and dementia better than those measured in late life. Midlife risk assessment may have greater predictive power because it may capture the cumulative impact of a lifetime of putative exposures. Additionally, some vascular risk factors, such as blood pressure and serum cholesterol, decline during the years immediately preceding the onset of dementia.[99,100] If the risk factors were measured in the years proximal to dementia onset, this drop in blood pressure and cholesterol would obscure the true relation between life-long hypertension or hypercholesterolemia and late life cognitive function.

Blood Pressure and Cholesterol

Finnish population-based studies report that elevated blood pressure and serum cholesterol levels measured in midlife (mean age, 50 years) predict onset of mild cognitive impairment (thought to be a marker of preclinical dementia),[101] and Alzheimer's disease 20 years later.[100,101] The association of midlife blood pressure with dementia in later life has been confirmed in men in the Honolulu-Asia aging study and among men and women in a Swedish cohort.[99,102]

Body Mass Index

Body mass index measured between 40 and 44 years of age is a strong predictor of subsequent Alzheimer's disease.[103] In the Cardiovascular Health Study, body mass index at age 50 was positively associated with dementia risk in later life, whereas body mass index measured after age 65 showed an inverse association with dementia risk.[104]

Midlife Diabetes Onset

Onset of diabetes before age 65, but not after it, predicts the development of mild cognitive impairment or dementia.[105,106] Diabetes duration of at least 10 years is also associated with a greater incidence of mild cognitive impairment.[105] A case-control twin study found that diabetes onset before age 65 more than doubled the risk of dementia, whereas onset after age 65 was not associated with incident dementia risk.[106]

SUMMARY

Perimenopause may have contemporary as well as long-term effects on cognitive function. The contemporaneous impact of perimenopause on cognition seems to be both transient (occurring only during perimenopause) and subtle. In both KIWI and SWAN, the only published longitudinal studies of measured cognitive performance during the menopause transition, an absence of improved test scores with repeated annual measurements, not a decline in test scores, was evident during perimenopause.

The presence of menopause transition symptoms could indirectly mediate the effect of the perimenopause on cognitive performance. In SWAN, the perimenopausal decrement in cognitive performance was not accounted for by vasomotor, depressive, anxiety, or disturbed sleep symptoms. Although several studies report no relation between performance on cognitive tests and self-reported hot flashes, 1 small study did find that moderate-to-severe objectively measured hot flashes, but not subjectively reported ones, were related to declines in verbal memory. Thus, the possibility that hot flashes contribute to the memory deficits observed in the menopausal transition remains open.

The increases in anxiety and depressive symptoms that accompany the perimenopausal transition have an independent effect on cognitive performance. This is consistent with basic science findings that the effects of estrogen on depression and anxiety are largely mediated by estrogen receptor-β effects on serotonin and HPA axis function. Additionally, higher baseline cortisol levels or greater cortisol reactivity could link hot flashes, depressive or anxiety symptoms with perimenopausal decrements in cognitive performance. While there is mounting evidence for a cortisol-stress-cognition link in older men and women, this pathway has not been directly explored in perimenopausal women.

Long term cognitive consequences of perimenopause may stem directly from the decline in estradiol level that accompanies this transition. Animal and human experimental models show that estradiol protects against the detrimental mood and cognitive changes that result from serotonin withdrawal. Similarly, estrogen defends against cognitive changes after cholinergic depletion in midlife women and middle aged female rats. These studies suggest that the loss of estrogen at midlife results in changes in cholinergic and serotonergic function which in turn contribute to mood problems and cognitive deficits.

Age and/or health status may be determinants of the impact of sex hormones on cognitive function. In both animal and human experimental models, estrogen benefits cognitive function early in the menopausal transition but not later in life. In observational studies, early estrogen use is associated with improved memory and hippocampal function later in life.

Worsened cardiovascular risk factors, which accompany the perimenopause, may be a pathway by which the menopausal transition affects cognitive function in older age. Cardiovascular risk factors, particularly those present in midlife, have been linked to cognitive decline and dementia in later life. Women with the highest levels of vascular risk factors during perimenopause maintain the highest risk levels after menopause, resulting in protracted exposure to a cardiovascular risk profile that may ultimately lead to dementia.

CLINICAL IMPLICATIONS

Information about the short and long-term effects of perimenopause on contemporary cognitive function and risk of future cognitive decline is scant—but is there anything that can be used to inform clinical practice? Albeit based on limited longitudinal data, it seems that there is a small (but probably perceptible to the woman) decrement in perimenopausal cognitive performance that resolves in postmenopause. This knowledge may be of use in counseling perimenopausal patients who raise concerns about memory dysfunction. Also noteworthy from a clinical perspective is that cognitive complaints during perimenopause may be the result of perimenopausal anxiety or depressive symptoms, thus clinicians should be alert to the potential memory-mood link. The perimenopause is also an opportune time to evaluate and treat modifiable cardiovascular risk factors, not only for primary prevention of cardiovascular disease but also because doing so may lessen the risk of cognitive decline or dementia. Finally, although several lines of evidence suggest that exogenous estrogens may result in beneficial cognitive outcomes when given in the perimenopause or early postmenopause, this notion of critical timing remains experimental.

RESEARCH DIRECTIONS

Longitudinal studies of measured cognitive performance during the menopause transition are scant; more are needed. Insights into the neurobiology of the perimenopause can be gained from future studies examining the effect of the perimenopause on the HPA axis in relation to cognition and mood. Further investigation of the critical timing hypothesis (and the related healthy cell bias hypothesis) is fundamental to our understanding of the care of perimenopausal women. Understanding of the cognitive biology of menopause will also be improved by making use of new animal models of the menopause transition, in which there is a gradual depletion of ovarian follicles, more closely mimic the biology of natural menopause in humans.

REFERENCES

1. Mitchell E, Woods N. Midlife women's attributions about perceived memory changes: Observations from the Seattle Midlife Women's Health Study. J Womens Health Gend Based Med 2001;10:351–62.
2. Gold EB, Sternfeld B, Kelsey JL, et al. Relation of demographic and lifestyle factors to symptoms in a multi-racial/ethnic population of women 40–55 years of age. Am J Epidemiol 2000;152:463–73.
3. McEwen BS. Invited review: estrogens effects on the brain: Multiple sites and molecular mechanisms. J Appl Physiol 2001;91:2785–801.
4. McEwen B. Estrogen actions throughout the brain. Recent Prog Horm Res 2002; 57:357–84.
5. Gleason CE, Cholerton B, Carlsson CM, et al. Neuroprotective effects of female sex steroids in humans: current controversies and future directions. Cell Mol Life Sci 2005;62:299–312.
6. Morrison JH, Brinton RD, Schmidt PJ, et al. Estrogen, menopause, and the aging brain: how basic neuroscience can inform hormone therapy in women. J Neurosci 2006;26:10332–48.
7. Brann DW, Dhandapani K, Wakade C, et al. Neutrophic and neuroprotective actions of estrogen: basic mechanisms and clinical implications. Steroids. 2007;72:381–405.
8. Hughes TF, Ganguli M. Modifiable midlife risk factors for late-life cognitive impairment and dementia. Curr Psychiatry Rev 2009;5:73–92.
9. Greendale GA, Wight RG, Huang MH, et al. Menopause-associated symptoms and cognitive performance: results from the study of women's health across the nation. Am J Epidemiol 2010;171:1214–24.
10. Donner N, Handa RJ. Estrogen receptor beta regulates the expression of tryptophan-hydroxylase 2 mRNA within serotonergic neurons of the rat dorsal raphe nuclei. Neuroscience 2009;163:705–18.

11. Weiser MJ, Wu TJ, Handa RJ. Estrogen receptor-beta agonist diarylpropionitrile: biological activities of R- and S-enantiomers on behavior and hormonal response to stress. Endocrinology 2009;150:1817–25.
12. Lund TD, Rovis T, Chung WC, et al. Novel actions of estrogen receptor-beta on anxiety-related behaviors. Endocrinology 2005;146:797–807.
13. Amin Z, Gueorguieva R, Cappiello A, et al. Estradiol and tryptophan depletion interact to modulate cognition in menopausal women. Neuropsychopharmacology 2006;31:2489–97.
14. Kugaya A, Epperson CN, Zoghbi S, et al. Increase in prefrontal cortex serotonin 2A receptors following estrogen treatment in postmenopausal women. Am J Psychiatry 2003;160:1522–24.
15. LeBlanc ES, Neiss MB, Carello PE, et al. Hot flashes and estrogen therapy do not influence cognition in early menopausal women. Menopause 2007;14:191–202.
16. Polo-Kantola P, Erkkola R. Sleep and the menopause. J Br Menopause Soc 2004;10:145–50.
17. Maki PM, Drogos LL, Rubin LH, et al. Objective hot flashes are negatively related to verbal memory performance in midlife women. Menopause 2008;15:848–56.
18. Meldrum DR, Defazio JD, Erlik Y, et al. Pituitary hormones during the menopausal hot flash. Obstet Gynecol 1984;64:752–6.
19. Kirschbaum C, Kudielka BM, Gaab J, et al. Impact of gender, menstrual cycle phase, and oral contraceptives on the activity of the hypothalamus-pituitary-adrenal axis. Psychosom Med 1999;61:154–62.
20. Newcomer JW, Selke G, Melson AK, et al. Decreased memory performance in healthy humans induced by stress-level cortisol treatment. Arch Gen Psychiatry 1999;56:527–33.
21. Lupien SJ, Gillin CJ, Hauger RL. Working memory is more sensitive than declarative memory in humans. Behav Neurosci 1999;113:420–30.
22. Seeman TE, McEwen BS, Singer BH, et al. Increase in urinary cortisol excretion and memory declines: MacArthur Studies of Successful Aging. J Clin Endocrinol Metab 1997;82:2458–65.
23. Greendale GA, Kritz-Silverstein D, Seeman T, et al. Higher basal cortisol predicts verbal memory loss in postmenopausal women: Rancho Bernardo Study. J Am Geriatr Soc 2000;48:1655–8.
24. Lupien SJ, de Leon M, de Santis S, et al. Cortisol levels during human aging predict hippocampal atrophy and memory deficits. Nat Neurosci 1998;1:69–73.
25. McEwen BS, Magarinos AM. Stress effects on morphology and function of the hippocampus. Ann N Y Acad Sci 1997;821:271–84.
26. Karlamangla AS, Singer BH, Chodosh J, et al. Urinary cortisol excretion as a predictor of incident cognitive impairment. Neurobiol Aging 2005;26(Suppl 1):80–4.
27. Kirschbaum C, Wust S, Hellhammer D. Consistent sex differences in cortisol responses to psychological stress. Psychosom Med 1992;54:648–57.
28. Kajantie E, Phillips DIW. The effects of sex and hormone status on the physiological response to acute psychosocial stress. Psychoneuroendocrinology 2006;31:151–78.
29. Symonds CS, Gallagher P, Thompson JM, et al. Effects of the menstrual cycle on mood, neurocognitive and neuroendocrine function in healthy premenopausal women. Psychol Med 2004;34:93–102.
30. Seeman TE, Singer B, Wilkinson CW, et al. Gender difference s in age-related changes in HPA axis reactivity. Psychoneuroendocrinology 2001;26:225–40.
31. Otte C, Hart S, Nevlan TC, et al. A meta-analysis of cortisol response to challenge in human aging: importance of gender. Psychoneuroendocrinology 2005;30:80–91.

32. Woods NF, Mitchell ES, Smith-DiJulio K. Cortisol levels during the menopausal transition and early postmenopause: observations from the Seattle Midlife Women's Health Study. Menopause 2009;16:708–18.

33. Woods NF, Carr MC, Tao EY, et al. Increased urinary cortisol levels during the menopausal transition. Menopause 2006;13:212–21.

34. LaCroix AZ, Chlebowski RT, Manson JE, et al; WHI Investigators. Health outcomes after stopping conjugated equine estrogens among postmenopausal women with prior hysterectomy: a randomized controlled trial. JAMA 2011;305:1305–14.

35. Salpeter SR, Walsh JM, Greyber E, et al. Brief report: coronary heart disease events associated with hormone therapy in younger and older women. A meta-analysis. J Gen Intern Med 2006;21:363–6.

36. Sherwin BB, Henry JF. Brain aging modulates the neuroprotective effects of estrogen on selective aspects of cognition in women: a critical review. Front Neuroendocrinol 2008;29:88–113.

37. Maki PM. Hormone therapy and cognitive function: is there a critical period for benefit? Neuroscience 2006;138:1027–30.

38. Maffucci JA, Gore AC. Age-related changes in hormones and their receptors in animal models of female reproductive senescence. In: Conn MP, editor. Handbook of models for human aging. San Diego: Academic Press and Elsevier; 2006. p. 533–52.

39. Dumas JA, Newhouse PA. The cholinergic hypothesis of cognitive aging revisited again: cholinergic functional compensation. Pharmacol Biochem Behav 2011 Mar 5 [Epub ahead of print].

40. Van Kempen TA, Milner TA, Waters EM. Accelerated ovarian failure: a novel, chemically induced animal model of menopause. Brain Res 2011;1379:176–87.

41. Acosta JI, Mayer LP, Braden BB, et al. The cognitive effects of conjugated equine estrogens depend on whether menopause etiology is transitional or surgical. Endocrinology 2010;151:3795–804.

42. Markowska AL, Savonenko AV. Effectiveness of estrogen replacement in restoration of cognitive function after long-term estrogen withdrawal in aging rats. J Neurosci 2002;22:10985–95.

43. Savonenko AV, Markowska AL. The cognitive effects of ovariectomy and estrogen replacement are modulated by aging. Neuroscience 2003;119:821–30.

44. Fader AJ, Johnson PE, Dohanich GP. Estrogen improves working but not reference memory and prevents amnestic effects of scopolamine of a radial-arm maze. Pharmacol Biochem Behav 1999;62:711–17.

45. Gibbs RB. Estrogen replacement enhances acquisition of a spatial memory task and reduces deficits associated with hippocampal muscarinic receptor inhibition. Horm Behav 1999;36:222–33.

46. Dumas J, Hancur-Bucci C, Naylor M, et al. Estradiol interacts with the cholinergic system to affect verbal memory in postmenopausal women: evidence for the critical period hypothesis. Horm Behav 2008;53:159–69.

47. Dumas J, Hancur-Bucci C, Naylor M, et al. Estrogen treatment effects on anticholinergic-induced cognitive dysfunction in normal postmenopausal women. Neuropsychopharmacology 2006;31:2065–78.

48. Craig MC, Fletcher PC, Daly EM, et al. Reversibility of the effects of acute ovarian hormone suppression on verbal memory and prefrontal function in pre-menopausal women. Psychoneuroendocrinology 2008;33:1426–31.

49. Craig MC, Fletcher PC, Daly EM, et al. Gonadotropin hormone releasing hormone agonists alter prefrontal function during verbal encoding in young women. Psychoneuroendocrinology 2007;32:1116–27.

50. Craig MC, Fletcher PC, Daly EM, et al. The interactive effect of the cholinergic system and acute ovarian suppression on the brain: an fMRI study. Horm Behav 2009;55:41–9.
51. Maki PM, Dennerstein L, Clark M, et al. Perimenopausal use of hormone therapy is associated with enhanced memory and hippocampal function later in life. Brain Res 2011;1379:232–43.
52. Erickson KI, Voss MW, Prakash RS, et al. A cross-sectional study of hormone treatment and hippocampal volume in postmenopausal women: evidence for a limited window of opportunity. Neuropsychology 2010;24:68–76.
53. Brinton RD. Investigative models for determining hormone therapy-induced outcomes in brain: evidence in support of a healthy cell bias of estrogen action. Ann N Y Acad Sci 2005;1052:57–74.
54. Resnick SM, Espeland MA, Jaramillo SA, et al. Postmenopausal hormone therapy and regional brain volumes: the WHIMS-MRI Study. Neurology 2009;72:135–42.
55. Espeland M, Rapp S, Shumaker S, et al. Conjugated equine estrogens and global cognitive function in postmenopausal women: Women's Health Initiative Memory Study. JAMA 2004;291:2959–68.
56. Tierney MC, Oh P, Moineddin R, et al. A randomized double-blind trial of the effects of hormone therapy on delayed verbal recall in older women. Psychoneuroendocrinology 2009;34:1065–74.
57. Fuh JL, Wang SJ, Lee SJ, et al. A longitudinal study of cognition change during early menopausal transition in a rural community. Maturitas 2006;53:351–62.
58. Meyer PM, Powell LH, Wilson RS, et al. A population-based longitudinal study of cognitive functioning in the menopausal transition. Neurology 2003;61:801–6.
59. Greendale GA, Huang MH, Wight RG, et al. Effects of the menopause transition and hormone use on cognitive performance in midlife women. Neurology 2009;72:1850–7.
60. Lamar M, Resnick SM, Zonderman AB. Longitudinal changes in verbal memory in older adults: distinguishing the effects of age from repeat testing. Neurology 2003;60:82–6.
61. Sowers MF, Crawford SL, Sternfeld B, et al. SWAN: a multicenter, multiethnic, community-based cohort study of women and the menopausal transition. In: Lobo RA, Kelsey J, Marcus R, editors. Menopause biology and pathobiology. San Diego: Academic Press; 2000. p. 175–88.
62. Smith A. Symbol digit modalities test. Los Angeles: Western Psychological Service; 1982.
63. Albert M, Smith LA, Scherr PA, et al. Use of brief cognitive tests to identify individuals in the community with clinically diagnosed Alzheimer's disease. Int J Neurosci 1991;57:167–78.
64. Wechsler D. A standardized memory scale for clinical use. J Psychol 1945;19:87–95.
65. Jonides J, Smith EE, Marsheutz C, et al. Inhibition in verbal working memory revealed by brain activation. Proc Natl Acad Sci U S A 1998;95:8410–3.
66. Maki PM, Sundermann E. Hormone therapy and cognitive function. Hum Reprod Update 2009;15:667–81.
67. Barrett-Connor E, Laughlin GA. Endogenous and exogenous estrogen, cognitive function, and dementia in postmenopausal women: evidence from epidemiologic studies and clinical trials. Semin Reprod Med 2009;27:275–82.
68. Randolph JF Jr, Zheng H, Sowers MR, et al. Change in follicle-stimulating hormone and estradiol across the menopausal transition: effect of age at the final menstrual period. J Clin Endocrinol Metab 2011;96:746–54.

69. Gold EB, Colvin A, Avis N, et al. Longitudinal analysis of the association between vasomotor symptoms and race/ethnicity across the menopausal transition: Study of Women's Health Across the Nation. Am J Public Health 2006;96:1226–35.

70. Bromberger JT, Meyer PM, Kravitz HM, et al. Psychologic distress and natural menopause: a multiethnic community study. Am J Public Health 2001;91:1435–42.

71. Bromberger JT, Matthews KA, Schott LL, et al. Depressive symptoms during the menopausal transition: the Study of Women's Health Across the Nation (SWAN). J Affect Disord 2007;103:267–72.

72. Kravitz HM, Zhao X, Bromberger JT, et al. Sleep disturbance during the menopausal transition in a multi-ethnic community sample of women. Sleep 2008;31:979–90.

73. Woods NF, Mitchell ES. Symptoms during the perimenopause: prevalence, severity, trajectory, and significance in women's lives. Am J Med 2005; 118(Suppl 12B):14–24.

74. Freeman EW, Sammel MD, Lin H, et al. Symptoms associated with menopausal transition and reproductive hormones in midlife women. Obstet Gynecol 2007;110: 230–40.

75. Cohen LS, Soares CN, Vitonis AF, et al. Risk for new onset of depression during the menopausal transition: the Harvard study of moods and cycles. Arch Gen Psychiatry 2006;63:385–90.

76. Freeman EW, Sammel MD, Lin H. Temporal associations of hot flashes and depression in the transition to menopause. Menopause 2009;16:728–34.

77. Young T, Rabago D, Zgierska A, et al. Objective and subjective sleep quality in premenopausal, perimenopausal, and postmenopausal women in the Wisconsin Sleep Cohort Study. Sleep 2003;26:667–72.

78. Zakzanis KK, Leach L, Kaplan E. On the nature and pattern of neurocognitive function in major depressive disorder. Neuropsychiatry Neuropsychol Behav Neurol 1998;11:111–9.

79. Wetherell JL, Reynolds CA, Gatz M, et al. Anxiety, cognitive performance, and cognitive decline in normal aging. J Gerontol B Psychol Sci Soc Sci 2002;57: 246–55.

80. Beaudreau SA, O'Hara R. Late-life anxiety and cognitive impairment: a review. Am J Geriatr Psychiatry 2008;16:790–803.

81. Eysenck MW, Derakshan N, Santos R, et al. Anxiety and cognitive performance: attentional control theory. Emotion 2007;7:336–53.

82. Matthews KA, Kuller LH, Sutton-Tyrrell K, et al. Changes in cardiovascular risk factors during the perimenopause and postmenopause and carotid artery atherosclerosis in healthy women. Stroke 2001;32:1104–11.

83. Launer LJ. Demonstrating the case that AD is a vascular disease: epidemiologic evidence. Ageing Res Rev 2002;1:61–77.

84. Decarli C. Vascular factors in dementia: an overview. J Neurol Sci 2004;226:19–23.

85. Breteler MM. Vascular risk factors for Alzheimer's disease: an epidemiologic perspective. Neurobiol Aging 2000;21:153–60.

86. Stampfer MJ. Cardiovascular disease and Alzheimer's disease: common links. J Intern Med 2006;260:211–23.

87. Schneider JA, Arvanitakis Z, Bang W, et al. Mixed brain pathologies account for most dementia cases in community-dwelling older persons. Neurology 2007;69:2197–204.

88. Snowdon DA, Greiner LH, Mortimer JA, et al. Brain infarction and the clinical expression of Alzheimer disease. The Nun Study. JAMA 1997;277:813–7.

89. Esiri MM, Nagy Z, Smith MZ, et al. Cerebrovascular disease and threshold for dementia in the early stages of Alzheimer's disease. Lancet 1999;354:919–20.

90. Riekse RG, Leverenz JB, McCormick W, et al. Effect of vascular lesions on cognition in Alzheimer's disease: a community-based study. J Am Geriatr Soc 2004;52: 1442–8.
91. Vermeer SE, Prins ND, den Heijer T, et al. Silent brain infarcts and the risk of dementia and cognitive decline. N Engl J Med 2003;348:1215–22.
92. Elias MF, Sullivan LM, D'Agostino RB, et al. Framingham stroke risk profile and lowered cognitive performance. Stroke 2004;35:404–9.
93. Au R, Massaro JM, Wolf PA, et al. Association of white matter hyperintensity volume with decreased cognitive functioning: the Framingham Heart Study. Arch Neurol 2006;63:246–50.
94. de Groot JC, de Leeuw FE, Oudkerk M, et al. Cerebral white matter lesions and cognitive function: the Rotterdam Scan Study. Ann Neurol 2000; 47:145–51.
95. Gunning-Dixon FM, Raz N. Neuroanatomical correlates of selected executive functions in middle-aged and older adults: a prospective MRI study. Neuropsychologia 2003;41:1929–41.
96. Prins ND, van Dijk EJ, den Heijer T, et al. Cerebral small-vessel disease and decline in information processing speed, executive function and memory. Brain 2005;128: 2034–41.
97. Tullberg M, Fletcher E, DeCarli C, et al. White matter lesions impair frontal lobe function regardless of their location. Neurology 2004;63:246–53.
98. Whitmer RA, Sidney S, Selby J, et al. Midlife cardiovascular risk factors and risk of dementia in late life. Neurology 2005;64:277–81.
99. Skoog I, Lernfelt B, Landahl S, et al. A 15-year longitudinal study of blood pressure and dementia. Lancet 1996;347:1141–5.
100. Notkola IL, Sulkava R, Pekkanen J, et al. Serum total cholesterol, apolipoprotein E4, and Alzheimer's disease. Neuroepidemiology 1998;17:14–20.
101. Kivipelto M, Helkala EL, Hanninen T, et al. Midlife vascular risk factors and late-life mild cognitive impairment: a population-based study. Neurology 2001;56:1683–9.
102. Launer LJ, Ross GW, Petrovitch H, et al. Midlife blood pressure and dementia: the Honolulu-Asia aging study. Neurobiol Aging 2000;21:49–55.
103. Whitmer RA, Gunderson EP, Quesenberry CP Jr, et al. Body mass index in midlife and risk of Alzheimer disease and vascular dementia. Curr Alzheimer Res 2007;4: 103–9.
104. Fitzpatrick AK, Kuller LH, Lopez OL, et al. Midlife and late-life obesity and the risk of dementia: cardiovascular health study. Arch Neurol 2009;66;336–42.
105. Roberts RO, Geda YE, Knopman DS, et al. Association of duration and severity of diabetes mellitus with mild cognitive impairment. Arch Neurol 2008;65:1066–73.
106. Xu W, Qui C, Gatz M, et al. Mid- and late-life diabetes in relation to the risk of dementia: a population-based twin study. Diabetes 2009;58;71–7.

Physical Activity and Health During the Menopausal Transition

Barbara Sternfeld, PhD[a],*, Sheila Dugan, MD[b]

KEYWORDS

• Physical activity • Menopause • Symptoms • Weight gain
• Bone loss

Habitual participation in physical activity results in many health benefits, including increased longevity, decreased risk of cardiorespiratory and metabolic diseases and some cancers (most notably colon and breast), maintenance of energy balance, and improved musculoskeletal, functional and mental health.[1] The extensive evidence base demonstrating these beneficial effects suggests that they apply to the adult population as a whole, women as well as men and older as well as younger. However, the question of whether physical activity attenuates any of the adverse health effects that frequently accompany the menopausal transition, such as occurrence of vasomotor symptoms (VMS), increases in weight and body fat, decreases in bone density, and changes in mood and somatic symptoms, has not been fully explored. In this article, we review the existing literature relevant to this question, drawing on findings from the Study of Women's Health Across the Nation (SWAN) and other studies of midlife women's health.

PHYSICAL ACTIVITY AND VMS

Considerable uncertainty still exists regarding the role of physical activity in reducing the risk of developing hot flashes and night sweats and the efficacy of physical activity as a treatment for VMS. The first analysis of this question in SWAN found an inverse association between physical activity and the occurrence of VMS, independent of potential confounding variables, based on cross-sectional data from the initial screening survey of over 16,000 women, ages 40 to 55, of varying menopausal status.[2] However, this result was not confirmed in 2 subsequent SWAN analyses conducted in the SWAN cohort, which found neither a cross-sectional relation at baseline between physical activity and VMS[3] nor a longitudinal relation over 5 years

[a] Division of Research, Kaiser Permanente, 2000 Broadway, Oakland, CA 94612, USA
[b] Department of Physical Medicine and Rehabilitation and Preventive Medicine, Rush University Medical Center, 1725 W. Harrison Street, Suite 970, Chicago, IL 60612, USA
* Corresponding author.
E-mail address: bxs@dor.kaiser.org

Obstet Gynecol Clin N Am 38 (2011) 537–566
doi:10.1016/j.ogc.2011.05.008
0889-8545/11/$ – see front matter © 2011 Elsevier Inc. All rights reserved.

obgyn.theclinics.com

of follow-up.[4] In both of these studies, physical activity was associated with fewer VMS in bivariate analyses, but the association did not persist after adjustment for confounders, particularly body mass index (BMI) and overall health. Complicating the picture in SWAN even further, a report by Gold et al[5] from the Daily Hormone Study, a substudy of SWAN, found that physical activity was associated cross-sectionally with increased risk of VMS, but only in the relatively small group of women (n = 134) who had low or medium levels of the progesterone metabolite, pregnanediol-glucuronide.[5]

Part of the explanation for the inconsistency in the SWAN findings is owing to differences in the assessment of physical activity. In the cross-sectional survey, physical activity was assessed by a single global question that asked respondents to compare their physical activity relative with others their age and gender. An evaluation of this question within the SWAN sample revealed that this question seemed to rank women reasonably accurately in terms of physical activity within their respective race/ethnic group, but did not result in the expected differences in physical activity across different race/ethnic groups.[6] Because the reporting of VMS varies by race/ethnicity, this global question may have led to a biased finding owing to differential misclassification. In the cohort study, physical activity was assessed with the Kaiser Physical Activity Survey,[7] which provides a much more detailed measure of activity across several domains, including household and care giving, recreational sports and exercise, and active living behaviors, such as walking to work. It is likely that the Kaiser Physical Activity Survey yields a less biased estimate, and, therefore, a more valid measure of association with any outcome of interest, including VMS.

On the other hand, the inconsistency in the SWAN findings regarding the relationship between physical activity and VMS reflects the inconsistency in the literature as a whole. Of the more than 30 studies that have addressed the question of physical activity and the risk of VMS, more than half have reported no association (**Table 1** provides a description of selected studies). The remaining suggest a generally protective, inverse relation while a small number (n = 3)[8–10] report increased VMS with higher levels of activity. The vast majority of these studies are observational and cross-sectional in design and suffer from many of the limitations common to this type of study, including heterogeneous study samples with regard to menopause status,[11–14] too few women with frequent and severe symptoms,[12,14,15] too few women participating in regular activity of at least moderate intensity,[9,16] a lack of adequate control over confounding variables,[8,11] and inability to establish temporality.[17] In addition, establishing comparability across studies is challenging, given the assessments of physical activity that range from a single global question[18,19] to detailed recalls of duration, frequency, and mode of activity that allow for creation of summary scores in terms of metabolic equivalent (MET)-hours or -minutes a week.[9,13,16,20–22] The differences in the assessment of symptoms, with some studies considering frequency, severity and/or bother as separate domains,[9,12] others combining those domains into a single measure,[21,23] and still others considering only frequency,[3,4,24] add to this challenge.

Perhaps the strongest evidence for a protective association between physical activity and VMS in the observational data comes from one of the few prospective analyses, the longitudinal Melbourne Women's Midlife Health Project, in which 438 women were followed over an 8-year interval.[20] Although physical activity was not associated with VMS in this cohort at baseline,[13] women who reported exercising every day at baseline were 49% less likely to report bothersome hot flashes during follow-up (odds ratio, 0.51; 95% confidence interval, 0.27–0.96). Furthermore, women whose exercise level decreased over the follow-up were more likely to experience bothersome hot flashes. In contrast, another longitudinal, observational

Table 1
Selected studies of physical activity and vasomotor symptoms

Observational Studies

Reference	Study Design	Sample	Physical Activity Measure	Symptom Measure	Other Variables	Main Findings
Collins et al, 1995[11]	Cross-sectional survey	Population-based sample of 1,324 Swedish women, 48 yrs old, varying menopausal status	Participation in regular exercise (yes/no)	Menopause Symptom Inventory (frequency of symptoms on scale of 1–5)	—	No relation between physical activity and vasomotor symptoms; inverse relation with negative mood, direct relation with well-being
Daley et al, 2007[15]	Cross-sectional survey	1,206 British women, ages 46–55, from 10 general practices, based on purposeful sampling for location, level of deprivation and practice size	Regularly active or not based on stage of readiness for change in moderate intensity activity 3 or more times a week for 20 minutes of longer each time	Vasomotor symptoms and 8 other domains of health related quality of life from Women's Health Questionnaire	—	No relation between physical activity and vasomotor symptoms; inverse relation with depressed mood and somatic symptoms
Elavsky and McAuley, 2005[12]	Cross-sectional survey	133 women, ages 44–60, varying menopausal status	Aerobics Center Longitudinal Study Physical Activity Survey	Menopause Symptom List (frequency and severity of 25 symptoms)	Self-esteem, life satisfaction	Significant inverse association between exercise frequency and frequency and severity of VMS, somatic and total symptoms

(continued on next page)

Table 1
(continued)

Observational Studies

Reference	Study Design	Sample	Physical Activity Measure	Symptom Measure	Other Variables	Main Findings
Gold et al, 2004[3], Gold et al, 2006[4]	Prospective cohort study	3,302 racially/ethnically diverse women, ages 42–52, initially in pre- or early peri-menopause	Ordinal ranking of total activity, as measured by Kaiser Physical Activity Survey	Occurrence and frequency of VMS in past 2 weeks	BMI, health status, other confounders	No association between physical activity and VMS, either at baseline or over time
Guthrie et al, 1995[13]	Cross-sectional survey	1,181 Australian women, ages 45–55, of varying menopausal status	MLTPA questionnaires, assessing frequency, duration and intensity of recreational activities in past year	Overall symptoms	BMI, self-rated health	No association between physical activity and vasomotor symptoms or psychological well-being; physical activity directly related to overall health
Guthrie et al, 2005[20]	Prospective cohort study	438 Australian women, ages 45–55, pre-menopausal at baseline	Frequency of exercise on 7 point ordinal scale	Hot flash index based on frequency and severity in past 2 weeks, frequency and bother of somatic symptoms	Health status, BMI, menopausal status, other confounding variables	Daily exercise at baseline significantly associated with 49% lower risk of developing VMS during follow-up
Li and Holm 2003[24]	Cross-sectional survey	239 post-menopausal women	Usual Physical Activity questionnaire	Women's health Assessment scale	Use of hormone therapy	Non-significant trend for active women to report fewer symptoms than inactive women, within HT stratum (use/no use)

(continued on next page)

Table 1
(continued)

Observational Studies

Reference	Study Design	Sample	Physical Activity Measure	Symptom Measure	Other Variables	Main Findings
Moilanen et al, 2010[14]	Population-based cross-sectional survey based on a national health examination survey	1,427 Finnish women, ages 45–64, varying menopausal status	Single ordinal question about level of recreational physical activity	Occurrence and bother of various vasomotor, somatic and mood symptoms	Lifestyle factors, medical conditions, other confounding variables	Low physical activity associated with significantly more psychological, somatic and vasomotor symptoms, relative to high physical activity, independently of confounders
Romani et al, 2009[8]	Population-based cross-sectional survey	639 pre- or early-peri-menopausal women from Baltimore	Three-level categorical variable regarding usual physical activity (light, moderate, or heavy) at work, home, and for recreation	Frequency, severity and duration of hot flashes	BMI	High level of physical activity associated with increased risk of moderate or severe hot flashes (OR = 2.88, 95% CI, 1.12-7.40 for moderate, OR = 4.16, 95% CI, 18.08, for heavy, p for trend = 0.02) relative to low level, and with non-significant increased risk for any hot flashes, daily hot flashes and hot flashes for more than a year

(continued on next page)

Table 1
(continued)

Observational Studies

Reference	Study Design	Sample	Physical Activity Measure	Symptom Measure	Other Variables	Main Findings
Slaven and Lee 1997[106], Study I and Study II	Cross-sectional	220 Australian women of varying menopausal status in Study I; 47 Australian women of varying menopausal status who were regular exercisers for Study II	Regular exercise defined as participation in aerobic activity at least twice a week for 30 minutes a time for last 3 months; exercisers assessed immediately prior to work-out	Women's Health Questionnaire	Profile of Mood States	Study I: No relation between physical activity and vasomotor symptoms; inverse relation with depressed mood, anxiety, fears, fatigue, tension, problems with memory and concentration, sexual dysfunction, sleep problems; direct relation with vigor and perceived attractiveness Study II: Fewer vasomotor and somatic symptoms reported following exercise class, independent of change in mood
Sternfeld et al, 1999[16]	Case-control	Cases defined as women 48–52 years old, 3–12 months since LMP with frequent vasomotor symptoms (n = 82), controls same chronological and biological age without vasomotor symptoms (n = 89)	Activity score based on intensity of activity and frequency; separate scores for recreational, occupational and household activity	Case definition based on frequency of VMS	Psychological and somatic symptoms	No relation between physical activity and case status; activity attenuated relation between psychological and vasomotor symptoms

(continued on next page)

Table 1
(continued)

Observational Studies

Reference	Study Design	Sample	Physical Activity Measure	Symptom Measure	Other Variables	Main Findings
Van Poppel and Brown 2008[22]	Prospective cohort study	3,300 mid-life women participating in 3rd and 4th surveys of the Australian Longitudinal Study on Women's Health	Change in physical activity based on frequency, duration and intensity of usual physical activity	Vasomotor symptoms, somatic and psychological symptoms, total symptom score	Change in weight	No association between change in physical activity with total symptoms, fasomotor or psychological symptoms; significant, but modest, inverse association with somatic symptoms; weight gain associated with increased total, vasomotor and somatic symptoms and weight loss association with reduction in total and vasomotor symptoms
Whitcomb et al, 2007[9]	Cross-sectional survey	512 peri- and post-menopausal women in Baltimore metropolitan area	Historical physical activity (frequency of participation in moderate and vigorous activities at different ages; activity at 35–39 used to examine long-term effects	History of frequency of hot flashes, summarized as any menopausal hot flashes, daily hot flashes and any moderate or severe hot flashes	History of HT, smoking, BMI	High activity associated with increased risk of moderate to severe hot flashes (adjusted OR = 1.77, p = 0.01) and daily hot flashes (OR = 1.77, p = 0.01), relative to minimal activity; those highly active during 5 year age period prior to LMP had increased risk for moderate to severe hot flashes and for daily hot flashes compared to minimal activity

(continued on next page)

Table 1 (*continued*)

Observational Studies

Reference	Study Design	Sample	Physical Activity Measure	Symptom Measure	Other Variables	Main Findings
Wilbur et al, 1990[128]	Cross-sectional	386 Australian women between ages 34–62 volunteering for bone density study, varying menopausal status	Energy expenditure in recreational, occupational, and housework activity, based on Minnesota Leisure Time Physical Activity survey (LTPA)	Kaufert and Syrotuik Symptom Index (VMS and general health symptoms)	Aerobic fitness	No relation between physical activity and vasomotor symptoms; inverse relation between recreational activity and somatic symptoms and other general health symptoms; direct relation between occupational activity and same outcomes

(continued on next page)

Table 1
(continued)

Intervention Studies

Reference	Study Design	Sample	Physical Activity Measure	Symptom Measure	Other Variables	Main Findings
Aiello et al, 2004[10]	RCT of exercise vs stretching controls	173 sedentary post-menopausal women, ages 50–75, 87 exercisers vs 86 in stretching control group	45 mins moderate-intensity exercise, 5 days/wk for 12 months, 3 months facility-based training and 9 months home-based training	Occurrence and severity of VMS and other symptoms, assessed at baseline, 3, 6, 9 and 12 months	Body fat, sex hormones	No significant differences in occurrence of symptoms; non-significant decrease in occurrence of memory problems in exercise group, non-significant increase in risk of moderate-severe hot flashes (OR = 2.8, 95% CI, 0.8–9.3)
Elavsky and McAuley, 2007[27]	RCT of exercise vs yoga vs control	164 inactive, symptomatic women, ages 42–58, 63 to exercise, 62 to yoga and 39 to control	4 month walking program 3 times a week for an hour, intensity starting at 50% heart rate reserve (HRR), increased to 60–75% HRR; 4 month Iyengar yoga class 2 times a week for 90 mins/class	Greene Climacteric Scale	Fitness, body composition, affect, depression, Utian Quality of Life	Non-significant decreases in VMS in exercise and yoga groups relative to controls; significant increases in positive affect in exercise and yoga groups relative to controls; change in fitness was significant predictor of change in symptoms

(continued on next page)

Table 1
(continued)

Intervention Studies

Reference	Study Design	Sample	Physical Activity Measure	Symptom Measure	Other Variables	Main Findings
Huang et al, 2010[25]	RCT of behavioral weight loss program	338 overweight or obese women with urinary incontinence, 226 to intervention group and 112 to structured education control group	Based on Diabetes Prevention Program and Look AHEAD to achieve 7%–9% weight loss, physical activity goal was to increase to 200 minutes of moderate intensity exercise, mostly brisk walking	Bothersomeness of VMS and other symptoms, assessed at baseline and 56 months	Weight, waist circumference	Of those reporting any symptoms at baseline (n = 99 in intervention and n = 55 in control group), intervention resulted in more than a 2-fold likelihood of improvement in bother of flushing, relative to control group (OR = 2.3 , 95% CI, 1.2-4.2), but this was attenuated to non-significance when adjusted for change in body size; decreases in weight and abdominal circumference significantly associated with improvement in reporting of hot flashes

(continued on next page)

Table 1
(continued)

Intervention Studies

Reference	Study Design	Sample	Physical Activity Measure	Symptom Measure	Other Variables	Main Findings
Kemmler et al, 2004[32]	RCT to reduce menopause related bone loss	137 women, ages 48–60 and 1–8 years post-menopause with low BMD; analysis based on 50 in exercise group, 31 in control group who completed study	264 months of exercise 4/wk (2 facility-based group exercise and 2 home-based individual training), 25 minutes/session, including warm-up, endurance, jumping, strength and flexibility exercises	Frequency of hot flashes, other somatic and mood symptoms	Bone density, strength, endurance, blood lipids	Hot flashes improved in both groups with no significant between group difference; improvements in mood and insomnia in exercise group significantly different from no change in control group; significant improvements in fitness, BMD, and blood lipids
Lindh-Astrand et al, 2003[28]	RCT	75 sedentary, naturally post-menopausal women, ages 48–63 with VMS	12 weeks of exercise classes twice a week for 60 minutes, plus additional session on own	Daily frequency and severity of VMS for two weeks at beginning and at end of 12 weeks, plus baseline and follow-up for for one week monthly during extended 24 week follow-up	Kupperman Index, quality of life, mood and general psychological wellbeing	Non-significant decrease in number and severity of hot flashes in exercisers from baseline to 12 weeks; significant pre-post declines in symptom scale

(continued on next page)

Table 1
(continued)

Intervention Studies

Reference	Study Design	Sample	Physical Activity Measure	Symptom Measure	Other Variables	Main Findings
McAndrew et al, 2009[31]	RCT designed to test three different approaches to promotion of physical activity	280 inactive, healthy women, 113 with symptoms at follow-up	12 month three arm design with one arm addressing stage and processes of change in physical activity behavior with tailored feedback (n = 95) vs,educational booklet based on social cognitive theory (n = 93) vs health-related print material on sleep and nutrition (control, n = 92)	MENQOL, administered at month 12 follow-up visit	Self-reported physical activity, depression, exercise self-efficacy, stress	Change in physical activity not associated with VMS; change in PA inversely associated with total symptoms, psychosocial and physical symptoms

(continued on next page)

Table 1
(continued)

Intervention Studies

Reference	Study Design	Sample	Physical Activity Measure	Symptom Measure	Other Variables	Main Findings
Moriyama et al, 2008[29]	2 by 2 RCT of exercise and estrogen therapy	44 hysterectomized women	6 months of moderate aerobic exercise for3 hrs/wk plus hormone therapy (n = 9), exercise and placebo (n = 11), HT and no activity (n = 14) and placebo and no activity (n = 11)	Kupperman index	Health-related quality of life (SF-12)	All groups had declines in symptoms; physical activity significantly associated with increases in physical functioning and decreases in bodily pain relative to no activity, regardless of drug or placebo assignment
Villaverde-Gutierrez et al, 2006[30]	Quasi-experimental (random group assignment, pre-post differences	48 sedentary Spanish women, ages 55–72	12 month program of endurance (50–85% maximum HR), strengthening, flexibility and relaxation exercises, twice a week in supervised classes (n = 24) vs control group (n = 24)	Kupperman Index	Health-related quality of life	Significant decrease in severe symptoms from 50% to 37.5% in exercise group and significant increase in control group; significant improvement in HRQOL in exercise group but decrease in controls

(continued on next page)

Table 1
(continued)

Observational Studies

Reference	Study Design	Sample	Physical Activity Measure	Symptom Measure	Other Variables	Main Findings
Ueda, 2004[26]	Non-randomized intervention	35 sedentary, symptomatic Japanese women, ages 40–60, 20 in intervention group vs 15 in control group	12 week exercise and menopause education program of one 90 minute class/wk (30 minute lecture, 60 minutes of either aerobic or resistance exercise), plus aerobic exercise twice a week on own	Kupperman index	Quality of life, attitudes towards exercise	22.5% decrease in overall Kupperman index in treatment group vs no change in controls, $p < 0.5$; 32% decrease psychosomatic symptoms in treatment group vs 3% increase in controls, $p < .05$; non-significant decrease in VMS in intervention group vs control group
Wilbur et al, 2005[23]	RCT	173 sedentary, healthy Caucasian and African American women, ages 45–65	24 week home-based moderate intensity walking program (50–74% maximal HR), 4 times/ week for 30 minutes at a time (n = 97) vs control (n = 66)	Frequency, severity and bother of VMS and other symptoms	BMI	Significant improvement in symptoms in both groups with no differences between groups; adherence to intervention led to significant improvement in sleep symptoms relative to controls

study, also of Australian women (but not the same cohort), failed to find any association between change in physical activity over time and reporting of VMS.[22]

In recent years, a number of intervention studies have tested the effect of physical activity (generally aerobic exercise and most often walking) on VMS. Here again, findings, summarized in the second half of Table 1, are inconsistent, with several reporting no effect,[23,25] one reporting a nonsignificant increase in hot flash severity in the exercisers compared with the controls,[10] and several reporting reductions in frequency and severity of VMS.[26–28] However, as with the observational studies, most of the trials also suffer from methodologic weaknesses, including very small sample sizes,[26,29–31] nonrandomized designs,[26,30,31] inadequately specified exercise dose,[31] and large loss to follow-up.[32] In one of the more carefully controlled trials, a 4-month intervention among 164 previously sedentary women randomized either to a walking group, yoga, or a control group[27] led to a decrease in VMS in both the walking and yoga arms relative to the control group, but the differences were not significant. In this study, change in symptoms seemed to be mediated by increases in physical fitness, such that women who had the greatest increase in fitness were most likely to have the greatest decrease in symptoms.[27]

Despite the equivocal evidence for a protective effect of physical activity on VMS, the hypothesis remains compelling, partly because physical activity is a generally beneficial intervention with few risks or side effects, partly because the hypothesis has not yet been adequately tested, and partly because there are plausible biological mechanisms by which activity could alleviate VMS. Although the etiology of the hot flash is still not fully understood, neuroendocrine processes at the level of the hypothalamus are implicated.[33] Physical activity, in turn, has a range of neuroendocrine responses that occur, both acutely, as a result of a single bout of exercise, and chronically, as a result of exercise training. Increases in brain norepinephrine and its metabolites occur in response to acute exercise,[34,35] but 24-hour urinary norepinephrine seems to decrease with training,[36] perhaps because of an increase in vagal tone. Decreases in resting heart rate and heart rate variability are a near universal response to aerobic exercise training[37,38] and are typically ascribed to increased vagal output and a resulting shift in autonomic balance in favor of the parasympathetic nervous system.[39]

Because stress seems to be a precipitating factor in hot flashes[40,41] and neuroendocrine substances, such as catecholamines and cortisol, are involved in the stress response and affect thermoregulation at the level of the hypothalamus,[42] hot flashes may result from an imbalance in the autonomic nervous system, in which the "stress-buffering" role of the parasympathetic nervous system is not adequate to counter the increased activation of the sympathetic nervous system.[43,44] If this is true, then the shift in that balance as a result of exercise training is a potential mechanism by which exercise could reduce the occurrence of VMS.

A second potential mechanism by which physical activity could have a favorable effect on the frequency or bother of VMS is through the release of endogenous opioids, particularly β-endorphins, that occurs in response to a single, sustained bout of vigorous exercise.[45–47] The evidence for a role of β-endorphins in the pathogenesis of the hot flash comes primarily from animal studies, in which administration of naloxone, an opiate antagonist, in the morphine-dependent rat, causes symptoms similar to those of the hot flash, including a sudden increase in peripheral tail temperature and an luteinizing hormone (LH) surge.[48,49] However, human experiments involving the infusion of naloxone in postmenopausal women have not consistently reduced the frequency of hot flashes or LH pulses,[50,51] and studies of plasma β-endorphin levels before hot flashes have been contradictory,[52,53] although plasma levels may not reflect the endorphin levels in the brain. It is not currently known whether β-endorphins are responsible for the so-called runner's high,[54] but the endogenous opioids are biochemically similar to exogenous opiates and have diverse physiologic effects, including temperature regulation (hypothermia), decreased sensitivity to pain, and decreased heart and respiratory rate, all of which could be responsible for a decrease in either frequency or bother of VMS.

Finally, physical activity could "distract" women from attention on their hot flashes by habituating them to the feelings of increased heat and heat dissipation through sweating that accompanies increases in physical effort and associating those feelings with behaviors that may make them feel good in other ways. This is similar to the "distraction" theory of how physical activity improves mental health and sense of well-being.[55] On the other hand, given the acute rise in core temperature that occurs with exercise, exercise might actually induce hot flashes, particularly if symptomatic women have a narrowed thermoregulatory zone that lowers their threshold for sweating.[56]

Given these plausible biological mechanisms and the absence of methodologically rigorous studies, it is still not possible to draw firm conclusions about the efficacy of physical activity as a treatment for VMS. Many questions remain unanswered: Does participation in regular physical activity matter at all in terms of frequency, severity, or bother of hot flashes or even length of time for which VMS persist? If so, does exercise make VMS better or worse? Does the "dose" of physical activity matter? Is more vigorous intensity exercise more effective than moderate intensity exercise, and are there any differences by mode of exercise (aerobic vs resistance exercise vs mind–body disciplines)? And if physical activity is effective, how does it work? Well-designed and sufficiently powered randomized trials are required to answer these questions adequately. The Menopause Symptoms: Finding Lasting Answers for Symptoms and Health Research Network is currently conducting such a trial, in which 112 previously sedentary women with frequent and bothersome hot flashes randomized to moderate-to-vigorous aerobic exercise for 12 weeks will be compared with 150 women in a usual activity control group. The findings from this carefully designed and controlled trial, in which women participate in facility-based, individual exercise training at a prescribed target heart rate and constant caloric expenditure, relative to body weight, should provide unique and definitive evidence regarding the efficacy of physical activity for treating VMS that has been lacking up to this point. It represents an important step forward in closing the gap in our knowledge regarding this question.

PHYSICAL ACTIVITY AND CHANGES IN BODY SIZE AND COMPOSITION

On-going adult weight gain[57,58] and the high prevalence of obesity[59,60] are issues that loom large for the population as a whole. They are of particular concern for women during the menopausal transition, when many may not only be gaining weight, but are also experiencing changes in body composition and fat distribution. A number of studies of midlife women find an annual rate of weight gain of about 0.5 kg or more,[61–65] but the evidence suggests that weight gain per se is more a function of aging than of the hormonal changes that define menopause.[61,62,64,66] This conclusion comes both from cross-sectional comparisons of weight in women of similar chronological age but varying menopausal status (premenopausal, early perimenopausal, late perimenopausal, or postmenopausal, and surgically menopausal), as well as from longitudinal studies that examine rate of weight change over time by change in menopausal status.

A number of different analyses in SWAN support this conclusion. For instance, a comparison of BMI among the more than 16,000 women who participated in the cross-sectional screening survey found no difference between premenopausal and postmenopausal women after adjusting for chronological age and other covariates.[67] Similarly, in a cross-sectional ancillary study of energy expenditure, body composition and menopausal status conducted at the Kaiser/UC Davis SWAN site at the 5-year follow-up visit for the SWAN longitudinal cohort, the median weight of the Chinese premenopausal and early perimenopausal women was not statistically different from that of the late perimenopausal and postmenopausal women [56.7 kg (interquartile range [IQR]), 50.3–61.5 vs 53.8 kg (IQR, 50.0–63.2), respectively; $P = .51$).[68] The median weight among the white women, although significantly higher than the Chinese, also did not differ by menopausal status [71.7 kg (IQR, 60.5–82.0) for premenopause and early perimenopause vs 68.2 kg (IQR, 56.9–79.0); $P = .21$). In addition, in the SWAN cohort as a whole, mean weight gain over 3 years of follow-up was 2.1 kg (standard deviation. 4.8) overall, and was not associated with menopausal status.[61]

In contrast, changes in body composition (increased fat mass and decreased lean mass) and in fat distribution (from a more gynoid pattern to a more android pattern) do seem to be influenced by the menopausal transition, as well as by chronological aging.[69–73] As discussed by Wildman and Sowers in this issue, a longitudinal analysis of 7-year changes in body composition, assessed by bioelectrical impedance at the Michigan SWAN site, showed substantial weight gain (3.4% or 2.9 kg over 6 years), significant increases in fat mass (10.1% or 3.4 kg), small but significant losses of skeletal muscle mass (1.06% or 0.23 kg), and a 6.2% (5.6 cm) increase in waist circumference.[74] The change in weight was linear, suggesting only an age effect, whereas the changes in fat mass and skeletal muscle mass were more curvilinear over time, suggesting a menopause effect. Interestingly, although change in body composition did not vary by menopausal stage, as defined by bleeding criteria, increases in fat mass and in waist circumference and decreases in skeletal muscle mass were significantly associated with increasing follicle-stimulating hormone levels, independent of age, indicating an independent and significant menopause effect.

Despite the seeming inevitability of these changes in weight, body composition, and fat distribution with age and menopause, physical activity may attenuate the impact of both of these factors. To begin with, more active individuals tend to be leaner than sedentary individuals at any given point in time,[75] which means that active midlife women have an advantage as they enter the menopausal transition in terms of starting out with a lower BMI, lower fat mass, greater lean mass, and less central adiposity. The site-specific Energy Expenditure SWAN study demonstrated this, particularly for the white women, in whom there was a strong, cross-sectional, inverse dose response relation between physical activity measured by accelerometry and both percent body fat and waist circumference.[68]

Second, physical activity may slow the rate of change of weight, both with menopause and over time. In a longitudinal analysis of the SWAN cohort, physical activity was inversely associated with changes in weight and waist circumference, independent of aging and change in menopausal status.[61] Women whose activity decreased the most experienced the greatest increases in weight and waist circumference, whereas those whose physical activity was essentially stable experienced much smaller increases (**Figs. 1** and **2**). This pattern was true for both sports and exercise and lifestyle physical activity.

In addition, physical activity, although not entirely preventing weight gain with age, may protect against the development of obesity. This conclusion is suggested by the observation in SWAN of a 9% decrease in risk of obesity (odds ratio, 0.91; 95% confidence interval, 0.84–0.98) over a 9-year follow-up associated with a one unit higher level of baseline total physical activity, after adjustment for numerous con-

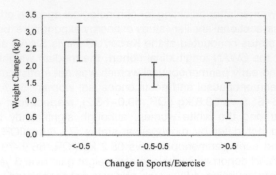

Fig. 1. Change in weight associated with change in sports and exercise, adjusted for multiple confounding variables.

founding factors.[76] Furthermore, a 1-unit increase in activity over time was independently associated with an even greater reduction in risk (odds ratio, 0.83; 95% confidence interval, 0.72–0.95). Finally, physical activity may protect against the accumulation not only of overall fat, but of intra-abdominal fat, which may be the most metabolically harmful type of fat. In a site-specific study conducted at the Chicago SWAN site, intra-abdominal fat, assessed by computed tomography, was significantly inversely associated with total physical activity (4.0 cm^2 for every 1-unit increase in physical activity score), independent of total percent fat and other covariates.[77] Compared with those women engaging in a level of physical activity approximating the current recommendations for general health (150 minutes a week of moderate intensity activity),[1] less active women had significantly greater amounts of intra-abdominal fat, regardless of menopausal status, but did not differ in terms of the level of subcutaneous abdominal fat (**Fig. 3**).

Other studies of midlife women confirm the protective role of physical activity against excess weight gain.[62,78] Most notably, in a recent analysis of weight changes over 13 years of follow-up, different levels of activity were examined to clarify the amount of physical activity required for prevention of unhealthful weight gain.[79] Although women expending 21 MET-hours or more a week (approximately equal to 60 minutes a day of moderate intensity activity) began at a lower weight than those expending between 7.5 and 21 and those expending fewer than 7.5 MET-hours per week (less than the recommended amount of 150 minutes a week of moderate

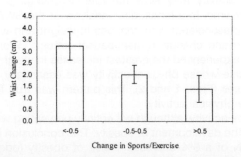

Fig. 2. Change in waist associated with change in sports and exercise, adjusted for multiple confounding variables.

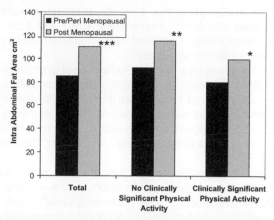

Fig. 3. Mean IAF associated with physical activity by menopausal status and level of physical activity approximating current guidelines.

intensity activity), the rate of weight gain in all 3 groups was essentially the same. However, in a fully adjusted model, the amount of weight gain was significantly greater in the 2 less active groups, relative to the most active group, particularly among women of normal weight to begin with. Finally, in the small group of women who maintained normal weight throughout the course of the study, the mean amount of physical activity was 21.5 MET-hours per week, which is equivalent to the recommendation for weight maintenance put forth by the Institute of Medicine in 2002 (60 minutes a day of moderate intensity activity).[80] These findings suggest the importance of sustaining relatively high levels of physical activity starting in young adulthood to maintain normal weight through middle age, menopause, and beyond.

PHYSICAL ACTIVITY AND BONE DENSITY

The impact of the menopausal transition on bone mineral density (BMD) and risk of osteoporotic fractures, along with the insights into this concern that have come from SWAN, is discussed elsewhere in this volume by Lo et al. Regular physical activity is among the primary determinants of BMD and is a key contributor to overall musculoskeletal health, because of the responsiveness of bone to the mechanical forces that physical activities places on it.[81] Both weight-bearing endurance activities, such as walking and running, and resistance exercises elicit this response, especially at the lumbar spine and femoral neck.[82-86] Although the increase in BMD observed in exercise intervention studies in response to physical activity is modest (about 1%–2%), animal studies have shown that this is accompanied by a large increase in the resistance of the bone to fracture.[1] This is in contrast with pharmacologic agents, in which the improvement in resistance of the bone is proportional to the improvement in BMD.[87]

The evidence for increased BMD in response to physical activity comes from a large number of cross-sectional studies,[88] exercise training studies,[89-91] and meta-analyses.[83,86,86,92-95] In SWAN, a baseline, cross-sectional analysis of the relation between domain-specific physical activity and BMD at the lumbar spine, femoral hip, and total hip concluded that home and care-giving activity was positively associated with BMD, independent of other types of activity and other confounding variables.[96] Spine and femoral BMD were both 1.7% greater in the highest tertile of home/care-giving activity than in the lowest tertile. Similarly, the highest tertile of sports and exercise was associated with 2.1% greater spine BMD and 2.6% greater femoral neck BMD than the lowest tertile. In contrast, neither lifestyle activity or occupational activity had a significant relation with BMD.

To date, the evidence is less clear about whether or not physical activity attenuates age-related loss of BMD.[1] Several prospective, observational studies suggest that higher levels of physical activity at baseline are independently associated with higher BMD many years later[97,98] and with less loss of BMD over time.[99,100] They also suggest that maintenance of regular physical activity over time results in attenuated bone loss, compared with reduced physical activity or consistently sedentary behavior.[97,98,101,102]

Few, if any, studies have specifically examined the role of physical activity on the rate of bone loss during the menopausal transition, a time when bone loss accelerates, relative to the premenopausal or later postmenopausal period. With 10 years of follow-up, during which time most of the SWAN cohort has transitioned to postmenopause, there is now adequate statistical power to address this question and such an analysis is currently underway.

PHYSICAL ACTIVITY AND OTHER SYMPTOMS IN MIDLIFE WOMEN

In addition to VMS, other symptoms, such as joint pain and stiffness, fatigue, difficulty concentrating, poor sleep, irritability, and depression, are quite prevalent among midlife women, even though they are not directly associated with the menopause.[103,104] In the SWAN cross-sectional survey, for instance, joint pain and stiffness were reported by more than 50% of the respondents, and difficulty sleeping was reported by just under 40%, although the prevalence of both of these complaints did not differ by menopausal status.[2] Nevertheless, these symptoms may adversely impact the health of midlife women and decrease functioning and overall quality of life. The benefits of physical activity for ameliorating somatic and mood symptoms are well-documented and suggest another way in which regular physical activity may preserve and improve health in perimenopausal women.

Somatic Symptoms, Bodily Pain, Physical Functioning, and Quality of Life

Many of the studies cited that explored the influence of physical activity on VMS also considered a variety of somatic symptoms, ranging from headaches and joint pain to heart palpitations. In general, the findings suggest an inverse relation between greater levels of physical activity and lower rates of somatic complaints and fewer difficulties with sleep.[11,23,105–108] In a relatively recent, cross-sectional analysis of menopause symptoms and lifestyle among Finnish women, for instance, women who were regularly active reported significantly fewer somatic symptoms and less pain, relative to women who were sedentary.[14] Similarly, in a large cross-sectional survey of physical activity, BMI, and health-related quality of life in British women, the mean somatic symptom score was 28% lower among active women.[15] In addition, in a longitudinal analysis based on 3300 Australian women, increases in physical activity over time were associated with decreases in somatic symptoms.[22] Similarly, in a randomized trial designed to increase physical activity behavior, women who increased their activity reported fewer total menopausal symptoms (measured by the MENQOL) at follow-up, although symptoms were not measured at baseline,[31] making it impossible to determine whether change in activity led to change in symptoms.

There is also considerable evidence that physical activity reduces feelings of bodily pain in general, and pain associated with osteoarthritis[109] and low back problems.[110] Several findings from SWAN reveal important relationships among bodily pain, menopausal status, and physical activity. At the baseline SWAN examination, the level of pain reported was higher among women in early perimenopause, relative to premenopause, but this difference did not remain after adjustment for multiple confounding variables.[111] Furthermore, a longitudinal analysis of the SWAN cohort over 7 years of follow-up demonstrated that women who were more physically active at midlife experienced less bodily pain over time regardless of change in menopausal status, sociodemographic status, or medical conditions.[112] In contrast, when pain was defined as a composite variable of aches and pains that included quantity of pain, interference from pain with work or sleep, stiffness and soreness, and low backaches or pain, postmenopausal women had significantly higher pain scores (more pain), relative to premenopausal women, even with adjustment for age, race/ethnicity, medical conditions, BMI, smoking, and depressive symptoms.[113] This study, unfortunately, did not also examine the impact of physical activity. However, a subsequent longitudinal SWAN analysis by this same investigator showed that higher baseline physical activity score was independently associated with a 7% increased likelihood of high physical role functioning and a 10% greater likelihood of a low bodily pain score.[114] Interestingly, the association between physical activity and physical role functioning seemed to be mediated by level of pain.

Evidence also suggests that physical activity improves physical function, not only in the elderly,[115,116] but also in the middle aged.[117] In SWAN, an analysis of the association between menopausal status and functional limitations based on the cross-sectional survey reported that almost 20% of the women reported some or substantial physical functioning limitations, and that the likelihood of physical limitations was significantly greater among postmenopausal women.[118] Although that analysis did not consider physical activity, a longitudinal follow-up of the SWAN women at the Chicago site observed that, although the transition through menopause was associated with a decline in grip and pinch strength, greater physical activity was the strongest predictor of increased grip and pinch strength.[119]

Finally, there is increasing evidence that physical activity enhances overall quality of life in the population as a whole as well as in patient populations, such as breast cancer survivors.[120] In the SWAN cohort, physical activity at baseline was significantly associated with reduced risk of impairment in health-related quality of life, as measured by the SF-12 for all 5 of the domains (role—physical, bodily pain, vitality, role—emotional, and social function),[111] as well as with lower risk of impairment in these domains over time,[112] independent of BMI, race/ethnicity, and other factors. Importantly, a recent randomized trial of several different doses of exercise conducted among sedentary postmenopausal women found a strong dose–response relation between volume of exercise and improvements in mental and physical aspects of quality of life, measured by the SF-36, and this finding was not accounted for by weight change.[121]

On the other hand, it is important to note that sports and exercise can cause acute activity-related musculoskeletal injuries, especially in deconditioned individuals or those with chronic injuries.[122] Obese individuals with knee osteoarthritis, for example, may experience transient increases in pain immediately after exercise that decreases later in the day to below initial levels.[123] These observations suggest a U-shaped dose–response curve for physical activity and pain, in which moderate activity decreases pain, relative to no or low activity, whereas excessive activity (for the specific individual) results in increased pain. In working with individual patients, it is important for clinicians to keep this possible U-shaped curve in mind.

Mood

Another significant benefit of regular physical activity is enhanced mental health, including protection against the onset of depressive and anxiety symptoms and disorders, reductions in existing symptoms of depression, anxiety and distress, and enhanced feelings of well-being.[1] This evidence comes both from population-based, prospective cohort studies, and from randomized clinical trials (for a review of specific studies, see the Report from Physical Activity Guidelines Advisory Committee[1]). Both psychological and physiologic mechanisms, including increased levels of neurotransmitters (specifically, dopamine and serotonin), and enhanced brain aminergic synaptic transmission,[124] increased endorphin secretion,[125] distraction from stressful stimuli,[55] and improved self-efficacy and self-esteem, may be responsible for these observed protective effects.[126]

Many of the studies of physical activity and symptoms in midlife women discussed previously also examined associations between physical activity and a range of mood states. Unlike the evidence regarding physical activity and VMS, the observational studies consistently show that physical activity is directly related to positive mood, vigor, and general well-being[11,12,15,105,107,127,128] and inversely related to negative symptoms, such as depression, anxiety, and perceived stress.[11,23,105–107] Evidence also suggests that increasing physical activity may improve mood and well-being, not only in midlife women with clinically meaningful symptoms of depression and anxiety, but in the general population as well. In the Melbourne Women's Midlife Health Project, change in physical activity over a 3-year follow-up period was positively related to change in well-being, although this was only a marginally significant finding.[129] Similarly, in an intervention study of sedentary midlife African-American women using a community-based walking program, adherence to walking was associated with lower depressive symptoms.[130] These observations are supported by randomized trials as well, which show that women in the exercise groups report improvements in mood symptoms, relative to controls.[26,27,30,31]

Still unaddressed is the issue of whether physical activity can attenuate the risk of depressive symptomatology or other negative mood states associated with the menopausal transition itself, particularly in susceptible women. In SWAN, within woman changes in menopausal status from premenopause onwards were independently associated with increased risk of a high level of depressive symptoms, suggestive of clinical depression, although the impact of these changes was of a lesser magnitude than that of various health-related and psychosocial factors, such as having VMS or experiencing stressful life events.[131] Although not undertaken to date, SWAN is in a position to examine whether physical activity is another factor independently associated with depressive symptoms and whether it may act as either a mediator or moderator of the effect of change in menopausal status. Hopefully, SWAN will, in the future, provide this type of insight into how lifestyle behavior might diminish the risk of mood changes during the menopause.

PHYSICAL ACTIVITY AND RISK OF BREAST CANCER

Cancer, particularly breast cancer, which has an increase in incidence rate after menopause, relative to premenopause, is another adverse outcome relevant to perimenopausal women that may be positively influenced by regular physical activity. A large body of observational studies suggests that women who are regularly active have a 25% to 30% lower risk of developing postmenopausal breast cancer than women who are inactive.[132] There is also a reduction in risk for premenopausal breast cancer, although the magnitude is less (about 20%–25%).[132] In addition, a growing body of literature suggests that physical activity after a breast cancer diagnosis and treatment is associated with lower rates of recurrence[133] and lower risk of all-cause mortality.[134,135] Potential mechanisms that may account for these observations include lower levels of circulating endogenous hormones, such as estrogen, sex hormone–binding globulin, and insulin-like growth factors, better maintenance of energy balance, and enhanced immune function.[136,137]

Although the SWAN cohort is too small to provide adequate numbers of breast cancer cases for any meaningful study of the disease, a SWAN ancillary study used measures of mammographic density, a powerful risk factor for breast cancer itself, and perhaps an intermediate marker of the disease, to examine the effect of hormonal status and sociodemographic, reproductive, and lifestyle factors on breast cancer risk among perimenopausal women. Both percent density and area of density were inversely associated with physical activity in all domains (sports/exercise, lifestyle activity, and home/care-giving activity), except for occupational activity, but these relationships were not significant after multiple adjustment for confounding factors.[138] Physical activity was also not associated with change in dense area over time, although it was inversely related to change in non-dense area.[139] Together, these findings do not provide any strong support for the hypothesis that the reduction in breast cancer risk associated with physical activity operates through the mechanism of mammographic density.

CLINICAL AND PUBLIC HEALTH IMPLICATIONS

Based on the SWAN findings described, and on many, many other studies,[1] physical activity is a potent tool for health promotion and disease prevention in perimenopausal women as well as in the population as a whole. Unfortunately, less than half of the population regularly participates in physical activity at even the minimal level required for health benefits, and adherence to physical activity guidelines is even lower among women ages 40 to 60.[140] This proportion may be even lower, depending on how physical activity is assessed.[141] This presents a clear mandate to clinicians and public health professionals alike. All clinicians should prescribe regular physical activity to their patients and should be prepared to discuss and problem solve with their patients the barriers that exist to becoming more physically active (for information and resources for the Exercise is Medicine initiative, go to www.exerciseismedicine.org). Public health professionals need to continue and enhance their ongoing efforts to promote physical activity among midlife women, particularly in women of minority race/ethnicity and women with disabilities and chronic health conditions. Even if regular physical activity does not prevent or treat VMS, the other health benefits that it confers on midlife women will ensure both a healthy menopausal transition and healthy aging.

REFERENCES

1. US Department of Health and Human Services, Office of Disease Prevention and Health Promotion. Physical Activity Guidelines Advisory Committee Report. Washington (DC): US Department of Health and Human Services, Office of Disease Prevention and Health Promotion; 2008.
2. Gold EB, Sternfeld B, Kelsey JL, et al. Relation of demographic and lifestyle factors to symptoms in a multi-racial/ethnic population of women 40-55 years of age. Am J Epidemiol 2000;152:463–73.
3. Gold EB, Block G, Crawford S, et al. Lifestyle and demographic factors in relation to vasomotor symptoms: baseline results from the Study of Women's Health Across the Nation. Am J Epidemiol 2004;159:1189–99.

4. Gold EB, Colvin A, Avis N, et al. Longitudinal analysis of the association between vasomotor symptoms and race/ethnicity across the menopausal transition: study of women's health across the nation. Am J Public Health 2006;96:1226–35.

5. Gold EB, Lasley B, Crawford SL, et al. Relation of daily urinary hormone patterns to vasomotor symptoms in a racially/ethnically diverse sample of midlife women: study of women's health across the nation. Reprod Sci 2007;14:786–97.

6. Sternfeld B, Cauley J, Harlow S, et al. Assessment of physical activity with a single global question in a large, multi-ethnic sample of midlife women. Am J Epidemiol 2000;152:678–87.

7. Sternfeld B, Ainsworth BE, Quesenberry CP. Physical activity patterns in a diverse population of women. Prev Med 1999;28:313–23.

8. Romani WA, Gallicchio L, Flaws JA. The association between physical activity and hot flash severity, frequency, and duration in mid-life women. Am J Hum Biol 2009;21:127–9.

9. Whitcomb BW, Whiteman MK, Langenberg P, et al. Physical activity and risk of hot flashes among women in midlife. J Womens Health (Larchmt) 2007;16:124–33.

10. Aiello EJ, Yasui Y, Tworoger SS, et al. Effect of a yearlong, moderate-intensity exercise intervention on the occurrence and severity of menopause symptoms in postmenopausal women. Menopause 2004;11:382–8.

11. Collins A, Landgren BM. Reproductive health, use of estrogen and experience of symptoms in perimenopausal women: a population-based study. Maturitas 1995; 20:101–11.

12. Elavsky S, McAuley E. Physical activity, symptoms, esteem, and life satisfaction during menopause. Maturitas 2005;52:374–85.

13. Guthrie JR, Smith AMA, Dennerstein L, et al. Physical activity and the menopause experience. Maturitas 1995;20:71–80.

14. Moilanen J, Aalto AM, Hemminki E, et al. Prevalence of menopause symptoms and their association with lifestyle among Finnish middle-aged women. Maturitas 2010; 67:368–74.

15. Daley A, MacArthur C, Stokes-Lampard H, et al. Exercise participation, body mass index, and health-related quality of life in women of menopausal age. Br J Gen Pract 2007;57:130–5.

16. Sternfeld B, Quesenberry CP Jr, Husson G. Habitual physical activity and menopausal symptoms: a case-control study. J Womens Health 1999;8:115–23.

17. Armstrong BK, White E, Saracci R. Principles of Exposure Measurement in Epidemiology. Oxford: Oxford University Press; 1994.

18. Gold EB, Sternfeld B, Kelsey JL, et al. Relation of demographic and lifestyle factors to symptoms in a multi-racial/ethnic population of women 40-55 years of age. Am J Epidemiol 2000;152:463–73.

19. Hyde RE, Inui TS, Kleinman K, et al. Differential association of modifiable health behaviors with hot flashes in perimenopausal and postmenopausal women. J Gen Intern Med 2004;19:740–6.

20. Guthrie JR, Dennerstein L, Taffe JR, et al. Hot flushes during the menopause transition: a longitudinal study in Australian-born women. Menopause 2005;12: 460–7.

21. Thurston RC, Joffe H, Soares CN, et al. Physical activity and risk of vasomotor symptoms in women with and without a history of depression: results from the Harvard Study of Moods and Cycles. Menopause 2006;13:553–60.

22. van Poppel MN, Brown WJ. "It's my hormones, doctor" – does physical activity help with menopausal symptoms? Menopause 2008;15:78–85.

23. Wilbur J, Miller AM, McDevitt J, et al. Menopausal status, moderate-intensity walking, and symptoms in midlife women. Res Theory Nurs Pract 2005;19:163–80.
24. Li S, Holm K. Physical activity alone and in combination with hormone replacement therapy on vasomotor symptoms in postmenopausal women. West J Nurs Res 2003;25:274–88.
25. Huang AJ, Subak LL, Wing R, et al. An intensive behavioral weight loss intervention and hot flushes in women. Arch Intern Med 2010;170:1161–7.
26. Ueda M. A 12-week structured education and exercise program improved climacteric symptoms in middle-aged women. J Physiol Anthropol Appl Human Sci 2004;23:143–8.
27. Elavsky S, McAuley E. Physical activity and mental health outcomes during menopause: a randomized controlled trial. Ann Behav Med 2007;33:132–42.
28. Lindh-Astrand L, Nedstrand E, Wyon Y, et al. Vasomotor symptoms and quality of life in previously sedentary postmenopausal women randomised to physical activity or estrogen therapy. Maturitas 2004;48:97–105.
29. Moriyama CK, Oneda B, Bernardo FR, et al. A randomized, placebo-controlled trial of the effects of physical exercises and estrogen therapy on health-related quality of life in postmenopausal women. Menopause 2008;15:613–8.
30. Villaverde-Gutierrez C, Araujo E, Cruz F, et al. Quality of life of rural menopausal women in response to a customized exercise programme. J Adv Nurs 2006;54:11–9.
31. McAndrew LM, Napolitano MA, Albrecht A, et al. When, why and for whom there is a relationship between physical activity and menopause symptoms. Maturitas 2009;64:119–25.
32. Kemmler W, Lauber D, Weineck J, et al. Benefits of 2 years of intense exercise on bone density, physical fitness, and blood lipids in early postmenopausal osteopenic women: results of the Erlangen Fitness Osteoporosis Prevention Study (EFOPS). Arch Intern Med 2004;164:1084–91.
33. Miller HG, Li RM. Measuring hot flashes: summary of a National Institutes of Health workshop. Mayo Clin Proc 2004;79:777–81.
34. Dunn A, Reigle T, Youngstedt S, et al. Brain norepinephrine and metabolites after treadmill training and wheel running in rats. Med Sci Sports Exerc 1996;28
35. Dunn AL, Dishman RK. Exercise and the neurobiology of depression. Exerc Sports Sci Rev 1991;19:41–98.
36. Rouveix M, Duclos M, Gouarne C, et al. The 24 h urinary cortisol/cortisone ratio and epinephrine/norepinephrine ratio for monitoring training in young female tennis players. Int J Sports Med 2006;27:856–63.
37. Sandercock GR, Bromley PD, Brodie DA. Effects of exercise on heart rate variability: inferences from meta-analysis. Med Sci Sports Exerc 2005;37:433–9.
38. Jurca R, Church TS, Morss GM, et al. Eight weeks of moderate-intensity exercise training increases heart rate variability in sedentary postmenopausal women. Am Heart J 2004;147:e21.
39. Jackson DM, Reilly JJ, Kelly LA, et al. Objectively measured physical activity in a representative sample of 3- to 4-year-old children. Obes Res 2003;11:420–5.
40. Swartzman LC, Edelberg R, Kemmann E. Impact of stress on objectively recorded menopausal hot flashes and on flush report bias. Health Psychol 1990;9:529–45.
41. Thurston RC, Blumenthal JA, Babyak MA, et al. Emotional antecedents of hot flashes during daily life. Psychosom Med 2005;67:137–46.
42. Rebar RW, Spitzer IB. The physiology and measurement of hot flushes. Am J Obstet Gynecol 1987;156:1284–8.

43. Berntson GG, Bigger JT Jr, Eckberg DL, et al. Heart rate variability: origins, methods, and interpretive caveats. Psychophysiology 1997;34:623–48.

44. Watkins LL, Grossman P, Krishnan R, et al. Anxiety and vagal control of heart rate. Psychosom Med 1998;60:498–502.

45. Boecker H, Sprenger T, Spilker ME, et al. The runner's high: opioidergic mechanisms in the human brain. Cereb Cortex 2008;18:2523–31.

46. Harber VJ, Sutton JR, MacDougall JD, et al. Plasma concentrations of beta-endorphin in trained eumenorrheic and amenorrheic women. Fertil Steril 1997;67:648–53.

47. Heitkamp HC, Huber W, Scheib K. Beta-endorphin and adrenocorticotrophin after incremental exercise and marathon running—female responses. Eur J Appl Physiol Occup Physiol 1996;72:417–24.

48. Simpkins JW, Katovich MJ, Song IC. Similarities between morphine withdrawal in the rat and the menopausal hot flush. Life Sci 1983;32:1957–66.

49. Simpkins JW, Katovich MJ. An animal model for pharmacologic evaluation of the menopausal hot flush. In: Notelovitz M, van Keep P, editors. Boston: MTP Press Ltd.; 1985. p. 213–51.

50. Lightman SL, Jacobs HS, Maguire AK, et al. Climacteric flushing: clinical and endocrine response to infusion of naloxone. Br J Obstet Gynaecol 1981;88:919–24.

51. DeFazio J, Verheugen C, Chetkowski R, et al. The effects of naloxone on hot flashes and gonadotropin secretion in postmenopausal women. J Clin Endocrinol Metab 1984;58:578–81.

52. Tepper R, Neri A, Kaufman H, et al. Menopausal hot flushes and plasma B-endorphins. Obstet Gynecol 1987;70:150–2.

53. Genazzani AR, Petraglia F, Facchinetti F, et al. Increase of proopiomelanocortin-related peptides during subjective menopausal flushes. Am J Obstet Gynecol 1984;149:775–9.

54. Dishman RK, O'Connor PJ. Lessons in exercise neurobiology: the case of endorphins. Ment Health Phys Act 2009;2:4–9.

55. Leith LM. Foundations of exercise and mental health. Morgantown (WV): Fitness Information Technology, Inc; 1994.

56. Freedman RR, Krell W. Reduced thermoregulatory null zone in postmenopausal women with hot flashes. Am J Obstet Gynecol 1999;181:66–70.

57. Lewis CE, Jacobs DR Jr, McCreath H, et al. Weight gain continues in the 1990s: 10-year trends in weight and overweight from the CARDIA study. Coronary Artery Risk Development in Young Adults. Am J Epidemiol 2000;151:1172–81.

58. Lewis CE, Smith DE, Wallace DD, et al. Seven-year trends in body weight and associations with lifestyle and behavioral characteristics in black and white young adults: the CARDIA study. Am J Public Health 1997;87:635–42.

59. Flegal KM, Carroll MD, Ogden CL, et al. Prevalence and trends in obesity among US adults, 1999–2000. JAMA 2002;288:1723–7.

60. Ogden CL, Carroll MD, Curtin LR, et al. Prevalence of overweight and obesity in the United States, 1999-2004. JAMA 2006;295:1549–55.

61. Sternfeld B, Wang H, Quesenberry CP Jr, et al. Physical activity and changes in weight and waist circumference in midlife women: findings from the Study of Women's Health Across the Nation. Am J Epidemiol 2004;160:912–22.

62. Owens JF, Matthews KA, Wing RR, et al. Can physical activity mitigate the effects of aging in middle-aged women? Circulation 1992;85:1265–70.

63. Sammel MD, Grisso JA, Freeman EW, et al. Weight gain among women in the late reproductive years. Fam Pract 2003;20:401–9.

64. Guthrie JR, Dennerstein L, Dudley EC. Weight gain and the menopause: a 5-year prospective study. Climacteric 1999;2:205–11.

65. Macdonald HM, New SA, Campbell MK, et al. Longitudinal changes in weight in perimenopausal and early postmenopausal women: effects of dietary energy intake, energy expenditure, dietary calcium intake and hormone replacement therapy. Int J Obes Relat Metab Disord 2003;27:669–76.

66. Wing RR, Matthews KA, Kuller LH, et al. Weight gain at the time of menopause. Arch Intern Med 1991;151:97–102.

67. Matthews KA, Abrams B, Crawford S, et al. Body mass index in mid-life women: relative influence of menopause, hormone use, and ethnicity. Int J Obes Relat Metab Disord 2001;25:863–73.

68. Sternfeld B, Bhat AK, Wang H, et al. Menopause, physical activity, and body composition/fat distribution in midlife women. Med Sci Sports Exerc 2005;37:1195–202.

69. Wang Q, Hassanger C, Ravn P, et al. Total and regional body-composition changes in early postmenopausal women: age-related or menopause-related. Am J Clin Nutr 1994;60:843–8.

70. Pasquali R, Casimirri F, Labate AM, et al. Body weight, fat distribution, and the menopausal status in women. the VMH collaborative group. Int J Obes Relat Metab Disord 1994;19:614–21.

71. Toth MJ, Tchernof A, Sites CK, et al. Effect of menopausal status on body composition and abdominal fat distribution. Int J Obes Relat Metab Disord 2000;24:226–31.

72. Ley CJ, Lees B, Stevenson JC. Sex- and menopause-associated changes in body-fat distribution. Am J Clin Nutr 1992;55:950–4.

73. Zamboni M, Armellini F, Milani MP, et al. Body fat distribution in pre- and post-menopausal women: metabolic and anthropometric variables and their inter-relationships. Int J Obes Relat Metab Disord 1992;16:495–504.

74. Sowers M, Zheng H, Tomey K, et al. Changes in body composition in women over six years at midlife: ovarian and chronological aging. J Clin Endocrinol Metab 2007;92:895–901.

75. DiPietro L. Physical Activity, Body Weight, and Adiposity: An Epidemiologic Perspective. Baltimore: Williams & Wilkins; 1995.

76. Sutton-Tyrrell K, Zhao X, Santoro N, et al. Reproductive hormones and obesity: 9 years of observation from the Study of Women's Health Across the Nation. Am J Epidemiol 2010;171:1203–13.

77. Dugan SA, Everson-Rose SA, Karavolos K, et al. Physical activity and reduced intra-abdominal fat in midlife African-American and white women. Obesity (Silver Spring) 2010;18:1260–5.

78. Brown WJ, Williams L, Ford JH, et al. Identifying the energy gap: magnitude and determinants of 5-year weight gain in midage women. Obes Res 2005;13:1431–41.

79. Lee IM, Djousse L, Sesso HD, et al. Physical activity and weight gain prevention. JAMA 2010;303:1173–9.

80. Institute of Medicine. Dietary Reference Intake for Energy, Carbohydrate, Fiber, Fat, Fatty Acids, Cholesterol, Protein, and Amino Acids (Macronutrients). Washington DC: National Academies Press; 2002.

81. American College of Sports Medicine position stand.Osteoporosis and exercise. Med Sci Sports Exerc 1995;27:i–vii.

82. Kelley G. Aerobic exercise and lumbar spine bone mineral density in postmenopausal women: a meta-analysis. J Am Geriatr Soc 1998;46:143–52.

83. Palombaro KM. Effects of walking-only interventions on bone mineral density at various skeletal sites: a meta-analysis. 2005;28:102–7.

84. Kelley GA, Kelley KS, Tran ZV. Exercise and bone mineral density in men: a meta-analysis. J Appl Physiol 2000;88:1730–6.

85. Martyn-St James M, Carroll S. Progressive high-intensity resistance training and bone mineral density changes among premenopausal women: evidence of discordant site-specific skeletal effects. Sports Med 2006;36:683–704.

86. Martyn-St James M, Carroll S. High-intensity resistance training and postmenopausal bone loss: a meta-analysis. Osteoporos Int 2006;17:1225–40.

87. McAteer ME, Niziolek PJ, Ellis SN, et al. Mechanical stimulation and intermittent parathyroid hormone treatment induce disproportional osteogenic, geometric, and biomechanical effects in growing mouse bone. Calcif Tissue Int 2010;86:389–96.

88. Beck BR, Shaw J, Snow CM. Physical activity and osteoporosis. In: Menopause. 2nd edition. San Diego: Academic Press; 2001.

89. Snow-Harter C, Bouxsein ML, Lewis BT, et al. Effects of resistance and endurance exercise on bone mineral status of young women: a randomized exercise intervention trial. J Bone Miner Res 1992;7:761–9.

90. Lohman T, Going S, Pamenter R, et al. Effects of resistance training on regional and total bone mineral density in premenopausal women: a randomized prospective study. J Bone Miner Res 1995;10:1015–24.

91. Friedlander AL, Genant HK, Sadowsky S, et al. A two-year program of aerobics and weight training enhances bone mineral density of young women. J Bone Miner Res 1995;10:574–85.

92. Kelley GA, Kelley KS, Tran ZV. Exercise and lumbar spine bone mineral density in postmenopausal women: a meta-analysis of individual patient data. J Gerontol A Biol Sci Med Sci 2002;57:M599–M604.

93. Kelley GA. Exercise and regional bone mineral density in postmenopausal women: a meta-analytic review of randomized trials. Am J Phys Med Rehabil 1998;77:76–87.

94. Wolff I, van Croonenborg JJ, Kemper HC, et al. The effect of exercise training programs on bone mass: a meta-analysis of published controlled trials in pre- and postmenopausal women. Osteoporos Int 1999;9:1–12.

95. Wallace BA, Cumming RG. Systematic review of randomized trials of the effect of exercise on bone mass in pre- and postmenopausal women. Calcif Tissue Int 2000;67:10–8.

96. Greendale GA, Huang MH, Wang Y, et al. Sport and home physical activity are independently associated with bone density. Med Sci Sports Exerc 2003;35:506–12.

97. Morseth B, Emaus N, Wilsgaard T, et al. Leisure time physical activity in adulthood is positively associated with bone mineral density 22 years later. The Tromso study. Eur J Epidemiol 2010;25:325–31.

98. Rikkonen T, Salovaara K, Sirola J, et al. Physical activity slows femoral bone loss but promotes wrist fractures in postmenopausal women: a 15-year follow-up of the OSTPRE study. J Bone Miner Res 2010;25:2332–40.

99. Gudmundsdottir SL, Oskarsdottir D, Indridason OS, et al. Risk factors for bone loss in the hip of 75-year-old women: a 4-year follow-up study. Maturitas 2010;67:256–61.

100. Puntila E, Kroger H, Lakka T, et al. Leisure-time physical activity and rate of bone loss among peri- and postmenopausal women: a longitudinal study. Bone 2001;29:442–6.

101. Tervo T, Nordstrom P, Neovius M, et al. Reduced physical activity corresponds with greater bone loss at the trabecular than the cortical bone sites in men. Bone 2009;45:1073–8.

102. Yasaku K, Ishikawa-Takata K, Koitaya N, et al. One-year change in the second metacarpal bone mass associated with menopause nutrition and physical activity. J Nutr Health Aging 2009;13:545–9.
103. Avis NE, Brockwell S, Colvin A. A universal menopausal syndrome? Am J Med 2005;118(Suppl 12B):37–46.
104. Sherman S, Miller H, Nerurkar L, et al. Research opportunities for reducing the burden of menopause-related symptoms. Am J Med 2005;118(Suppl 12B):166–71.
105. Nelson DB, Sammel MD, Freeman EW, et al. Effect of physical activity on menopausal symptoms among urban women. Med Sci Sports Exerc 2008;40:50–8.
106. Slaven L, Lee C. Mood and symptom reporting among middle-aged women: the relationship between menopausal status, hormone replacement therapy, and exercise participation. Health Psychol 1997;16:203–8.
107. Dennerstein L, Smith AMA, Morse C. Psychological well-being, mid-life and the menopause. Maturitas 1994;20:1–11.
108. Dunn AL, Trivedi MH, Kampert JB, et al. Exercise treatment for depression: efficacy and dose response. Am J Prev Med 2005;28:1–8.
109. Hughes SL, Seymour RB, Campbell R, et al. Impact of the fit and strong intervention on older adults with osteoarthritis. Gerontologist 2004;44:217–28.
110. Rainville J, Hartigan C, Martinez E, et al. Exercise as a treatment for chronic low back pain. Spine J 2004;4:106–15.
111. Avis NE, Ory M, Matthews KA, et al. Health-related quality of life in a multiethnic sample of middle-aged women: Study of Women's Health Across the Nation (SWAN). Med Care 2003;41:1262–76.
112. Avis NE, Colvin A, Bromberger JT, et al. Change in health-related quality of life over the menopausal transition in a multiethnic cohort of middle-aged women: Study of Women's Health Across the Nation. Menopause 2009;16:860–9.
113. Dugan SA, Powell LH, Kravitz HM, et al. Musculoskeletal pain and menopausal status. Clin J Pain 2006;22:325–31.
114. Dugan SA, Everson-Rose SA, Karavolos K, et al. The impact of physical activity level on SF-36 role-physical and bodily pain indices in midlife women. J Phys Act Health 2009;6:33–42.
115. Kaplan GA, Strawbridge WJ, Camacho T, et al. Factors associated with change in physical functioning in the elderly: a six year prospective study. Journal of Aging and Health 1993;5:140–53.
116. Sternfeld B, Ngo L, Satariano WA, et al. Associations of body composition with physical performance and self-reported functional limitation in elderly men and women. Am J Epidemiol 2002;156:110–21.
117. Huang Y, Macera CA, Blair SN, et al. Physical fitness, physical activity, and functional limitation in adults aged 40 and older. Med Sci Sports Exerc 1998;30:1430–5.
118. Sowers M, Pope S, Welch G, et al. The association of menopause and physical functioning in women at midlife. J Am Geriatr Soc 2001;49:1485–92.
119. Kurina LM, Gulati M, Everson-Rose SA, et al. The effect of menopause on grip and pinch strength: results from the Chicago, Illinois, site of the Study of Women's Health Across the Nation. Am J Epidemiol 2004;160:484–91.
120. Mandelblatt JS, Luta G, Kwan ML, et al. Associations of physical activity with quality of life and functional ability in breast cancer patients during active adjuvant treatment: the Pathways Study. Breast Cancer Res Treat. 2011 Apr 8 [Epub ahead of print].
121. Martin CK, Church TS, Thompson AM, et al. Exercise dose and quality of life: a randomized controlled trial. Arch Intern Med 2009;169:269–78.
122. Garrick JG, Requa RK. Sports and fitness activities: the negative consequences. J Am Acad Orthop Surg 2003;11:439–43.

123. Focht BC, Ewing V, Gauvin L, et al. The unique and transient impact of acute exercise on pain perception in older, overweight, or obese adults with knee osteoarthritis. Ann Behav Med 2002;24:201–10.

124. Weicker H, Struder HK. Influence of exercise on serotonergic neuromodulation in the brain. Amino Acids 2001;20:35–47.

125. Janal MN, Colt EW, Clark WC, et al. Pain sensitivity, mood and plasma endocrine levels in man following long-distance running: effects of naloxone. Pain 1984;19:13–25.

126. Paluska SA, Schwenk TL. Physical activity and mental health: current concepts. Sports Med 2000;29:167–80.

127. Wilbur J, Holm K, Dan A. The relationship of energy expenditure to physical and psychologic symptoms in women at midlife. Nurs Outlook 1992;40:269–76.

128. Wilbur J, Dan A, Hedricks C, et al. The relationship among menopausal status, menopausal symptoms, and physical activity in midlife women. Fam Community Health 1990;13:67–78.

129. Guthrie JR, Dudley EC, Dennerstein L, et al. Changes in physical activity and health outcomes in a population-based cohort of mid-life Australian-born women. Aust N Z J Public Health 1997;21:682–7.

130. Holm K, Dan A, Wilbur J, et al. A longitudinal study of bone density in midlife women. Health Care Women Int 2002;23:678–91.

131. Bromberger JT, Schott LL, Kravitz HM, et al. Longitudinal change in reproductive hormones and depressive symptoms across the menopausal transition: results from the Study of Women's Health Across the Nation (SWAN). Arch Gen Psychiatry 2010;67:598–607.

132. Sternfeld B, Lee I-M. Physical activity and cancer: the evidence, the issues and the challenges. In: Lee I-M, editor. Physical Activity and Health Epidemiologic Methods and Studies. New York: Oxford University Press; 2009.

133. Holmes MD, Chen WY, Feskanich D, et al. Physical activity and survival after breast cancer diagnosis. JAMA 2005;293:2479–86.

134. Sternfeld B, Weltzien E, Quesenberry CP Jr, et al. Physical activity and risk of recurrence and mortality in breast cancer survivors: findings from the LACE study. Cancer Epidemiol Biomarkers Prev 2009;18:87–95.

135. Irwin ML, McTiernan A, Manson JE, et al. Physical activity and survival in postmenopausal women with breast cancer: results from the Women's Health Initiative. Cancer Prev Res (Phila) 2011;4:522–9.

136. McTiernan A, Ulrich C, Slate S, et al. Physical activity and cancer etiology: associations and mechanisms. Cancer Causes Control 1998;9:487–509.

137. Lee I-M. Exercise and physical health: cancer and immune function. Res Q Exerc Sport 1995;66:286–91.

138. Oestreicher N, Capra A, Bromberger J, et al. Physical activity and mammographic density in a cohort of midlife women. Med Sci Sports Exerc 2008;40:451–6.

139. Conroy SM, Butler LM, Harvey D, et al. Physical activity and change in mammographic density: the Study of Women's Health Across the Nation. Am J Epidemiol 2010;171:960–8.

140. Centers for Disease Control and Prevention (CDC). Prevalence of physical activity, including lifestyle activities among adults—United States, 2000-2001. MMWR Morb Mortal Wkly Rep 2003;52:764–9.

141. Troiano RP, Berrigan D, Dodd KW, et al. Physical activity in the United States measured by accelerometer. Med Sci Sports Exerc 2008;40:181–8.

Sleep During the Perimenopause: A SWAN Story

Howard M. Kravitz, DO, MPH[a],*, Hadine Joffe, MD, MSc[b]

KEYWORDS

• Aging • Menopausal transition • Perimenopause
• Psychosocial • Reproductive hormones • Sleep

Is there evidence for a perimenopausal sleep disorder? Krystal and colleagues[1] raised this question in considering factors associated with sleep disruption among midlife women that could be uniquely attributed to the menopausal transition, encompassing the perimenopausal and early postmenopausal years. In recent years, many reviews[1–4] addressing the topic of perimenopausal sleep have been published.

Why the burgeoning interest? Women's life cycles have long been defined by their reproductive capacity. Circa 1900, the average life expectancy was only about 50 years, shorter than the average age at menopause.[5] Some things have not changed. The average age at menopause remains approximately 51 years. But, with improved health and sanitation conditions, medical care, and lifestyle choices, current survival trends indicate that women have a life expectancy of about 80 years.[6] Thus, on average, women now live more than one third of their lifetime, almost 30 years, beyond the menopausal transition.

Recognizing this trend, attention during the past couple decades has been directed increasingly toward health problems that are either unique to or more common in women than in men. Gender differences have been recognized in sleep and its disorders (such as sleep apnea and periodic limb movement disorder). Across a woman's reproductive life span, sleep is influenced by a wide variety of intrinsic (eg, circadian and endocrinologic) and extrinsic (eg, psychosocial) factors. Despite the fact that sleep complaints are approximately twice as prevalent among women of all ages compared with men, most sleep research has been conducted with men and factors unique to women have been ignored.[7]

Disclosure: See last page of article.
[a] Departments of Psychiatry and Preventive Medicine, Rush University Medical Center, 2150 West Harrison Street – Room 275, Chicago, IL 60612, USA
[b] Department of Psychiatry, Center for Women's Mental Health, Massachusetts General Hospital, Harvard Medical School, 185 Cambridge Street, Suite 2000, Boston, MA 02114, USA
* Corresponding author.
E-mail address: hkravitz@rush.edu

Obstet Gynecol Clin N Am 38 (2011) 567–586
doi:10.1016/j.ogc.2011.06.002
0889-8545/11/$ – see front matter © 2011 Elsevier Inc. All rights reserved.

Perimenopause, the period encompassing the years of menstrual irregularities and the 12 months immediately following, marks the transition from reproductive to nonreproductive life. The median age of onset of the perimenopause is in the mid-to-late forties and typically lasts 2 to 10 years, with a median duration of 4 years.[8]

A significant proportion of women experience perimenopause as a particularly challenging period of life for preserving good sleep. To date, relatively few publications have addressed the effects of perimenopause, compared with those associated with the postmenopause, on sleep and its related physiologic changes. According to the National Institutes of Health State-of-the-Science Panel's Conference Statement on the Management of Menopause-Related Symptoms,[9] "(W)omen seem to have more sleep disturbances as they progress through the menopausal stages. The prevalence of sleep disturbance varies from 16% to 42% in premenopause, from 39% to 47% in perimenopause, and from 35% to 60% in postmenopause." These estimates included surgically as well as naturally menopausal women. At that time, longitudinal data on the prevalence of sleep difficulty during the menopausal transition from ongoing longitudinal studies were not yet available.[10]

Despite observations of increased incidence of sleep disturbances and disorders during perimenopause, the cause(s) remains unclear. Disentangling the effects of gender and aging, 2 important but nonmodifiable factors, is not a simple matter. In a meta-analysis based on literature published between 1960 and 2003, Ohayon and associates[11] examined sleep across the lifespan. Men and women had similar associations between sleep measures and aging. Larger effects of age on changes in objective (polysomnographic) sleep measurements of total sleep time, sleep efficiency, percentage of stage 1 sleep, and REM latency were observed in women than in men. Women also had longer total sleep time and sleep latency, more slow wave sleep, and less stage 2 sleep than similarly aged men. However, many studies excluded middle-aged subjects, maximizing age differences in sleep variables between the young and elderly. More complex analysis of progression from young and middle-aged and from middle-aged and elderly subjects conducted in this meta-analysis showed that age progression for all sleep variables was much less marked than simple comparisons of young and elderly subjects suggested.

Woods and Mitchell[12] developed a model to examine the effects of other symptoms on sleep using data from the Seattle Midlife Women's Health Study. In addition to age, factors in their model that are likely to affect sleep symptoms include those unique to the menopausal transition, such as menopausal transition stage, vasomotor symptoms (eg, hot flashes, night sweats), endogenous reproductive hormone levels, and exogenous hormone use. Other pertinent symptoms not specific to the transition but perhaps more relevant during this phase of women's life cycle include depressed mood, anxiety, back aches, and joint pains. Stress- and health-related and lifestyle factors also contribute to sleep disturbance.

How these factors are inter-related remains an important but unresolved question. Krystal and co-workers[1] suggested, for example, that behavioral conditioning of vasomotor-initiated insomnia, which was triggered initially by night sweats but persisted after both the night sweats and their directly associated sleep disturbances resolved, was a possible explanation for perimenopausal sleep disruption. Based on a review of population surveys, they suggested that a mood or anxiety disorder specifically associated with menopausal hormonal changes was a less likely explanation for sleep disruption during perimenopause. Dennerstein and colleagues[13] examined the influence of hormonal changes on a variety of health outcomes in the Melbourne Women's Midlife Health Project, a prospective population-based study of Australian-born women assessed annually for 9 years while traversing the menopausal transition. "Trouble sleeping" was an item from a symptom checklist measuring frequency/severity in the previous 2 weeks. The prevalence of this symptom increased across the transition and was not significantly alleviated by hormone therapy, consistent with Krystal and co-workers's[1] earlier observation that perimenopausal and postmenopausal insomnia does not respond consistently to hormonal therapy, though it was indirectly related to decreasing estradiol (E2) levels, via vasomotor symptoms.[13] Moreover, sleep problems negatively affected self-rated health as well as mood and well-being. Taken together, these data suggest that sleep problems can be influenced by mood as well as other health-related symptoms and behaviors during this phase of life.

On the other hand, Freeman and colleagues,[14] using data from the Penn Ovarian Aging Study, a younger population-based cohort (35–47 years and premenopausal at enrollment), also analyzed data from 9 years of annual assessments. The prevalence of poor sleep (43%–53% in this cohort) increased only slightly across the menopausal transition and was not significantly associated with menopausal stage, nor was this symptom associated with E2 levels. Instead, poor sleep was associated with lower levels of inhibin B, which declined during the early transition period, and with a history of depression.

Against this backdrop of these somewhat contradictory observations, we focus this review on data from a well-characterized, multiethnic community cohort participating in the Study of Women's Health Across the Nation (SWAN) and the ancillary SWAN Sleep Study, and describe what we have learned about sleep thus far from the SWAN studies. Our goal is to emphasize the importance of simply asking women seen in clinical settings about their sleep as they traverse this life cycle stage because sleep problems are common and they warrant clinical attention because of the impact of sleep disturbance on quality-of-life and health outcomes. Where applicable, SWAN findings are compared with research related to sleep during perimenopause available from other large, epidemiologic studies on the menopausal transition that have been conducted during the past 20 years.

MEASURING SLEEP SYMPTOMS AND THEIR PREVALENCE: EARLY EPIDEMIOLOGIC STUDIES OF SLEEP AND METHODOLOGIC CONSIDERATIONS

Among the early published epidemiologic studies on insomnia, Karacan and associates[15] randomly sampled 1,645 adults and reported that approximately 24% of women reported having trouble with sleeping "sometimes" and 15% reported "often or all the time," compared with 19% and 11%, respectively, of men. In particular, rates were higher in respondents who were female, older, African American, unpartnered (widowed, separated, or divorced), or of lower socioeconomic status. Although trouble falling asleep was the most prevalent complaint, breakdown by age showed that staying asleep and waking too early were more prominent among those 40 years and older. In a gender-by-age analysis, Bixler and colleagues[16] observed that a significantly larger number of women older than 50 years reported difficulty with falling asleep and early morning awakening. Karacan and co-workers[15] attributed their findings to age-related changes, but also suggested that older individuals may "take problems to bed with them." Thus, social and behavioral factors must be considered in addition to biological and physiologic factors.

Self-reported sleep disturbances increase during midlife, with prevalences in women diverging markedly from those reported by men. Cirignotta and colleagues[17] noted that there seemed to be a critical age, around 45 years, when insomnia (defined as sleeping well without sleeping pills "rarely" or "never") becomes a particularly frequent occurrence in women (**Fig. 1**). Initial unadjusted estimates from the SWAN

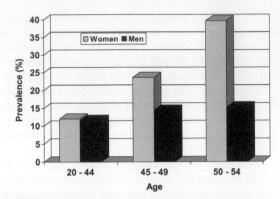

Fig. 1. Age-related gender differences in self-reported sleep problems. (*Data from* Cirignotta F, Mondini S, Zucconi M, et al. Insomnia: an epidemiological survey. Clin Neuropharmacol 1985;8(Suppl 1):S49–S54.)

Cross-sectional Study (n = 16,065) indicated that 37.3% (n = 4,632) of 12,425 women aged 40 to 55 years reported difficulty sleeping.[18]

At this juncture, 2 points require clarification and should be kept in mind throughout our discussion. First, what is "sleep difficulty" and, second, how is it measured? In general, the definition is quite broad and diverse. Individuals report perceived sleep disturbance, their subjective experiences, rather than objectively measured sleep patterns. Ohayon and colleagues[19] defined 4 categories of "insomnia" prevalence estimates: (1) Insomnia symptoms, (2) insomnia symptoms accompanied by daytime consequences (eg, low mood, reduced function), (3) dissatisfaction with sleep quality or quantity, and (4) a diagnostic entity (insomnia diagnosis). Thus, depending on the operational criteria used, "insomnia" prevalence varied approximately 5- to 8-fold: from 30% to 48% if simply based on acknowledgment of a sleep problem (eg, yes/no in the past 1–2 weeks) to 6% with the most restrictive diagnostic criteria (eg, the *Diagnostic and Statistical Manual of Mental Disorders*, Fourth Edition, Text Revision,[20] which requires symptoms plus daytime consequences such as fatigue or evidence of impaired functioning persisting for ≥1 month).

With regard to objective measurement of sleep, advances in our understanding of sleep and its relationship to health and other physiologic functions have been achieved through use of polysomnography (PSG). Sleep laboratory studies conducted in well-controlled environments in which sleep and other physiologic functions can be precisely measured have been considered the "gold standard" for recording sleep. However, this objective method "is expensive, time-consuming and necessarily limited in its capacity to generate epidemiological type data for a large population of individuals."[15]

To lessen participant burden and expense in large epidemiologic studies, wrist actigraphs have been used to collect objective sleep data. Actigraphy involves the use of a wristwatch-like device with a highly sensitive accelerometer to digitally record an integrated measure of motor activity. By this means, rest–activity cycles are analyzed to identify sleep–wake periods, although it must be acknowledged that "rest" does not necessarily mean "sleep." Actigraphy has been used in to monitor sleep in epidemiologic studies such as the Coronary Artery Risk Development in Young Adults Study[21] and the Women's Health Initiative.[22] Whereas actigraphy, compared with PSG, is less intrusive and does not require a technician's presence to monitor recordings, it has a tendency to both underestimate sleep when it is significantly fragmented (eg, sleep apnea) and overestimate sleep in individuals who lie quietly immobile in bed while awake. Although it has been demonstrated that individuals with insomnia and apnea tend to underestimate how much they sleep while monitored polysomnographically, Lauderdale and associates[23] have observed that actigraphy tends to underestimate self-reported sleep duration.

Despite potential limitations of survey methods, such as biased reporting by insomniacs, self-report questionnaires can provide information that cannot be provided by laboratory analysis, such as daytime consequences of sleep symptoms and (dis)satisfaction with sleep quantity and/or quality. Okun and co-workers[24] used SWAN Sleep Study data to test the validity of the Insomnia Symptom Questionnaire. This a new instrument, which was developed based on established diagnostic criteria to capture the multidimensionality of insomnia, showed high specificities (>90%) and identified an insomnia prevalence of 9.8% in this SWAN subcohort of 266 premenopausal, perimenopausal, and postmenopausal women. This prevalence was similar to that described in the general population when insomnia was diagnosed based on symptoms and daytime consequences (9%–15%)[19] and among Korean premenopausal, perimenopausal, and postmenopausal women reporting sleep difficulties at least 3 times per week (14.3%).[25] As Karacan and associates[15] concluded, "(T)he ultimate criterion as to what constitutes a good night's sleep may be a subjective one." Questionnaires like the Insomnia Symptom Questionnaire can be easily implemented to describe the prevalence of insomnia symptoms in a large population.

In the SWAN Sleep Study, an ancillary study of the parent SWAN, 370 women were recruited from 4 of the 7 sites (Chicago, Illinois; Detroit area, Michigan; Oakland, California; and Pittsburgh, Pennsylvania). Participants underwent an extensive assessment of their sleep, beginning with 3 nights of home-monitored PSG during the first 3 days of the protocol, up to 35 days (1 cycle) of actigraphy monitoring and sleep diaries, and questionnaires related to sleep, lifestyle, and mood.[26] Analyses currently are being conducted to evaluate relationships among indices of sleep duration and continuity measured by PSG, actigraphy and sleep diaries (Hall and colleagues, unpublished data). With these data, we are able to evaluate complex relationships between menopausal characteristics (eg, hormones, hot flashes), sleep [eg, quantitative electroencephalogram (EEG), heart rate variability during sleep], race/ethnicity, socioeconomic status, lifestyle factors (eg, smoking, exercise), and mood (depression, anxiety, stress), which will advance our understanding of how these measurements relate to each other in midlife women.[26]

Manber and Armitage[7] described a number of other factors that complicate the study of sleep in women. These issues are particularly relevant to studying sleep during the perimenopause/menopausal transition. These include (1) the confounding effect of menstrual phase; (2) timing of the surge of luteinizing hormone, ovulation, estrogen and progesterone peaks, and menstruation, which vary from cycle to cycle as well as within and across women; (3) variability in timing of sleep measurements relative to the cycle; and (4) how many intervals in which to subdivide the menstrual cycle. In the following sections, we present data from analyses of both questionnaire and polysomnogram data collected in Core SWAN and the SWAN Sleep Study that examine sleep during the perimenopause and in which we have tried to address these complicating factors that have not been accounted for in the majority of studies examining sleep disturbance in midlife women.

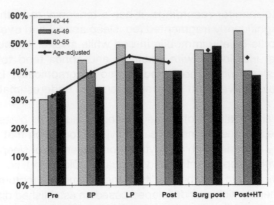

Fig. 2. Cross-sectional age-adjusted prevalence of sleep difficulty across the menopausal transition. EP, early perimenopausal; LP, late perimenopausal; Post, postmenopausal; Pre, premenopausal; Post + HT, postmenopausal and using hormonal therapy (HT; this is the only group that includes HT users); Surg post, surgically postmenopausal. (*Data from* Kravitz HM, Ganz PA, Bromberger J, et al. Sleep difficulty in women at midlife: a community survey of sleep and the menopausal transition. Menopause. 2003;10:19–28.)

RESULTS OF SWAN SLEEP STUDIES ADDRESSING SELF-REPORTED SLEEPING DIFFICULTIES
Cross-Sectional Studies

From November 1995 through October 1997, a community-based survey of women's health and menopausal symptoms was conducted at each of the 7 SWAN sites (n = 16,065). Women were asked whether, over the past 2 weeks, they had experienced difficulty sleeping. Difficulty sleeping was reported by 37.7% of 12,603 women (78.5% of those participating in this cross-sectional survey) 40 to 55 years old, who completed the sleep item and whose menopausal status could be classified by bleeding criteria (ie, not taking reproductive hormones for ≥3 months) or were surgically menopausal.[27]

Age-adjusted prevalences as well as age differences by menopausal status are illustrated in **Fig. 2.** Prevalences increased from premenopause to late perimenopause and plateaued through postmenopause, decreasing slightly in age-adjusted analyses. Late perimenopausal and surgically menopausal groups were most likely to report difficulty sleeping. Within each group, the trend was for higher rates of sleeping problems in the younger age group in all but the premenopausal (and surgically menopausal) group. This observation is remarkable in light of the relatively narrow age range examined and suggests that women beginning the menopausal transition at a younger age may experience more frequent and/or severe sleep symptoms. These cross-sectional data also suggest that age may be important but not the main determinant of the menopause–sleep relationship.

A key aim of SWAN is to examine race/ethnic differences in a diverse cohort of women traversing the menopausal transition.[28] Among the race/ethnic groups included in SWAN, prevalences for difficulty sleeping ranged from lowest (28.2%) in Japanese women to highest (40.3%) in Caucasian women, with Chinese (31.6%), Hispanic (38.0%) and African-American (35.5%) women in between. Within each race/ethnic group, some deviance from the overall trends across menopausal transition stages may be due at least in part to relatively smaller race/ethnic sample sizes, particular among the Asian groups.

Multivariate analyses demonstrated that a number of additional variables were significantly associated with difficulty sleeping, as observed in other studies. Most notably, vasomotor and psychological (depression, anxiety) symptoms, self-perceived health, quality of life, health behaviors, and arthritis were important contributors. Results were similar when women with vasomotor symptoms were excluded. The major difference was that the magnitude of self-reported sleep difficulty within the surgically menopausal group was reduced to a level similar to that of the premenopausal group. Age was not a significant covariate in any of these analyses, perhaps related to our sample's relatively narrow age range. Thus, these data suggest that sleep difficulties peak at late perimenopause and remain elevated in postmenopause, even in the absence of vasomotor symptoms. These results support the notion that a sizable number of women experience sleep problems during the perimenopause and that the association is not fully explained by vasomotor symptoms.

In another SWAN analysis, which focused on variables associated with vasomotor symptoms, Thurston and colleagures[29] examined correlates of "vasomotor symptom bother" beyond symptom frequency. Separate analyses were conducted, controlling for frequency of either hot flashes or night sweats, as well as a number of other variables associated with bothersomeness of either of these 2 vasomotor symptoms. In both sets of analyses, sleep problems (defined as self-reported symptoms of falling or staying asleep or waking early ≥3 nights a week) had the strongest influence on bother secondary to night sweats and second strongest influence (after African-American race) on bother related to hot flashes. Their findings, suggesting bidirectionality in the association between sleep disturbance and vasomotor symptoms, indicate that, in addition to being a consequence of vasomotor symptoms, sleep problems can influence the extent to which vasomotor symptoms are bothersome.

Psychosocial factors also may be important contributors to perimenopausal sleep problems. Hall and associates[30] showed that lower income is a correlate of perceived sleep difficulty (trouble falling asleep or waking up repeatedly or earlier than planned), or restless sleep. Financial strain, measured as "somewhat or very hard to pay for basics," partially mediated this relationship between low income and sleep difficulty.

Relationship factors also were examined cross-sectionally. Troxel and colleagues[31] looked at marital happiness in relation to sleep disturbance (difficulty falling asleep, waking up repeatedly or early than planned, and restless sleep). Happily married women, compared with women reporting lower marital happiness, endorsed fewer sleep disturbances. This association was found in the Caucasian group and, to a lesser extent, in the African-American group, but because of small numbers, could not be examined in the other racial/ethnic (Hispanic, Chinese, or Japanese) groups.

Although we should be cautious in drawing conclusions about directionality and causation owing to the cross-sectional nature of these analyses, these analyses have provided us with important insights regarding sleep in perimenopausal women. The results confirmed findings from other studies that self-reported sleep disturbances increase through late perimenopause and are higher in surgically menopausal women not using hormone therapy, that there are racial/ethnic differences in sleep difficulties, and that vasomotor, health, and psychosocial factors also contribute. What cross-sectional studies do not tell us is what is the effect of becoming perimenopausal or postmenopausal on sleep. To try to answer this question, we need to look at longitudinal studies.

Longitudinal Studies

SWAN longitudinal analyses have examined data collected through 7 years of annual follow-up.[32] Separate analyses were conducted for each of the 3 types of sleep disturbances: trouble falling asleep, waking up several times, and waking up earlier

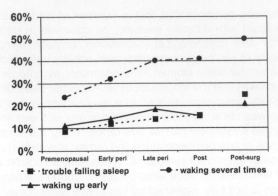

Fig. 3. Prevalence of sleep difficulty across menopausal transition during longitudinal follow-up (average rates for each menopausal stage; n = 3,045). Data are reported separately for 3 types of sleep problems occurring 3 or more nights per week in the previous 2 weeks: trouble falling asleep, waking up several times during the night, and waking up earlier than planned. (*Data from* Kravitz HM, Zhao X, Bromberger JT, et al. Sleep disturbance during the menopausal transition in a multi-ethnic community sample of women. Sleep 2008;31:979–90.)

than planned. Sleep disturbance was considered present if it was reported as present for at least 3 nights weekly in the past 2 weeks. Three aspects of the transition were examined as predictors of sleep disturbance: transition stage by bleeding criteria, vasomotor symptoms, and reproductive hormones [follicle-stimulating hormone (FSH), E2].

Fig. 3 shows the progression of sleep problems as women traversed the transition (not all women had transitioned to postmenopausal). At baseline assessment, 30.8% of the 3,045 women included in this analysis had at least 1 type of sleep difficulty on 3 or more nights per week in previous 2 weeks. Waking during the night was by far the most prevalent type of sleeping problem, but trouble falling and staying asleep also increased significantly during the transition compared with remaining premenopausal. Only early morning awakening decreased during postmenopause.

Fig. 4 shows the effects of hormone therapy. Hormone therapy seemed to benefit both naturally and surgically postmenopausal women, particularly for alleviating problems falling asleep. Postmenopausal women receiving hormone therapy did not differ significantly from premenopausal women (all confidence intervals include 1; see **Fig. 4**). On the other hand, exogenous hormone use provided no significant benefit for premenopausal and perimenopausal women, compared with premenopausal women not using hormone therapy, particularly for trouble falling asleep or early morning awakening (odds ratio >1; confidence intervals do not include 1). Comparing postmenopausal women using hormones with those not using hormones indicates a clear benefit for those who were naturally postmenopausal for both falling asleep and staying asleep, but not for early morning wakening. For surgically postmenopausal women, hormone therapy helped only for trouble falling asleep.

These longitudinal analyses show that vasomotor symptoms have a very clear adverse effect on sleep (**Fig. 5**). Women experiencing these symptoms report significantly more of each of the 3 sleep disturbances, and do so in a dose-dependent fashion. Those experiencing symptoms on more nights per week were more likely to report a sleep disturbance than those without vasomotor symptoms, ranging from 31% to 37% more likely if vasomotor symptoms occurred for 1 to 5

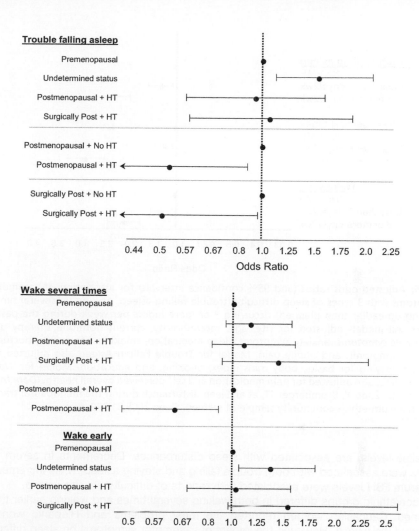

Fig. 4. Adjusted odds ratios (and 95% confidence intervals) for each of the 3 sleep difficulties in premenopausal/perimenopausal ("undetermined status"), naturally postmenopausal and surgically postmenopausal ("surgically post") women using hormone therapy (+ HT) compared with premenopausal women not using HT, and naturally and surgically postmenopausal women using HT compared with their counterparts not using HT. All 3 sleep models adjusted for site, age, race/ethnicity, current HT, depressive and anxiety symptoms, sleep medications, smoking, life events, nocturia, physical symptoms, and bodily pain. Model for Trouble Falling Asleep (*top*) also adjusted for financial strain, body mass index, smoking, and education. Model for Wake Several Times (*bottom*) also adjusted for pain medications and self-reported overall health. (*Data from* Kravitz HM, Zhao X, Bromberger JT, et al. Sleep disturbance during the menopausal transition in a multi-ethnic community sample of women. Sleep 2008;31:979–90.)

days in the past 2 weeks to 116% to 193% more likely if they occurred on 6 to 14 days.

Fig. 6 shows the associations between E2 and FSH, respectively, and sleep disturbances. The results indicate that only changes in hormone levels, but not

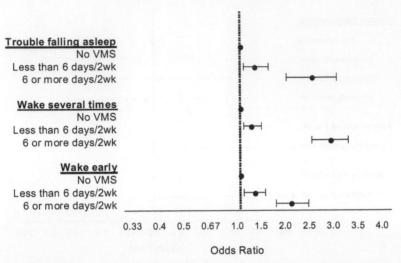

Fig. 5. Adjusted odds ratios (and 95% confidence intervals) for association of vasomotor symptoms with 3 types of sleep difficulty (trouble falling asleep, waking up several times, waking up earlier than planned) occurring 3 or more nights per week during the past 2 weeks. All models adjusted for site, age, race/ethnicity, current hormone therapy use, depressive symptoms, anxiety symptoms, sleep medication, smoking, life events, nocturia, physical symptoms, and bodily pain. Model for Trouble Falling Asleep also adjusted for difficulty paying for basics, body mass index, smoking, and education. Model for Wake Several Times also adjusted for pain medication and self-perceived overall health. (*Data from* Kravitz HM, Zhao X, Bromberger JT, et al. Sleep disturbance during the menopausal transition in a multi-ethnic community sample of women. Sleep 2008;31:979–90.)

baseline levels, are associated with sleep disturbances. Decrements in serum E2 levels were associated with both trouble falling and staying asleep, while increments in serum FSH levels were associated with reports of difficulty staying asleep.

Race/ethnic groups differed in both waking several times and waking earlier than planned. Caucasian women reported the most problems and Hispanic women reported the fewest. However, the impact of vasomotor symptoms on sleep differed among race/ethnic groups only for waking early, and associations between sleep difficulties and menopausal status did not vary among the race/ethnic groups.

Thus, longitudinal analyses in sleeping difficulties confirmed the findings of differences between menopausal transition stages and that, while vasomotor symptoms play an important role, they are not the only determinant of perimenopausal sleep disturbances. The associations with hormone levels was less robust in this study involving annual blood levels of E2 and FSH. Finally, hormone therapy (alone) may not improve sleep quality for all women or at all stages of the transition.

Daily Hormone Study

Gracia and associates[33] observed that, although reproductive hormone trends have been described, bleeding patterns still are used to define menopausal status because no clear cutoffs in hormone levels have distinguished women by menopause status. Differences among studies in the associations between hormone levels and sleep symptoms during the menopausal transition may be due to the complex nature of the relationship between these sex steroids and sleep as well as differences in cohorts

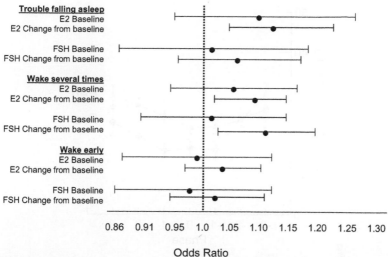

Fig. 6. Adjusted odds ratios (and 95% confidence intervals) for association of 3 types of sleep difficulty (trouble falling asleep, waking up several times, waking up earlier than planned, all occurring 3 or more nights per week during the past 2 weeks) with E2 levels (increased sleep difficulty associated with lower levels) and FSH levels (increased sleep difficulty associated with higher levels). All 3 sleep models adjusted for site, age, race/ethnicity, current hormone therapy use, blood draw in cycle day 2 to 5 window, depressive symptoms, anxiety symptoms, sleep medication, smoking, life events, nocturia, physical symptoms, and bodily pain. Models for Wake Several Times also adjusted for number of medical conditions. (*Data from* Kravitz HM, Zhao X, Bromberger JT, et al. Sleep disturbance during the menopausal transition in a multi-ethnic community sample of women. Sleep 2008;31:979–90.)

studied and methods used.[7] Single annual hormone sampling may have limited ability to provide information about the underlying hormone dynamics that occur during the menopausal transition. Thus, differences among studies in relationships between sleep symptoms and perimenopausal hormonal changes may be due to limitations of the hormone/sleep analyses with annual/infrequent sampling.

To address the association between hormone levels and self-reported trouble sleeping, we analyzed data from SWAN's Daily Hormone Study (DHS).[34] The DHS[35–37] included a subset of 848 women in SWAN aged 43 to 53 years and represented all SWAN racial/ethnic groups. These premenopausal and early perimenopausal women collected their first morning urine specimen and completed a bedtime diary daily for a single menstrual cycle or 50 days (whichever came first) annually. Data for this analysis were obtained from 630 (92.6%) of the 680 women with evidence of luteal activity (women presumed to have ovulatory cycles), as determined by a substantial increase in pregnanediol glucuronide (PdG) excretion during the cycle. Urine was assayed for luteinizing hormone, FSH, E2 metabolites (estrone conjugates, E1c), and PdG, and sleep was measured with a single diary item, "Trouble sleeping? (yes/no)."

Fig. 7 shows the differences in sleep outcomes by menstrual cycle phase (early, middle, and late follicular or luteal, and day of luteal transition) and day-by-day. As expected, the day-by-day analysis shows more variability, and within each of the 2 groups significantly more women reported trouble sleeping on days at the beginning (early follicular phase) or end (late luteal phase) of their cycle; sleep was best at

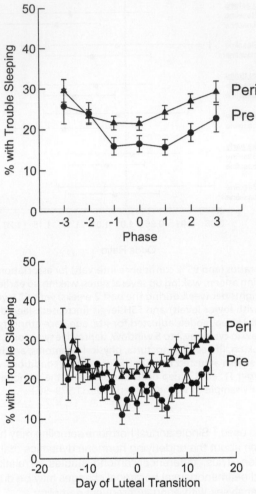

Fig. 7. Comparison of daily report of self-reported trouble sleeping across 1 menstrual cycle, by phase of cycle (*top*) and day-by-day (*bottom*), both centered on day of luteal transition. *Circles* represent the premenopausal group (Pre) and *triangles* represent the early perimenopausal group (Peri). In phase of the cycle, 0 is the day of luteal transition, −1 (days −1 to −5), −2 (days −6 to −10), −3 (days −11 to −15) correspond to late, mid, and early follicular phase, respectively, and +1 (days 1–5), +2 (days 6–10), +3 (days 11–15) correspond to early, mid, and late luteal phase, respectively. (Bottom figure *adapted from* Kravitz HM, Janssen I, Santoro N, et al. Relationship of day-to-day reproductive hormone levels to sleep in midlife women. Arch Intern Med 2005; 165:2370–6; with permission. Copyright © 2005 American Medical Association. All rights reserved.)

mid-cycle. Across the whole cycle, early perimenopausal women were 29% more likely to report trouble sleeping compared with premenopausal group. Separate analyses were conducted for each group to determine which hormone(s) were associated with trouble sleeping. Among premenopausal women there was an 11.1% increase in the likelihood of trouble sleeping for each log-unit increment in FSH level, whereas among early perimenopausal women there was a 9.5% increment in the likelihood of trouble sleeping for each log-unit increment in PdG level. These associations between changes in reproductive hormone levels across the menstrual cycles and difficulty sleeping were observed independent of the effects of vasomotor and mood symptoms on sleep.

Thus, we learned from the SWAN DHS that sleep problems are more prevalent across a menstrual cycle among perimenopausal than a similarly aged group of premenopausal women and that the prevalence of sleep difficulties varies across cycle phase, with more premenopausal and perimenopausal women reporting problems at the beginning and end of the cycle and fewer reporting problems at mid-cycle. Premenopausal women had more problems in association with higher FSH levels, which were higher than expected in premenopausal women in the early follicular phase. Perimenopausal women experienced more problems in concert with higher levels of the progesterone metabolite PdG in the luteal phase. Finally, the associations between hormone levels and trouble sleeping remained significant even after accounting for the contributions of mood and vasomotor symptoms to sleep symptoms.

THE SWAN SLEEP STUDY
Overview

The SWAN Sleep Study is an ancillary study conducted at 4 of SWAN's 7 sites (Rush University Medical Center, the University of California Davis/Kaiser, University of Michigan, and the University of Pittsburgh). The baseline study, Sleep I, used a multidimensional and multi-method approach to characterize (1) sleep disturbances in the perimenopause and (2) the effects of psychobiological factors on the meno-pause–sleep relationship in 370 women. In Sleep II, the follow-up study, 348 (94%) of the 370 Sleep I women participated in a shorter but similar protocol. Participants in the SWAN Sleep study were recruited from the Core SWAN cohort. Sleep I and II procedures were conducted during Core SWAN follow-up years 5 to 7 (2003–2005) and years 8 to 10 (2006–2008), respectively. Thus, the Sleep Study was enriched by up to 10 years of data on the participants' previous health and functioning.

The Sleep Study I protocol was conducted across an entire menstrual cycle or 35 days, whichever was shorter. Study participants included 328 premenopausal and perimenopausal women and a small group (n = 42) of postmenopausal women. Three days of in-home PSG was performed during women's early follicular phase (if still menstruating, otherwise scheduled at the participant's convenience); sleep diary, actigraphy, and event monitor recordings of vasomotor symptoms were collected throughout the cycle, along with questions on sleep quality, daytime sleepiness, mood, and stress. The Sleep II protocol included the same measures, but PSG sleep data were collected on only 2 nights, and actigraphy and sleep diary collections were shortened to 14 days. There were 3 to 4 years between the 2 assessments, to allow sufficient numbers of women to transition into postmenopause to test study aims.

Longitudinal assessment of sleep during the menopausal transition was conducted to evaluate Spielman's[38] model of the development of acute and chronic sleep disturbances and its consequences for health status. Whereas acute sleep disturbances reflect the combined effects of predisposing and precipitating factors, chronic sleep disturbances are maintained by perpetuating factors, which may develop in response to acute sleep disturbances. Moreover, these data may help to identify potential adverse effects of sleep disturbances on health status during early post-menopause as we continue annual assessments of the SWAN cohort. Thus far, data have been published from Sleep I only, and are summarized below.

Sleep I

Of the 370 women recruited, 178 were Caucasian, 134 were African American, and 58 were Chinese, and they ranged in age from 48 to 59 years. Hall and colleagues[39] examined race/ethnic differences in sleep and whether socioeconomic status measures were associated with these differences. On a measure of self-reported sleep quality, the Pittsburgh Sleep Quality Index (PSQI),[40] 66% of the Sleep Study cohort had scores exceeding the cutpoint for clinically significant complaints (PSQI score >5; possible range, 0–21; mean = 6.6; SD = 2.4). Moreover, PSQI scores were significantly higher for African Americans, but not Chinese women, than for Caucasians, indicating worse sleep quality. PSG sleep measures showed shorter sleep duration and indicators of sleep continuity demonstrated more disturbed sleep (longer sleep latency, more wakefulness after sleep onset, lower sleep efficiency) in African Americans compared with both the Caucasian and Chinese groups.

With regard to socioeconomic factors, financial strain, but not educational level, was associated with decreased sleep quality (PSQI) and lower sleep efficiency (on PSG), independent of race. Thus, race–sleep relationships did not differ according to whether a woman had earned a college or advanced degree or whether she reported financial strain, perhaps because too few of the Sleep Study women were of low socioeconomic status.[39]

Spectral analysis of the EEG, also known as quantitative EEG and completed as part of the PSG, may be a more sensitive procedure for analyzing EEG signals recorded during sleep and detecting subtle sleep EEG disturbances than traditional manual sleep stage scoring. As such, quantitative EEG can provide additional information about sleep quality. Hall and co-workers[39] examined 2 quantitative EEG sleep measures, delta and beta power. The slow wave EEG of non–rapid eye movement sleep, stage 3 and 4 (delta EEG), reflects deep, restful sleep, with higher delta EEG power indicating more slow wave sleep. Beta EEG power reflects cortical arousal level during sleep; higher power in the beta EEG band has been associated with psychological stress and insomnia. Consistent with the self-reported and PSG findings in this sample, beta EEG power was higher in African Americans, but not Chinese women, compared with Caucasians. Both delta EEG power and PSG measures of stage 3 and 4 sleep were lower in African Americans and Chinese compared with Caucasians. These sophisticated analyses of measured sleep quality support racial differences in sleep observed using both standard PSG measures and reports of poor sleep quality.

Clinical disorders of sleep were also examined in Sleep I. Clinically significant levels of sleep apnea and periodic leg movements were observed in a substantial proportion of the sample; 20% had apnea plus hypopnea values above 15 events per hour of sleep, and 8% had periodic leg movements with arousal values above 10 events per hour of sleep.[39] The mean apnea–hypopnea index (AHI) was 10.4 events per hour of sleep and the mean periodic leg movements with arousal index was 3.9 events per hour of sleep. In contrast, the estimated prevalence of AHI greater than 15 events per hour of sleep in similarly aged middle-aged women (50–60 years) in the Wisconsin Sleep Cohort was 4.0%.[41] Young and colleagues[42] reported that menopausal status was associated with AHI level, which increased across the menopausal transition, after controlling for age, body mass index (BMI), and lifestyle factors. The mean BMI at baseline of Young and associates' cohort was 30.1 mg/kg^2,[41] similar to that reported by Hall and co-workers[39] (29.96 mg/kg^2). Thus, an explanation for the difference in AHI between the SWAN Sleep Study and the Wisconsin Sleep Cohort Study, which were conducted approximately a decade apart, is not immediately clear.

Possible contributing factors could include differences in sample demographics and in sleep recording and apnea scoring procedures as well as the fact that the SWAN Sleep Study was conducted in-home, whereas the Wisconsin Sleep Cohort Study used an in-laboratory protocol. Although sleep apnea[43] and periodic leg movements[44] can affect sleep duration and continuity measures in perimenopausal and postmenopausal women, we found no racial differences in either of these sleep pathologies in our sample, suggesting that sleep disorders are unlikely to explain racial differences seen on sleep EEG analyses.

Analyses of SWAN Sleep Study data have shown the association of sleep disorders with other health conditions. These data show that indices of sleep-disordered breathing (including sleep apnea, oxygen desaturation event frequency, and percent of total sleep time with oxygen saturation levels of ≤90%), may be risk factors for cardiometabolic disorders in perimenopausal women. Matthews and colleagues[45] examined associations between inflammation and pro-coagulation biomarkers (C-reactive protein, fibrinogen, factor VIIc, and plasminogen activator inhibitor-1), and measures of PSG sleep and sleep-disordered breathing. Regression analyses revealed that each of these 4 inflammatory and coagulation indices were associated with indicators of sleep-disordered breathing after adjusting for a variety of covariates, including BMI [41% of the sample were categorized as obese (BMI ≥ 30 kg/m^2)]. In adjusted models, AHI and oxygen desaturation indices (desaturation event frequency and percent of total sleep with oxygen saturation of ≤90%) were significantly associated with all biomarkers except factor VIIc (only the association with desaturation frequency was significant). These observations suggest that inflammation and pro-coagulation processes may be an important pathway connecting sleep-disordered breathing and cardiometabolic disorders in women. Analyses exploring racial variation showed that African Americans with elevated inflammatory markers had shorter sleep duration and lower sleep efficiency.

Of particular importance for clinicians is that the cross-sectional associations of sleep with race/ethnicity, financial strain, and marital happiness, and of sleep-disordered breathing indices with inflammatory and coagulation indices, were obtained in community samples of midlife women, rather than women referred because of sleep problems. In addition, the study findings were based on in-home sleep assessments and were adjusted for potential confounders of the association. Whereas inflammation and coagulation may provide a pathway that connects sleep characteristics with risk for cardiometabolic disorders, longitudinal assessment of the impact of the menopause transition, reproductive hormones, vasomotor symptoms, and other factors on sleep, and of the associations between sleep disorders and sleep patterns with inflammation and other cardiometabolic risk factors, is needed to more clearly delineate the temporal relationship of sleep with inflammation and other menopause-related and health outcomes. Longitudinal analyses involving Sleep II data and continued follow-up of the cohort are underway.

Although longitudinal analyses involving changes in sleep and other factors between the Sleep I and Sleep II studies are not yet available, several analyses of Sleep I data have been conducted that examine the associations between sleep and subject characteristics collected as part of the overall SWAN study during the years preceding and following the Sleep I study. One example of such an analysis examines the longitudinal changes in the sex steroid hormones and gonadotropins in relation to measures of sleep duration, continuity, and architecture. The SWAN Sleep Study benefits from the standardized collection of hormone data obtained in the years before and after the sleep studies, which allow for changes in gonadotropins to be examined in relationship to sleep parameters.

Sowers and associates[46] examined associations between objectively and subjectively measured sleep characteristics and endogenous levels of serum FSH, E2, or testosterone (T), or changes in these levels, over the preceding 5- to 7-year time period. A number of interesting sleep–perimenopause relationships were revealed. In adjusted analyses, a greater rate of increase in FSH from the baseline value to the time of the Sleep Study was associated with significantly longer sleep duration and higher delta (slow wave) sleep percent on the PSG, and a perception of worse sleep quality. On the other hand, women who had a slower rate of FSH change had significantly lower sleep efficiency. However, the FSH cutpoint of 40 mIU/mL, which is commonly used to denote the transition to postmenopause, was not associated with the sleep measures being evaluated.

In contrast with associations observed between changes in FSH and sleep, sleep measures did not reflect changing levels of E2 preceding the sleep studies, although a higher baseline E2 was associated with a slightly poorer sleep quality 7 years later. Relatively limited change in T occurred across the visits preceding the Sleep Study. However, the E2/T ratio, which may reflect the increasing androgenemia associated with progression of the transition, was reduced progressively across the menopausal transition stages. A lower E2/T ratio preceding the Sleep Study was significantly associated with less time awake after sleep onset, indicating better sleep consolidation. Notably, menopausal status (based on variability in menstrual bleeding) was not associated with any sleep measure when any of the serum hormones were in the analytic model, indicating that the hormone levels may be a better predictor of sleep than menopausal stage per se. Similarly, Young and co-workers[43] observed that PSG-measured sleep was not worse in perimenopausal or postmenopausal women, compared with premenopausal women, although perimenopausal and postmenopausal women reported experiencing more sleep dissatisfaction.

Our results suggest that measures of a more rapid rate of progress through the menopause transition, as indicated by the trajectory of FSH change (rate of change over time), together with objective measures of sleep, may be clinically useful for validating sleep complaints in perimenopausal women. However, the cost-benefit of using PSG for this purpose remains to be evaluated.

Sleep also has a social context. Extending previous work with the SWAN cohort, showing that marital happiness was associated with higher sleep quality in women,[31] Troxel and colleagues[47] explored whether the marital or cohabiting relationship, current and/or past, is associated with sleep, as measured both subjectively (PSQI) and objectively (PSG and actigraphy). Analyses of women's relationship histories over the 6 to 8 years before the sleep study showed advantages in sleep for women who were consistently partnered versus women who were unpartnered throughout this interval, or those who had lost or gained a partner over that time course.

For those who gained a partner, there were discrepancies in the effects of sleeping with a partner on subjective versus objective sleep measures. Whereas women who had gained a partner were similar to consistently married women in terms of subjective sleep quality and PSG measures of sleep continuity and architecture, their differences, and the discrepancies in subjective versus objective sleep parameters in regard to the effects of sleeping with a partner, suggest that although the presence of a bed partner can negatively affect objective measures of sleep, participants prefer to sleep with the partner despite objective costs vis-à-vis sleep.

These findings make unique contributions toward our understanding of how a positive relationship transition, the gain of a new partner, is associated with better sleep in midlife women. Thus, asking questions regarding relationships need to be part of a sleep history in women, particularly during this period of social as well as biological transition.

SUMMARY

Converging evidence supports the existence of perimenopausal sleep disturbances, rather than a single specific disorder, as distinct phenomena that exist independent from other factors that are common in this population and likely to influence sleep (vasomotor symptoms, mood disturbance, sleep apnea). Moreover, the perimenopausal transition is a plausible determinant of worsening sleep in midlife women. In addition to the hormone changes underlying the perimenopause, a diverse variety of factors, both directly related (eg, vasomotor symptoms) and unrelated to the transition (eg, age-related sleep changes, sleep apnea, mood disturbance, and relationship and co-sleeping habits), contribute to sleep disturbances in the menopausal transition.[12-14,32] SWAN data show that the menopausal transition is related to self-reported difficulty sleeping, independent of age,[27] indicating that age is not the primary determinant of the perimenopause–sleep relationship. As another source of sleeping difficulty in perimenopausal women, SWAN and other studies have shown that vasomotor symptoms are strongly associated with poor sleep quality.[2,27] However, subgroup analyses restricted to women without vasomotor symptoms continue to find an association between the perimenopause and poor sleep quality, albeit a weaker association, providing evidence that the perimenopause–sleep relationship is not entirely explained by vasomotor symptoms.[27] We have also found,[32] as shown in **Fig. 4**, that exogenous sex steroid hormones (alone) may be an insufficient intervention for improving sleep quality, except in naturally and surgically postmenopausal women.

Although the perimenopause is clearly associated with sleep dissatisfaction, objective measures of sleep patterns and sleep disorders must also be analyzed to characterize the relations among sleep symptoms, vasomotor symptoms, physical and emotional health consequences, aging, and menopause. Ongoing SWAN Sleep Study analyses will address these issues to more fully distinguish whether the perimenopause–sleep relationship exists independent of age, vasomotor, mood, and other health conditions.

Sleep disturbances are associated with increased health care costs and many negative health outcomes, such as decreased quality of life, poor work performance, and mood and anxiety symptoms. Sleep apnea prevalence, which seems to be higher in SWAN participants than in other epidemiologic studies that include community middle-aged women not selected for any particular health problems, increases in middle-aged women and may affect cardiovascular disease risk.

Characterizing sleep and its psychobiological and psychosocial correlates is vital for identifying factors that may ease menopause-related sleep disturbances and their impact on health status in midlife women of differing racial and ethnic groups. The menopausal transition is an important time for change in risk for sleep disturbances and their associated health consequences. The SWAN Sleep Study provides a unique opportunity to collect longitudinal data on multiple high-quality objective and subjective measures of sleep in a multi-ethnic cohort of midlife women. Sleep I has provided baseline data on menopausal-related sleep disturbances, and these measures have been evaluated in conjunction with longitudinal measures drawn from the Core SWAN study. Anticipated results from Sleep II will provide further insights into the course of sleep across the menopause transition.

DISCLOSURE

Funding for the SWAN Sleep Study is from the National Institute on Aging (Grants AG019360, AG019361, AG019362, AG019363). Support for this manuscript was also provided in part by National Institute of Mental Health (5R01MH082922; H. Joffe, PI). The content of this manuscript is solely the responsibility of the authors and does not necessarily represent the official views of the NIA, NINR, ORWH or the NIH. The authors also acknowledge the graphics assistance of Dr Imke Janssen in preparing **Fig. 7**.

Dr Joffe discloses that over the past 12 months she has served as a co-investigator on clinical trials supported by Bayer HealthCare Pharmaceuticals, Forest Laboratories, and GlaxoSmithKline, and served as a consultant to Sunovion.

REFERENCES

1. Krystal AD, Edinger J, Wohlgemuth, et al. Sleep in peri-menopausal and post-menopausal women. Sleep Med Rev 1998;2:243–53.
2. Joffe H, Massler A, Sharkey KM. Evaluation and management of sleep disturbance during the menopausal transition. Semin Reprod Med 2010;28:404–21.
3. Moline ML, Broch L, Zak R, et al. Sleep in women across the life cycle from adulthood through menopause. Sleep Med Rev 2003;7;155–77.
4. Parry BL, Martinez LF, Maurer EL, et al. Sleep, rhythms and women's mood. Part II. Menopause. Sleep Med Rev 2006;10:197–208.
5. Soules MR, Bremner WJ. The menopause and climacteric: endocrinologic basis and associated symptomatology. J Am Geriatr Soc 1982;30:547–61.
6. Kochanek KD, Xu J, Murphy SL, et al. Deaths: preliminary data for 2009. Natl Vital Stat Rep 2011;59:1–68.
7. Manber R, Armitage R. Sex, steroids, and sleep: a review [published correction appears in Sleep 2000;23:145–9]. Sleep 1999;22:540–55.
8. McKinlay SM, Brambilla DJ, Posner JG. The normal menopause transition. Maturitas 1992;14:103–15.
9. NIH State-of-the-Science Panel. National Institutes of Health State-of-the-Science conference statement: management of menopause-related symptoms. Ann Intern Med 2005;142:1003–13.
10. Woods NF, Mitchell ES. Symptoms during the perimenopause: prevalence, severity, trajectory, and significance in women's lives. Am J Med 2005;118(Suppl 12B):14S–24S.
11. Ohayon MM, Carskadon MA, Guilleminualt C, et al. Meta-analysis of quantitative sleep parameters from childhood to old age in healthy individuals: developing normative sleep values across the human lifespan. Sleep 2004;27:1255–73.
12. Woods NF, Mitchell ES. Sleep symptoms during the menopausal transition and early postmenopause: observations from the Seattle Midlife Women's Health Study. Sleep 2010;33:539–49.
13. Dennerstein L, Lehert P, Guthrie JR, et al. Modeling women's health during the menopausal transition: a longitudinal analysis. Menopause 2007;14:53–62.
14. Freeman EW, Sammel MD, Lin H, et al. Symptoms associated with menopausal transition and reproductive hormones in midlife women. Obstet Gynecol 2007;110:230–40.
15. Karacan I, Thornby JI, Anch M, et al. Prevalence of sleep disturbance in a primarily urban Florida county. Soc Sci Med 1976;10:239–44.
16. Bixler EO, Kales A, Soldatos CR, et al. Prevalence of sleep disorders in the Los Angeles metropolitan area. Am J Psychiatry 1979;136:1257–62.

17. Cirignotta F, Mondini S, Zucconi M, et al. Insomnia: an epidemiological survey. Clin Neuropharmacol 1985;8(Suppl 1):S49–S54.
18. Gold EB, Sternfeld B, Kelsey JL, et al. Relation of demographic and lifestyle factors to symptoms in a multi-racial/ethnic population of women 40-55 years of age. Am J Epidemiology. 2000;152:463–73.
19. Ohayon MM. Epidemiology of insomnia: what we know and what we still need to learn. Sleep Med Rev. 2002;6:97–111.
20. American Psychiatric Association. Diagnostic and statistical manual of mental disorders. 4th edition, Text Revision. Washington DC: American Psychiatric Association; 2000.
21. Lauderdale DS, Knutson KL, Yan LL, et al. Objectively measured sleep characteristics among early-middle-aged adults: the CARDIA study. Am J Epidemiol 2006;164:5–16.
22. Kripke DF, Langer RD, Elliott JA. Mortality related to actigraphic long and short sleep. Sleep Med 2010;12:28–33.
23. Lauderdale DS, Knutson KL, Yan LL, et al. Self-reported and measured sleep duration: how similar are they? Epidemiology 2008;19:838–45.
24. Okun ML, Kravitz HM, Sowers MF, et al. Psychometric evaluation of the Insomnia Symptom Questionnaire: a self-report measure to identify chronic insomnia. J Clin Sleep Med 2009;5:41–51.
25. Shin C, Lee S, Lee T, et al. Prevalence of insomnia and its relationship to menopausal status in middle-aged Korean women. Psychiatry Clin Neurosci 2005;59:395–402.
26. Hall M, Kravitz HM, Gold E, et al. Sleep during the menopausal transition in a multi-ethnic cohort: feasibility and preliminary results [abstract: 0350]. Sleep 2005; 28(Suppl):A119.
27. Kravitz HM, Ganz PA, Bromberger J, et al. Sleep difficulty in women at midlife: a community survey of sleep and the menopausal transition. Menopause 2003;10: 19–28.
28. Sowers MF, Crawford SL, Sternfeld B, et al. SWAN: a multicenter, multiethnic, community-based cohort study of women and the menopausal transition. In: Lobo R, Marcus R, Kelsey J, editors. Menopause: biology and pathobiology. Orlando: Academic Press Inc; 2000. p. 175–88.
29. Thurston RC, Bromberger JT, Joffe H, et al. Beyond frequency: who is most bothered by vasomotor symptoms? Menopause 2008;15:841–7.
30. Hall M, Bromberger J, Matthews K. Socioeconomic status as a correlate of sleep in African-American and Caucasian women. Ann N Y Acad Sci 1999;896:427–30.
31. Troxel WM, Buysse DJ, Hall M, et al. Marital happiness and sleep disturbances in a multi-ethnic sample of middle-aged women. Behav Sleep Med 2009;7:2–19.
32. Kravitz HM, Zhao X, Bromberger JT, et al. Sleep disturbance during the menopausal transition in a multi-ethnic community sample of women. Sleep 2008;31:979–90.
33. Gracia CR, Sammel MD, Freeman EW, et al. Defining menopause status: creation of a new definition to identify the early changes of the menopausal transition. Menopause 2005;12:128–35.
34. Kravitz HM, Janssen I, Santoro N, et al. Relationship of day-to-day reproductive hormone levels to sleep in midlife women. Arch Intern Med 2005; 165:2370–6.
35. Santoro N, Crawford SL, Allsworth JE, et al. Assessing menstrual cycles with urinary hormone assays. Am J Physiol Endocrinol Metab 2003;284:E521–30.
36. Santoro N, Lasley BL, McConnell D, et al. Body size and ethnicity are associated with menstrual cycle alterations in women in the early menopausal transition: the Study of Women's Health Across the Nation (SWAN) Daily Hormone Study. J Clin Endocrinol Metab 2004;89:2622–31.

37. Weiss G, Skurnick JH, Goldsmith LT, et al. Menopause and hypothalamic-pituitary sensitivity to estrogen. JAMA 2004;292:2991–6 [published correction appears in JAMA 2005;293:163].
38. Spielman AJ. Assessment of insomnia. Clin Psychol Rev 1986;6:11–25.
39. Hall MH, Matthews KA, Kravitz HM, et al. Race and financial strain are independent correlates of sleep in mid-life women: the SWAN Sleep Study. Sleep 2009;32:73–82.
40. Buysse DJ, Reynolds CF, Monk TH, et al. The Pittsburgh Sleep Quality Index: a new instrument for psychiatric practice and research. Psychiatry Res 1989;28:193–213.
41. Young T, Palta M, Dempsey J, et al. The occurrence of sleep-disordered breathing among middle-aged adults. N Engl J Med 1993;328:1230–5.
42. Young T, Finn L, Austin D, et al. Menopausal status and sleep disordered breathing in the Wisconsin Sleep Cohort Study. Am J Respir Crit Care Med 2003;167:1181–5.
43. Young T, Rabago D, Zgierska A, et al. Objective and subjective sleep quality in premenopausal, perimenopausal, and postmenopausal women in the Wisconsin Sleep Cohort Study. Sleep 2003;26:667–72.
44. Polo-Kantola P, Rauhala E, Erkkola R, et al. Estrogen replacement therapy and nocturnal periodic limb movements: a randomized controlled trial. Obstet Gynecol 2001;97:548–54.
45. Matthews KM, Zheng H, Kravitz HM, et al. Are inflammatory and coagulation biomarkers related to sleep characteristics in mid-life women?: Study of Women's Health Across the Nation Sleep Study. Sleep 2010;33:1649–55.
46. Sowers MF, Zheng H, Kravitz HM, et al. Sex steroid hormone profiles are related to sleep measures from polysomnography and the Pittsburgh Sleep Quality Index. Sleep 2008;31:1339–49.
47. Troxel WM, Buysse DJ, Matthews KA, et al. Marital/cohabitation status and history in relation to sleep in midlife women. Sleep 2010;33:973–81.

The Perimenopause and Sexual Functioning

Nancy E. Avis, PhD[a], Robin Green, PSYD[b]

KEYWORDS

• Perimenopause • Sexual functioning

Sexual functioning is an important component of women's lives and has increasingly received public health, pharmaceutical, and medical attention.[1] More than 75% of the middle-aged women in the Study of Women's Health Across the Nation (SWAN) reported that sex was moderately to extremely important to them.[2] Sexual functioning, however, declines with age,[1,3–7] leading to much debate about the contribution of menopause to sexual activity and functioning among women.

The standard epidemiologic definition of natural menopause as 12 consecutive months of amenorrhea in the absence of surgery or other pathologic or physiologic cause (eg, pregnancy, lactation) that would terminate menstruation, has been consistently used over many years.[8] Perimenopause, however, has been less consistently defined. A frequently used epidemiologic definition is menses within the past 12 months, with changes in regularity or no menstrual cycle in the past 3 to 11 months.[9,10] However, some studies have classified women as postmenopausal after only 6 months of amenorrhea, whereas others combine premenopausal and perimenopausal or perimenopausal and postmenopausal women for analysis. More recent research has distinguished between early and late perimenopause based on a more rigorous, consensus-based staging system for reproductive aging in women—the Stages of Reproductive Aging Workshop (STRAW).[11] This group recommended classifying early perimenopausal as experiencing cycle changes in regularity in the past year and late perimenopausal as no menses in previous 3 months, but menses within the previous 11 months. The present article covers research related to the perimenopause in which early and late perimenopause are distinguished and research where it is not. We do not address women who have had a surgical menopause because they would be either considered postmenopausal (if the surgery occurred after menopause) or their status would be unclassifiable if their surgery occurred before menopause (since most studies are unable to determine whether or not ovaries were removed).

[a] Department of Social Sciences and Health Policy, Division of Public Health Sciences, Wake Forest University School of Medicine, Medical Center Boulevard, Winston-Salem, NC 27157, USA
[b] Department of Obstetrics, Gynecology and Women's Health, Albert Einstein College of Medicine, 1300 Morris Park Avenue, Bronx, NY 10461, USA
E-mail address: navis@wakehealth.edu.

Obstet Gynecol Clin N Am 38 (2011) 587–594
doi:10.1016/j.ogc.2011.05.009
0889-8545/11/$ – see front matter © 2011 Elsevier Inc. All rights reserved.

ASPECTS OF SEXUAL FUNCTIONING

Sexual functioning is generally studied in terms of satisfaction, frequency of activity (intercourse, masturbation), desire (including interest and sexual thoughts or fantasies), arousal, attitudes toward sexuality, and difficulties such as pain during intercourse and problems reaching orgasm. These reflect the characterization of sexual functioning in terms of libido and potency.[12,13] Libido includes sexual interest, desire, drive, motivation, and pleasure. Potency is the physiologically measurable event during sexual arousal/activity—the sexual response.[14] Whereas postmenopausal declines in ovarian hormone production and reproductive atrophy may increase the incidence of dyspareunia and vaginal dryness (one measure of potency), it is less clear how menopause affects sexual interest or libido.[12]

SEXUAL FUNCTIONING AND PERIMENOPAUSE

Early cross-sectional studies among general populations of women did not show clear associations between the perimenopause and sexual functioning. Although some studies found lower sexual interest among perimenopausal or postmenopausal women compared with premenopausal women[15–17] other studies did not find associations between menopause status and sexual functioning.[18–20] These earlier studies, however, used differing measures of sexual functioning, sampling, and definitions of perimenopause.

Cross-Sectional Research

More recent research has focused on broader aspects of sexual functioning and more detailed definitions of menopausal status. The Massachusetts Women's Health Study was a community-based, prospective study that examined a wide range of aspects of sexual functioning among 200 women.[21] Women were defined as perimenopausal if they had experienced menstrual bleeding within the previous 12 months, but not within the past 3 months. In cross-sectional analyses of this cohort, unadjusted analyses showed that perimenopausal women, compared with premenopausal women, reported feeling less arousal than when they were in their 40s, but did not differ on any other of the sexual functioning outcomes: A belief that interest in sexual activity declines with age, frequency of sexual intercourse, satisfaction with one's sexual relationship, frequency of sexual desire, difficulty reaching orgasm, or pain during or after intercourse. After adjusting for age and a range of other variables, results showed that perimenopausal women reported significantly less frequency of sexual desire than premenopausal women, but did not differ on the other outcomes.

The Melbourne Women's Midlife Health Project was a prospective, population-based study of Australian-born women begun in 1991. Cross-sectional data from the initial baseline study of 2001 women aged 45 to 55 had only 4 questions related to sexual functioning: Changes in sexual interest over the past year, reasons for changes, occurrence of sexual intercourse, and unusual pain on intercourse.[15] Although postmenopausal women reported a decline in sexual interest over the past year, perimenopausal women did not differ from premenopausal women.

The SWAN is among the largest community-based studies that includes a broad range of sexual functioning domains and relevant covariates. SWAN is a multiethnic, observational cohort study of the menopausal transition in 3302 women at 7 sites across the United States.[22] Baseline eligibility criteria included age 42 to 52 years, intact uterus and at least 1 ovary, not currently using exogenous hormones affecting ovarian function, at least 1 menstrual period in the previous 3 months, and self-identification with a site's designated racial/ethnic group. By study design, almost half of the sample was white (47%) with the other half consisting of African-American (28%), Hispanic (8.7%), Chinese (7.5%), and Japanese (8.5%) women.

Sexuality outcome variables were measured at each study visit using a 20-item questionnaire designed to address sexual activity and function in women with and without partners. Variables of interest fall into the domains of importance of sex, sexual desire, frequency of activities (sexual intercourse and masturbation) and physical pleasure, emotional satisfaction with partner, arousal, and pain. All study women were asked how important sex was in their lives, how often they felt desire in the past 6 months to engage in any form of sexual activity (either alone or with a partner), frequency of engaging in masturbation in the past 6 months, and whether they had engaged in sexual activities with a partner in the last 6 months. Respondents who reported having engaged in sexual activities with a partner in the last 6 months were asked about frequency of sexual intercourse, arousal during sexual activity, and degree of emotional satisfaction and physical pleasure from their relationship with a partner. Women who reported having sexual intercourse in the past 6 months were also asked about frequency of vaginal or pelvic pain during intercourse.

Baseline analyses comparing premenopausal and early perimenopausal women (defined as menses occurring in the past 3 months but reported as less predictable) found that early perimenopausal women reported greater pain with intercourse than premenopausal women.[23] This association was found even after adjustment for vaginal dryness, age, and other covariates. Perimenopausal women were about 40% more likely to report having frequent pain during intercourse than premenopausal women. The 2 groups did not differ on frequency of sexual intercourse, desire, arousal, or physical or emotional satisfaction.

Longitudinal Research

Cross-sectional studies are limited in their ability to distinguish changes in sexual functioning owing to menopause or aging and to examine changes over the menopausal transition. Several longitudinal studies have provided a clear advantage over the prior body of cross-sectional literature. The longitudinal component of the Melbourne Women's Midlife Health Project recruited 438 women from the initial baseline sample who were premenopausal or early perimenopausal for follow-up.[3] Eight annual assessments with blood sampling for hormone levels were conducted. Sexual functioning was assessed by the Personal Experiences Questionnaire, which measures feelings for partner, sexual responsivity (arousal, orgasm, enjoyment), frequency of sexual activities, libido, partner problems, and vaginal dryness/dyspareunia. Early perimenopause was defined as a change in menstrual frequency and late perimenopause was determined when women reported at least 3 months of amenorrhea but fewer than 12 months of amenorrhea. Hormone therapy users were analyzed in a separate category. Analyses examined changes from premenopause and early perimenopause (combining these 2 groups of women) to late perimenopause, and compared late perimenopause to postmenopause. Results showed that from premenopause/early perimenopause to late perimenopause, reports of sexual responsivity declined, feelings for partner declined and partner problems increased. From late perimenopause to postmenopause, there were further declines in sexual responsivity, libido, and frequency of sexual activities along with an increase in vaginal dyspareunia and partner problems. To control for the effect of aging, this study compared changes in sexual functioning among women who transitioned from one menopausal stage to another with sexual functioning among women who remained premenopausal or postmenopausal during these 7 years. These analyses showed that both of these groups also reported significant declines in sexual responsivity, suggesting that this domain is adversely affected by aging as much as by the menopause transition itself.

The Penn Ovarian Aging Study is a longitudinal study of a population-based cohort of 436 women (half African American and half Caucasian) recruited from 1996 to 1997 when the women were aged 35 to 47. Women received 10 study assessments over a 9-year period. Gracia et al[24] reported on sexual functioning data collected over a 3-year period at study assessments 8 through 10. Sexual functioning was assessed by the Female Sexual Function Index, a 19-item measure that includes the domains of desire, arousal, lubrication, orgasm, satisfaction, and pain. Menopausal status was adapted from the STRAW staging system of reproductive aging.[11] In both unadjusted results, and models adjusting for age and a range of other variables, sexual dysfunction increased significantly among late transition women, but not women early in the transition. Analyses of specific domains of sexual functioning revealed that lubrication and orgasm scores significantly decreased early in the transition, whereas arousal, lubrication, orgasm, and pain all decreased late in the transition.

The Medical Research Council National Survey of Health and Development is a longitudinal study of the health of individuals in England, Scotland, and Wales born in 1946. Since 1992, when cohort members were age 47, a questionnaire has been sent annually to 1778 women. Mishra and Kuh[25] reported on sexual functioning data collected from 1993 to 2000. Sexual functioning was measured in terms of perceived change in sex life and difficulties with sexual intercourse. Perimenopausal status was defined as between 3 and 12 months of amenorrhea or irregular periods within the preceding 12 months (this combines the early and late perimenopause categories of the STRAW staging system for reproductive aging in women[11]). Women who had a hysterectomy or were on hormone therapy were classified separately. Analyses were based on menopausal transition categories over 2 consecutive years. Interestingly, women who remained perimenopausal reported a significantly greater change in sex life and difficulties with intercourse, whereas women who transitioned from premenopause to perimenopause were not significantly different from women who remained premenopausal. Women who reported vaginal dryness were more likely to report worse sexual functioning.

The SWAN reported on 6 years of follow-up data in their cohort of 3302 women.[26] At each study visit, menopausal status was classified as premenopausal (menses in the previous 3 months with no change in menstrual regularity in preceding year), early perimenopausal (menses in the previous 3 months and changes in regularity in past year), late perimenopausal (no menses in the previous 3 months but menses in the previous 11 months), or postmenopausal (≥12 months of amenorrhea). Women who reported having taken hormone therapy in the previous 12 months were classified as current hormone therapy users, whereas past users were classified as former hormone therapy users.

Covariates included age, menopausal factors (hot flashes, night sweats, vaginal dryness, use of lubricants during intercourse), social factors (race/ethnicity, education, marital status, change in relationship status, having children at home), health and lifestyle factors (self-reported health, alcohol consumption, body mass index, and cigarette smoking), and psychological factors (attitudes toward aging and menopause, anxiety, depressive symptoms, and importance of sex). In analyses adjusting for these covariates, early perimenopausal women were significantly more likely to report more frequent masturbation and greater pelvic pain, consistent with cross-sectional results. Late perimenopausal women reported significantly less sexual desire than premenopausal women.

Taken together, these studies suggest that increased pain during sexual inter-course may occur early in the perimenopause, independent of aging. Decreases in sexual desire may occur later in the perimenopause, which might also be a result of chronically increased pain or increases in partner problems.

Perimenopause seems to be a time of increasing pain during intercourse and diminished sexual interest. The increase in masturbation during early perimenopause is an interesting finding and may be related to the concurrent increase in painful intercourse. The decline in masturbation after menopause may be related to the concurrent decline in desire, suggesting a plausible causal pattern underlying declines in sexual functioning, because increases in pain may lead to lowered sexual desire. The vulvovaginal epithelium is rich in estrogen receptors, and estrogens are a necessity for urogenital maturation, maintenance, and genital vascular congestion during arousal. Lower estrogen levels in the late transition may lead to decreased vascular engorgement and vaginal secretions during sex, resulting in a diminished sense of pleasure from subjective arousal and a disruption in the intimacy-based sexual response cycle.

The lack of an association between the menopause transition and frequency of sexual intercourse or satisfaction with partner suggests that these domains of sexual function are not directly related to the menopause transition.

FACTORS OTHER THAN MENOPAUSE STATUS

Psychosocial and aging factors are often reported as more important determinants than ovarian function of sexual functioning among mid-aged women.[19,20,27,28] Some of these factors include the availability of a partner,[20,24,27,29] previous sexual behavior and enjoyment,[29] the relationship quality,[23,30,31] psychological function,[19,21,24,31] general physical health,[20,21] and race/ethnicity.[23,32]

The Massachusetts Women's Health Study found that health was a significant variable related to all aspects of sexual functioning.[21] Depression and more psycho-logical symptoms were related to lower satisfaction, frequency, and desire. Interest-ingly, smoking was related to less desire and lower frequency of sexual intercourse. This finding is consistent with other research on the negative effects of smoking on sex steroid levels.[33–35]

In the longitudinal cohort of the Melbourne Women's Midlife Health Project, prior level of sexual function and relationship factors were more important than hormonal determinants of sexual function.[31] The most important factors (in decreasing order of importance) influencing domains of libido and sexual responsiveness were prior level sexual functioning, change in partner status, feelings for partner, and estradiol levels. Frequency of sexual activities was not influenced by estradiol level, but was predicted by prior level of sexual function, change in partner status, feelings for partner, and level of sexual response.

Longitudinal results from SWAN found that health, psychological functioning and the importance of sex were related to all sexual function outcomes.[26] Age, race/ethnicity, marital status, change in relationship, and vaginal dryness were also associated with sexual function. Vaginal dryness was an important factor associated with masturbation, pain, arousal, physical pleasure, and emotional satisfaction. Racial/ethnic differences were found for all domains. Chinese and Japanese women reported less importance ascribed to sex, and less desire, masturbation, arousal, and more pain, whereas African-American women reported greater importance ascribed to sex, frequency, and pain, but less arousal, emotional satisfaction, and physical pleasure than did Caucasian women. Age and changes in relationship were related to all outcomes except pain. Women who had a new relationship reported higher importance, desire, arousal, frequency, and emotional satisfaction, whereas women who lost a relationship reported more masturbation, and less arousal, frequency, emotional satisfaction, and physical pleasure.

In summary, this large, community-based study of middle-aged women found a decrease in sexual desire, an increase in painful intercourse beginning in the late perimenopause, and a temporary increase in masturbation during the early perimenopause. These changes were independent of chronologic aging, menopausal symptoms, and health, social, and psychological factors. In adjusted analyses, the menopausal transition was unrelated to arousal, frequency of sexual activity, physical pleasure, or satisfaction with partner. Although vasomotor symptoms were largely unrelated to sexual functioning, vaginal dryness was highly associated with pain and lower arousal, emotional satisfaction, and physical pleasure. The most important variable related to sexual functioning was the importance of sex, which was highly related with all outcomes. Psychological status, physical health, and relationship status were also important.

Taken as a whole, research has shown some changes in sexual functioning beginning at the perimenopause that are primarily related to vaginal dryness, but other factors such as a woman's prior sexual functioning, physical and mental health, and partner's health are equally, or possibly more, important.

CLINICAL IMPLICATIONS AND APPROACH TO TREATMENT

Sexual functioning during the perimenopause is complex and influenced by hormonal and nonhormonal factors. The strong associations of psychological status, physical health, and social factors with sexual function underscore the clinical imperative to explore and address these factors when discussing women's concerns regarding sexual dysfunction. The very strong association of the importance of sex with all domains of sexual function suggests that asking patients about the importance of sex may be a cornerstone of the management of the sexual concerns of midlife women.

There is a paucity of research on the treatment of sexual dysfunction and/or sexual problems specifically in the perimenopause. To date, there have been no clinical trials that focus exclusively on sexual dysfunction in perimenopausal women. A few trials have been conducted among postmenopausal women. Studies of estrogen therapy, whether oral, transdermal, or vaginal among postmenopausal women, have demonstrated positive effects on vaginal pain and dryness,[36–39] but not other aspects of sexual functioning.

REFERENCES

1. Laumann EO, Paik A, Rosen RC. Sexual dysfunction in the United States: prevalence and predictors. JAMA 1999;281:537–44.
2. Cain VS, Johannes CB, Avis NE, et al. Sexual functioning and practices in a multiethnic study of midlife women: baseline results from SWAN. J Sex Res 2003;40:266–76.
3. Dennerstein L, Dudley EC, Burger H. Are changes in sexual functioning during midlife due to aging or menopause? Fertil Steril 2001;76:456–60.
4. Dennerstein L, Hayes RD. Confronting the challenges: epidemiological study of female sexual dysfunction and the menopause. J Sex Med 2005;(Suppl 3):118–32.
5. Hällstrom T, Samuelsson S. Changes in women's sexual desire in middle life: the longitudinal study of women in Gothenburg. Arch Sex Behav 1990;19:259–68.
6. Kinsey AC, Pomeroy WB, Martin CW. Sexual behavior in the human female. Philadelphia: WB Saunders; 1953.

7. Avis NE. Sexual function and aging in men and women: community and population-based studies. J Gend Specif Med 2000;3:37–41.
8. World Health Organization. Research on the menopause in the 1990s, WHO technical services report series no. 866 82. Geneva: World Health Organization; 1996.
9. Brambilla D, McKinlay S, Johannes C. Defining the perimenopause for application in epidemiologic investigations. Am J Epidemiol 1994;140:1091–5.
10. Cooper GS, Baird DD. The use of questionnaire data to classify peri- and premeno-pausal status. Epidemiology 1995;6:625–8.
11. Soules MR, Sherman S, Parrott E, et al. Executive summary: Stages of Reproductive Aging Workshop (STRAW). Fertil Steril 2001;76:874–8.
12. Davidson JM. Sexual behavior and its relationship to ovarian hormones in the menopause. Maturitas 1985; 7:193–201.
13. Iddenden DA. Sexuality during the menopause. Med Clin North Am 1987;71:87–94.
14. Masters W, Johnson V. Human sexual response. Boston: Little Brown; 1966.
15. Dennerstein L, Smith AMA, Morse CA. Sexuality and the menopause. J Psychosom Obstet Gynecol 1994;15:59–66.
16. Hällstrom T. Sexuality in the climacteric. Clin Obstet Gynecol 1977;4:227–39.
17. Hunter M, Battersby R, Whitehead M. Relationships between psychological symptoms, somatic complaints and menopausal status. Maturitas 1986;8:217–28.
18. Dennerstein L, Dudley EC, Hopper JL, et al. Sexuality, hormones and the menopausal transition. Maturitas 1997;26:83–93.
19. Hawton K, Gath D, Day A. Sexual function in a community sample of middle-aged women with partners: effects of age, marital, socioeconomic, psychiatric, gynecological, and menopausal factors. Arch Sex Behav 1994;23:375–95.
20. Køster A, Garde K. Sexual desire and menopausal development. Maturitas 1993;16: 49–60.
21. Avis NE, Stellato R, Crawford S, et al. Is there an association between menopause status and sexual functioning? Menopause 2000;7:297–309.
22. Sowers M, Crawford S, Sternfeld B, et al. Design, survey sampling and recruitment methods of SWAN: a multi-center, multi-ethnic, community-based cohort study of women and the menopausal transition. In: Lobo RA, Kelsay J, Marcus R, editors. Menopause: biology and pathobiology. San Diego: Academic Press; 2000. p. 175–88.
23. Avis NE, Zhao X, Johannes CB, et al. Correlates of sexual function among multi-ethnic middle-aged women: results from the Study of Women's Health Across the Nation (SWAN). Menopause 2005;12:385–98.
24. Gracia CR, Freeman EW, Sammel MD, et al. Hormones and sexuality during transition to menopause. Obstet Gynecol 2007;109:831–40.
25. Mishra G, Kuh D. Sexual functioning throughout menopause: the perceptions of women in a British cohort. Menopause 2006;13:880–90.
26. Avis NE, Brockwell S, Randolph JF, et al. Longitudinal changes in sexual functioning as women transition through menopause: results from the Study of Women's Health Across the Nation. Menopause 2009;16:442–52.
27. Leiblum S, Bachmann G, Kemmann E, et al. Vaginal atrophy in the postmenopausal woman. The importance of sexual activity and hormones. JAMA 1983;249:2195–8.
28. Hagstad A. Gynecology and sexuality in middle-aged women. Women Health 1988; 13:57–80.
29. Pfeiffer E, Verwoerdt A, Davis GC. Sexual behavior in middle life. Am J Psychiatry 1972;128:1262–7.
30. Cawood EH, Bancroft J. Steroid hormones, the menopause, sexuality and well-being of women. Psychol Med 1996;26:925–36.

31. Dennerstein L, Lehert P, Burger H. The relative effects of hormones and relationship factors on sexual function of women through the natural menopausal transition. Fertil Steril 2005;84:174–80.
32. Dennerstein L, Lehert P. Women's sexual function, lifestyle, mid-age, and menopause in 12 European countries. Menopause 2004;11:778–85.
33. Greendale G, Hogan P, Shumaker S. Sexual functioning in postmenopausal women: the Postmenopausal Estrogen/Progestin Interventions (PEPI) trial. J Women's Health 1996;5:445–58.
34. Johnston CC Jr, Hui SL, Witt RM, et al. Early menopausal changes in bone mass and sex steroids. J Clin Endocrinol Metab 1985;61:905–11.
35. Michnovicz JJ, Bradlow HL. Dietary and pharmacological control of estradiol metabolism in humans. Ann N Y Acad Sci 1990;595:291–9.
36. Huang A, Yaffe K, Vittinghoff E, et al. The effect of ultralow-dose transdermal estradiol on sexual function in postmenopausal women. Am J Obstet Gynecol 2008;198: 265–7.
37. Wiklund I, Karlberg J, Mattsson LA. Quality of life of postmenopausal women on a regimen of transdermal estradiol therapy: a double-blind placebo-controlled study. Am J Obstet Gynecol 1993;168:824–30.
38. Nathorst-Boos J, von SB, Carlstrom K. Elective ovarian removal and estrogen replacement therapy— effects on sexual life, psychological well-being and androgen status. J Psychosom Obstet Gynaecol 1993;14:283–93.
39. Gast MJ, Freedman MA, Vieweg AJ, et al. A randomized study of low-dose conjugated estrogens on sexual function and quality of life in postmenopausal women. Menopause 2009;16:247–56.

Menstruation and the Menopausal Transition

Siobán D. Harlow, PhD*, Pangaja Paramsothy, MPH

KEYWORDS

- Menstruation • Menstrual cycle • Menopause
- Perimenopause

In broad strokes, the nature of change in menstrual bleeding patterns as women approach and transition through the menopause were well defined more than 40 years ago by the classic menstrual calendar studies of Treloar and colleagues,[1] Vollman,[2] and others.[3,4] Our current attribution of menopause, defined retrospectively after 12 months of amenorrhea have been observed and derived from the ground-breaking paper on the probability of natural menopause after age 40, is based on the Treloar data (now referred to as TREMIN).[5] However, these early studies told us little about subpopulation differences in the menopausal experience, nor did they provide clear insights into the specific bleeding changes that mark the onset of the transition. Over the past 15 years, a more nuanced understanding of the range and variability of women's experience has begun to emerge from the several longitudinal cohort studies of the midlife that have had women maintain menstrual calendars as they transition from premenopause to postmenopause, including the multisite, multiethnic Study of Women's Health Across the Nation (SWAN).[6–12]

The classic studies demonstrated that menstrual characteristics change across the reproductive lifespan, with the population mean menstrual cycle length and variability declining as women age from 20 to 40 years. Before menopause, population variability in menstrual cycle length increases,[1,2] with the transition to menopause being characterized by an increased frequency of both very long and very short cycles. This pattern of change in menstrual cycle characteristics has been confirmed in smaller clinical studies of predominantly Caucasian women,[13,14] as well as in the more recent cohort studies where midlife women have maintained menstrual calendars.[6–12] The Massachusetts Women's Health Study (MWHS) found that, among women over the age of 50, short menstrual cycles and short bleeding/spotting episodes occurred more frequently during early perimenopause and menstrual cycles of 90 days or longer occurred later in the transition.[15] Increasingly longer menstrual cycles generally signal proximity to the final menstrual period (FMP). The Melbourne

Department of Epidemiology, University of Michigan, 1415 Washington Heights, Room 5208, Ann Arbor, MI 48109-2029, USA
* Corresponding author.
E-mail address: harlow@umich.edu

Obstet Gynecol Clin N Am 38 (2011) 595–607
doi:10.1016/j.ogc.2011.05.010
0889-8545/11/$ – see front matter © 2011 Elsevier Inc. All rights reserved.

Women's Midlife Health Project (MWMHP) reported that menstrual cycle length increased in the last 20 menstrual cycles before the FMP compared with earlier menstrual cycles.[16] The SWAN Daily Hormone Study also observed that short menstrual cycles (<21 days) were common in early perimenopause, with both short and long menstrual cycles more likely to be anovulatory.[17]

Treloar[18] was the first to define the concept of a menopausal transition and to estimate age at onset of the transition based on visual inspection of the menstrual history of 291 women during the 12 years preceding the FMP. He estimated the median age of entry into the transition to be 45.5 years, with a median duration of the transition of 4.8 years. The concept of late perimenopause was introduced by Brambilla and colleagues[19] to predict the likelihood, based on interview questions, that a woman would be postmenopausal at subsequent interviews. Based on data from the MWHS, they estimated the median age at entry into the late perimenopause, defined as a self-report of 3 to 11 months of amenorrhea, to be 47.5 years.[8]

Clinicians have long been aware that women's menopausal experiences differ markedly, and that the classic patterns described above capture the experience of many but not all women. In 1 clinical study, 12% of women experienced sudden amenorrhea,[20] whereas another study documented women's self-report of experiencing regular cycles until the onset of menopause.[21] Recently, several studies have begun to examine subpopulation variability in the experience of the menopausal transition. The limited data to date corroborate this clinical understanding, identifying subgroups of women whose menstrual patterns differ from the normative pattern described by Treloar and colleagues, and assessing factors associated with differences in timing of the transition and in women's experience of changes in cycle characteristics. Using the TREMIN data, the first author of this paper and colleagues modeled within-woman change in menstrual cycle variability after age 35 and calculated that the menopausal transition lasts from 6 to 10 years after the onset of increased variability, depending on a woman's characteristic menstrual patterns before and during the transition as well as on the age at onset of the transition.[21] Approximately 15% of women experienced minimal change in their menstrual characteristics before the FMP. In another analysis of TREMIN data, Gorrindo and colleagues[22] proposed that women's menstrual patterns could be categorized into 5 subtypes based on several key features related to mean and variability across the lifespan. Although they did not explicitly assess changes at the time of transition, they noted that in addition to the most common pattern (where menstrual cycle lengths increase as menopause approached), about 25% of women seemed to have no or minimal change in menstrual cycle variability or mean length before their FMP.[22] In SWAN, longer menstrual cycles as well as more variable menstrual cycles are associated with a shorter time to FMP.[23]

Menstrual cycle characteristics during the menopausal transition differ, to some extent, by age at menopause. Women with later menopause have longer mean cycle lengths and greater variability 2 years before menopause than women with earlier menopause,[5] with differences most notable at the extremes of menopausal age. Women with later menopause have also been found to have longer cycles throughout reproductive life[24] and in the 9 years before menopause.[25]

BLEEDING MARKERS OF THE EARLY AND LATE MENOPAUSAL TRANSITION

At the turn of the millennium, the stages of ovarian aging were not yet understood. Recognizing the importance of clearly defining the stages of reproductive aging as well as of identifying valid, reliable, and clinically useful criteria for the onset of each stage of the menopausal transition, the Stages of Reproductive Aging Workshop

(STRAW) was convened in 2001. Based on a consensus discussion of scientific evidence, STRAW recommended that reproductive life be characterized by 7 stages.[26] Before menopause, reproductive life was divided into the reproductive years (3 stages) and the transition years (2 stages). Postmenopausal years (2 stages) follow the FMP. Given limitations at that time in the scientific understanding of ovarian aging and in the availability of valid, reliable, and widely available assays, STRAW staging criteria were limited to menstrual markers and qualitative changes in follicle-stimulating hormone (FSH). STRAW characterizes entry into the early transition by increased levels of FSH and increased variability in menstrual cycle length, defined as menstrual cycle length of more than 7 days different from normal. Entry into the late transition was characterized by the continued elevation of FSH and the occurrence of 2 or more skipped cycles or amenorrhea of 60 days or more.

STRAW's recommended staging approach is conceptually consistent with prior definitions of the menopausal transition; however, the proposed bleeding criteria for the early and late transition included important departures from then current clinical and research practice. Following STRAW, the ReSTAGE Collaboration conducted empirical analyses to assess the validity and reliability of STRAW's menstrual criteria in four cohort studies including SWAN, TREMIN, the MWMHP, and the Seattle Midlife Women's Health Study (SMWHS).[27] Their findings supported and clarified many of the STRAW recommendations.

Specifically, based on results from the MWHS,[19] SWAN[10] and other longitudinal cohort studies of midlife women[6] have used amenorrhea of 90 days or more as their criterion for entry into the late stage of the menopausal transition, the definition commonly used in clinical practice. STRAW's recommendation to use a shorter duration of amenorrhea, specifically 60 or more days, was based on emerging results from menstrual calendar data in TREMIN,[28] the SMWHS,[9] and the MWMHP[16] studies. Each of these studies observed that a somewhat shorter interval of amenorrhea was equally predictive of the approach of the FMP and less likely to misclassify the subpopulation of women who do not experience extended episodes of amenorrhea before their FMP as late perimenopausal when they were in fact already postmenopausal. The SWMHS had recommended occurrence of a skipped cycle as a criterion for onset of the late menopausal transition,[9] the MWMHP had recommended the 42-day running range (difference between the longest and shortest cycle across 10 cycles) as a criterion,[16] and a reanalysis of TREMIN had recommended a 60-day cycle.[28]

Re-STAGE analyses demonstrated that, across the four cohort studies, an episode of amenorrhea of 60 days or longer cycle occurred on average 0.5 to 1.5 years earlier than an episode of amenorrhea of 90 days or longer, although in roughly one third of the women the first occurrence of a 60-day or longer cycle was in fact 90 days or longer.[29] In contrast, a remarkable concordance was noted between the age at occurrence of each of the other proposed criterion. For example, in 65% to 74% of women, a 60-day or longer cycle occurred on the exact same bleeding episode as a running range more than 42 days and occurred within 1 year of each other in 86% to 94% of women. After age 40, the median time from occurrence of these bleeding markers of late transition to FMP was on average 1.5 to 2.3 years for at least 90-days of amenorrhea and 2.6 to 3.3 years for the other 3 bleeding markers. All the proposed bleeding markers of late transition identified women who were closer to achieving their FMP compared with women who had not yet experienced these menstrual changes.

Based on these findings and the fact that 90 or more days of amenorrhea was not observed in 10% to 20% of women across the four studies, whereas 60 or more days of amenorrhea was observed in 90% to 100% of women, ReSTAGE recommended using 60 or more days of amenorrhea after age 40 as the bleeding criterion for onset of the late menopausal transition.[27] Occurrence of 60 or more days of amenorrhea is also the most easily identified description—by women, clinicians, and researchers—of the menstrual phenomenon of interest. Evaluation of the association between these bleeding criteria and changes in serum FSH levels suggests that the 60-day criterion correlates well with underlying hormonal changes that characterize the transition.[30] In the clinical setting, among women age 40 to 44 years old, requiring the repeated occurrence of an episode of amenorrhea of at least 60 days may help to distinguish women who are in fact in late menopause from women who are experiencing an aberrant long cycle secondary to life stress or other environmental insults.[31] In SWAN and MWMHP, a single annual early follicular phase serum FSH level was less predictive of proximity to the FMP than occurrence of an episode of amenorrhea of at least 60 days, but given an episode of amenorrhea, women with higher serum FSH concentrations were more likely to achieve their FMP than women with lower levels of FSH.[30] Notably, although experience of hot flashes is a marker of the late menopausal transition in the absence of information about occurrence of 60-day cycles or FSH level, it adds no information about the proximity of the FMP when information on these other, latter markers of the transition are available.[30]

Bleeding criteria for entry into the early transition have been more controversial,[9,16,28] because the bleeding changes that mark initial onset of the transition tend to be more subtle, often being apparent to women before they can be easily assessed by a clinician or researcher. Most longitudinal cohort studies to date, including SWAN and the MWMHP, have relied on women's self-report of changes in menstrual function, with no clear definition of what constituted "change" or "irregularity." Following results from the SMWHS,[9] STRAW proposed that the criterion for defining the increased variability that marks entry into the early menopausal transition be a "change in cycle length of 7 or more days from normal."[2] After evaluating several proposed menstrual criteria for the early transition, including those proposed by the MWMHP (the occurrence of more than 2 menstrual cycles outside the 21 to 35 day range over 10 cycles),[16] the SMWHS (the occurrence of a 7 or more day difference in length between consecutive menstrual cycles that repeated within the next 12 months),[9] and TREMIN (standard deviation in menstrual cycle length greater than 6 or 8 days or a 45 day menstrual cycle),[28] ReSTAGE suggested that a change in cycle length of 7 or more days may be the most appropriate criterion for onset of the early menopausal transition.[32]

ReSTAGE found that across the 4 cohort studies, a persistent 7 or more day difference in consecutive menstrual cycles occurred earliest and was the only proposed criterion that occurred consistently earlier than 60 days of amenorrhea.[32] After age 40, the median time from occurrence of a persistent 7 or more day difference in consecutive cycle lengths to FMP was 5 to 8 years. Annual measures of serum FSH were strongly associated with occurrence of each of the bleeding criteria, although at any given FSH value, associations were highest for the persistent 7 or more day difference in menstrual cycle length. Thus, ReSTAGE's empirical findings supported the STRAW recommendation that this relatively small but marked change in menstrual cycle length be used as the bleeding criterion for early transition. Recently published data from SWAN[33] and the Michigan Bone Health and Metabolism Study[12] on trajectories of change in FSH from late reproductive life through the FMP indicate that the initial rise in FSH occurs on average about 7 years before the FMP, which is consistent with the timing of onset of the early transition defined by the 7 or more day difference in cycle length criterion.

Other investigators[7,34–36] have provided additional evidence regarding the validity of STRAW's proposed criteria based on their association with predicted changes in hormone profiles. The Penn Ovarian Aging Study has demonstrated that small changes and single occurrences of change in menstrual cycle length are associated with change in inhibin-B and FSH levels.[7] Efforts are continuing to identify the most useful menstrual marker of the onset of early menopausal transition. Several recent studies suggest that declines in inhibin-B and anti-Mullerian hormone may prove the most useful markers of onset of the early transition.[11,37,38]

The STRAW criteria are now widely considered the gold standard for staging ovarian aging. However, STRAW specifically excluded 7 categories of women, including those with chronically irregular menstrual cycles or hysterectomies, smokers and women with a body mass index (BMI) of more than 30 kg/m^2.[26] Emerging data from SWAN and other studies suggest that although smoking and body size influence endocrine levels and the timing of transition, these factors do not alter the pattern or stages of ovarian aging.[33,39–44]

Defining menopausal status in women who have had a hysterectomy and in women with endocrine or medical conditions that may have an impact on menstrual bleeding patterns is more challenging. The Women's Ischemia Syndrome Evaluation study proposed an algorithm based on age, time since last menses, surgery history, and serum hormone values to classify women as perimenopausal or postmenopausal in their population of women.[45] When applied to the SWAN cohort, substantial concordance with SWAN's menstrually based classifications was observed, but further development of this algorithm is needed to distinguish between early and late perimenopause. Recent advances in our understanding of trajectories of change in FSH, estradiol (E2), anti-Mullerian hormone, and inhibin-B should facilitate development of such an algorithm.

Polycystic ovarian syndrome (PCOS) is characterized by oligomenorrhea. Current evidence suggests that women with PCOS have more antral follicles and higher serum anti-Mullerian hormone than control women,[46] which implies that women with PCOS may have increased ovarian reserve and a later age at menopause.[47] Ongoing analyses focused on identifying subtypes of change in menstrual patterns as women approach the menopausal transition and FMP, like that reported by Gorrindo and colleagues,[22] should help to clarify how best to stage women with this condition and others who do not menstruate regularly. Distinguishing amenorrhea secondary to weight loss and nutritional compromise from onset of the late transition or menopause can be particularly complex in women with chronic medical conditions, such as HIV/AIDS. Recent studies have also demonstrated lower FSH levels in HIV-infected women, secondary to use of opiates, and elevated E2 among women treated with HAART.[48]

Developing clear, easily observable, and easily communicable criteria for menopausal staging is of particular importance to ensure that women, clinicians, and researchers are describing the same phenomenon, because women currently seem to rely only partially on menstrual characteristics to define their menopausal status.[49] In an early SWAN study of the correspondence between women's attributions and SWAN's classification of menopausal status, menstrual patterns explained about half the variance between menstrually based and self-defined menopause status, with older women classifying themselves as later in the transition. Notably, women with vasomotor symptoms tended to self-designate themselves as being in transition regardless of their menstrual patterns.

In the MWMHP, information on self-reported change in frequency improved prediction of proximity to the FMP, because more than half the women reporting change became postmenopausal within 4 years, compared with only a small proportion of those reporting no change.[50]

CHARACTERISTICS OF MENSTRUAL BLEEDING

Another hallmark of the menopausal transition is change in the amount and duration of menstrual flow. Increased duration of menstruation as well as heaviness of bleeding episodes have been reported in clinical studies, population based-surveys, and cohort studies of midlife women.[4,51–53] The classic study of menstrual blood loss volume documented that 50-year-old women bled about 6 mL more than women aged 20 to 45, whereas heavy bleeding is experienced most commonly by women approaching the FMP, as indicated by the 90th percentile of menstrual blood loss being 133 mL in women aged 50, versus 86 to 88 mL for women aged 30 to 45.[54] A similar result was found in a recent study that quantified blood loss across 2 bleeding episodes in Australian women aged 21 to 55 years. Although mean blood loss did not differ during the late menopausal transition, the range of menstrual blood loss was significantly greater among women in late transition.[52] Consistent with data on the relationship between high E2 and increased blood loss, Hale and colleagues found that menstrual blood loss in excess of 200 mL was associated in ovulatory cycles with high E2 levels,[33,55] as well as with the late menopausal transition itself.[52] In a population-based menstrual calendar study of Danish women, onset of irregular cycles as women entered the menopausal transition was associated with increased variability in the duration of bleeding, increased frequency of spotting, bleeds lasting 10 or more days, and increased variability in women's subjective reports of the amount of menstrual flow.[56]

The SWAN Daily Hormone Study has examined menstrual characteristics in early perimenopausal women.[17] Consistent with Hale, in the SWAN Daily Hormone Study self-reported heavy bleeding was less frequent after anovulatory cycles than following ovulatory cycles, with 20% of cycles being anovulatory cycles.[17] However, both short (1–3 days) and long (>8 days) duration of menstrual bleeding were associated with anovulation. Self-reports of heavy bleeding were associated with obesity and self-reported leiomyomata, but were unrelated to steroid hormone concentrations. Ethnic differences in heavy bleeding were not apparent after adjustment for self-reported leiomyoma and BMI.

FACTORS THAT INFLUENCE MENSTRUAL CHARACTERISTICS DURING THE MENOPAUSAL TRANSITION

Although few studies have examined factors that influence menstrual cycle characteristics during the menopausal transition, available data indicate that factors known to influence menstrual cycle length as well as the amount and duration of menstrual flow throughout reproductive life[57] also influence population differences in bleeding patterns at the end of reproductive life. Research from SWAN and other studies has focused on factors that influence differences in hormone levels and hormone trajectories. Those data are summarized elsewhere in this volume.

Ethnicity

Data on racial and ethnic differences in menstrual bleeding patterns remains relatively limited. Studies of postmenarchal girls have found that Caucasian girls have longer menstrual cycle lengths and longer menstrual bleeding, but are less likely to report heavy bleeding than African-American girls.[58,59] The Semiconductor Health Study and the Women's Reproductive Health Study found, based on menstrual calendar data, that Asian women had adjusted menstrual cycle lengths that were approximately 2 days longer than cycles for Caucasian women.[60,61] In 1 European study that utilized retrospective questionnaire data, Caucasian women reported having mean cycle lengths that were a half day longer than non-Caucasian women.[62] Studies of ethnic differences in the perimenopause have primarily examined timing and hormone parameters, and not menstrual characteristics. In the Harvard Study of Moods and Cycles, women of color had an earlier entry into perimenopause than white women,[63] whereas in the Penn Ovarian Aging Study, African-American women started the menopausal transition earlier than Caucasian women, but no ethnic difference was observed in timing of transition to later stages.[64] In contrast, SWAN reported that older age was associated with a higher hazard ratio for menopause among African-American, Japanese, and Chinese women than among Caucasian women.[23] As discussed in detail elsewhere in this volume, ethnic differences in hormone profiles across the menopausal transition have been observed in SWAN; however, in the SWAN Daily Hormone Study ethnic differences were not observed in the characteristics of menstrual bleeding episodes.[17]

Body Size

Both low and high BMI are well known to influence menstrual cycle characteristics.[57] Low BMI has been associated with longer menstrual cycle length in postmenarchal girls[59] and young adult women.[65,66] Higher BMI has also been associated with longer menstrual cycle length.[61,62,66–68] In the Michigan Bone Health and Metabolism Study, the lowest body fat mass deciles and the highest body fat mass deciles were associated with longer menstrual cycle length.[66] BMI has been associated with bleeding duration and heaviness of flow. Low BMI has been associated with longer bleeding duration.[58,69,70] High BMI has been associated with shorter bleeding duration.[58,65,71,72] The Michigan Bone Health and Metabolism Study did not find an association with bleeding duration and BMI.[73] In a Danish study of premenopausal and perimenopausal women, obesity was associated with a higher frequency of flooding.[56] In the SWAN DHS,[43] heavier women had shorter cycles than women with BMI of less than $25 kg/m^2$, but obesity was also associated with an increased number of heavy bleeding days.[17] The Harvard Study of Moods and Cycles found the age-adjusted incidence rate of perimenopause to be 1.58 times higher among obese women as compared with normal weight women.[63] However, the Penn Ovarian Aging Study did not find an association between BMI and entry into any stage of menopause.[64] Similarly, SWAN has not found an association between BMI and age at or proximity to the FMP.[23,74]

Medical Conditions

Although less frequently examined, evidence suggests that medical conditions also impact menstrual characteristics, and consideration of such conditions may be particularly relevant during the menopausal transition as the burden of chronic illness increases. Endocrine disorders including diabetes have been associated with an earlier age at menopause.[75] In SWAN, diabetes has been associated with premature ovarian failure[76] and with earlier age at menopause.[74] Diabetes may also be associated with longer menstrual cycles,[68,77] as well as with longer bleeding duration and heavier bleeding episodes.[77] In the SWAN Daily Hormone Study, women with diabetes had longer menstrual cycles than nondiabetic women[17]; however, no difference was found in the duration or amount of menstrual bleeding. Abnormal thyroid function has also been linked with menstrual dysfunction and women with a history of Grave's disease were more likely to report long cycles.[68] An early descriptive study of women with hyperthyroidism found the more severe the disease, the less menstrual blood flow. The same study found that women with hypothyroidism had higher frequencies of menorrhagia.[78] In SWAN, higher baseline thyroid stimulating hormone levels were associated with increased duration of menstrual bleeding.[79] However, in the SWAN Daily Hormone Study, thyroid conditions were not associated with menstrual cycle characteristics.[17] Although some evidence suggests that uterine leiomyomas are associated with abnormal bleeding and menstrual cycle length, the evidence is contradictory.[80–84] In the SWAN DHS/menstrual calendar study, fibroids were associated with shorter menstrual cycle length, but longer bleeding duration and heavier bleeding episodes.[17] Menorraghia may also be secondary to use of oral anticoagulants.[85]

Cigarette Smoking

Studies on the impact of tobacco smoking on menstrual characteristics are inconsistent, with some studies suggesting an association with shorter menstrual cycle lengths[62,68,86] and others finding no difference.[60,65,73,87] Smoking has been associated with both shorter[86,87] and longer bleeding duration,[73] and increased amount of bleeding.[87] In the SWAN Daily Hormone Study, smoking history was not independently associated with cycle length, bleeding duration, or heavy bleeding.[17] However, current smoking was associated with earlier age at and closer proximity to the FMP.[23,74] In the Penn Ovarian Aging Study, smoking was also associated with an increased probability of transition into each stage of the menopausal transition, such that smokers had a shorter transition than nonsmokers.[64]

CLINICAL IMPLICATIONS

Although the classic description of the menopausal transition[18] as a stage first marked by increased variability in menstrual cycle lengths followed by increasing frequency of very long cycles until permanent amenorrhea occurs describes the experience of the majority of women, marked differences occur in the magnitude of change in women's menstrual experience. Approximately 15% to 25% of women experience minimal or no change in menstrual regularity before their FMP. Short cycles are most frequent in the early transition, whereas long cycles are most frequent in the late transition, with older age at menopause associated with longer menstrual cycles, both during the transition and throughout reproductive life. The duration and amount of blood loss during the menopausal transition is more variable, and women are most likely to experience excessive blood loss during this reproductive life stage, particularly during the late transition. Excessive bleeding is most often associated with ovulatory cycles in this reproductive phase, although spotting and bleeding for longer than 8 days are associated with anovulatory cycles. Heavy bleeding during the transition is more common in obese women and women with leiomyomas.

Onset of the early transition is best characterized by a noticeable change in menstrual cycle lengths after age 40, defined as a persistent difference in consecutive menstrual cycles of 7 or more days, which occurs on average 6 to 8 years before the FMP. Onset of the late transition is best characterized by an episode of 60 or more days of amenorrhea, which occurs on average 2 years before the FMP. Evidence suggests that the STRAW stages are applicable to women who smoke and to women of all body sizes; however, identifying onset of the menopausal transition and the FMP may be difficult in women with chronic diseases associated with nutritional compromise, or in women using medications that alter hormone profiles (such as HIV-infected women taking HAART). PCOS seems to be associated with a later age at menopause. More research is needed to assess how women with PCOS experience the menopausal transition. Clinicians should pay careful attention to medical factors, including both medical conditions and medical treatments, that may increase menstrual blood loss or alter menstrual cycle characteristics sufficiently to obscure the onset of the menopausal transition or the FMP when treating women in the midlife.

REFERENCES

1. Treloar AE, Boynton RE, Behn BG, et al. Variation of the human menstrual cycle through reproductive life. Int J Fertil 1967;12:77–126.
2. Vollman RF. The degree of variability of the length of the menstrual cycle in correlation with age of woman. Gynaecologia 1956;142:310–4.
3. Chiazze L Jr, Brayer FT, Macisco JJ Jr, et al. The length and variability of the human menstrual cycle. JAMA 1968;203:377–80.
4. Matsumoto S, Mogami Y, Ohkuri S. Statistical studies on menstruation; a criticism on the definition of normal menstruation. Gunma J Med Sci 1962;11:294–318.
5. Wallace RB, Sherman BM, Bean JA, et al. Probability of menopause with increasing duration of amenorrhea in middle-aged women. Am J Obstet Gynecol 1979;135: 1021–4.
6. Dudley EC, Hopper JL, Taffe J, et al. Using longitudinal data to define the perimenopause by menstrual cycle characteristics. Climacteric 1998;1:18–25.
7. Gracia CR, Sammel MD, Freeman EW, et al. Defining menopause status: creation of a new definition to identify the early changes of the menopausal transition. Menopause 2005;12:128–35.
8. McKinlay SM, Brambilla DJ, Posner JG. The normal menopause transition. Am J Hum Biol 1992;4:37–46.
9. Mitchell ES, Woods NF, Mariella A. Three stages of the menopausal transition from the Seattle Midlife Women's Health Study: toward a more precise definition. Menopause 2000;7:334–49.
10. Sowers M, Crawford S, Sternfeld B, et al. SWAN: a multicenter, multiethnic, community-based cohort study of women and the menopausal transition. In: Lobo RA, Kelsey J, Marcus R, editors. Menopause: biology and pathobiology. San Diego: Academic Press; 2000. p. 175–88.
11. Sowers MR, Eyvazzadeh AD, McConnell D, et al. Anti-mullerian hormone and inhibin B in the definition of ovarian aging and the menopause transition. J Clin Endocrinol Metab 2008;93:3478–83.
12. Sowers MR, Zheng H, McConnell D, et al. Follicle stimulating hormone and its rate of change in defining menopause transition stages. J Clin Endocrinol Metab 2008;93: 3958–64.
13. Klein NA, Illingworth PJ, Groome NP, et al. Decreased inhibin B secretion is associated with the monotropic FSH rise in older, ovulatory women: a study of serum and follicular fluid levels of dimeric inhibin A and B in spontaneous menstrual cycles. J Clin Endocrinol Metab 1996;81:2742–5.
14. Santoro N, Brown JR, Adel T, et al. Characterization of reproductive hormonal dynamics in the perimenopause. J Clin Endocrinol Metab 1996;81:1495–501.
15. Johannes CB, Crawford SL, Longcope C, et al. Bleeding patterns and changes in the perimenopause: a longitudinal characterization of menstrual cycles. Clinical Consultations in Obstetrics and Gynecology 1996;8:9–20.
16. Taffe JR, Dennerstein L. Menstrual patterns leading to the final menstrual period. Menopause 2002;9:32–40.
17. Van Voorhis BJ, Santoro N, Harlow S, et al. The relationship of bleeding patterns to daily reproductive hormones in women approaching menopause. Obstet Gynecol 2008;112:101–8.
18. Treloar AE. Menstrual cyclicity and the pre-menopause. Maturitas 1981;3:249–64.

19. Brambilla DJ, McKinlay SM, Johannes CB. Defining the perimenopause for application in epidemiologic investigations. Am J Epidemiol 1994;140:1091–5.

20. Seltzer VL, Benjamin F, Deutsch S. Perimenopausal bleeding patterns and pathologic findings. J Am Med Womens Assoc 1990;45:132–4.

21. Mansfield PK, Carey M, Anderson A, et al. Staging the menopausal transition: data from the TREMIN Research Program on Women's Health. Womens Health Issues 2004;14:220–6.

22. Gorrindo T, Lu Y, Pincus S, et al. Lifelong menstrual histories are typically erratic and trending: a taxonomy. Menopause 2007;14:74–88.

23. Santoro N, Brockwell S, Johnston J, et al. Helping midlife women predict the onset of the final menses: SWAN, the Study of Women's Health Across the Nation. Menopause 2007;14:415–24.

24. Lisabeth L, Harlow S, Qaqish B. A new statistical approach demonstrated menstrual patterns during the menopausal transition did not vary by age at menopause. J Clin Epidemiol 2004;57:484–96.

25. den Tonkelaar I, te Velde ER, Looman CW. Menstrual cycle length preceding menopause in relation to age at menopause. Maturitas 1998;29:115–23.

26. Soules MR, Sherman S, Parrott E, et al. Executive summary: Stages of Reproductive Aging Workshop (STRAW). Fertil Steril 2001;76:874–8.

27. Harlow SD, Crawford S, Dennerstein L, et al. Recommendations from a multi-study evaluation of proposed criteria for staging reproductive aging. Climacteric 2007;10:112–9.

28. Lisabeth LD, Harlow SD, Gillespie B, et al. Staging reproductive aging: a comparison of proposed bleeding criteria for the menopausal transition. Menopause 2004;11:186–97.

29. Harlow SD, Cain K, Crawford S, et al. Evaluation of four proposed bleeding criteria for the onset of late menopausal transition. J Clin Endocrinol Metab 2006;91:3432–8.

30. Randolph JF Jr, Crawford S, Dennerstein L, et al. The value of follicle-stimulating hormone concentration and clinical findings as markers of the late menopausal transition. J Clin Endocrinol Metab 2006;91:3034–40.

31. Taffe JR, Cain KC, Mitchell ES, et al. "Persistence" improves the 60-day amenorrhea marker of entry to late-stage menopausal transition for women aged 40 to 44 years. Menopause 2010;17:191–3.

32. Harlow SD, Mitchell ES, Crawford S, et al. The ReSTAGE Collaboration: defining optimal bleeding criteria for onset of early menopausal transition. Fertil Steril 2008;89:129–40.

33. Randolph JF Jr, Zheng H, Sowers MR, et al. Change in follicle-stimulating hormone and estradiol across the menopausal transition: effect of age at the final menstrual period. J Clin Endocrinol Metab 2011;96:746–54.

34. Burger HG, Hale GE, Dennerstein L, et al. Cycle and hormone changes during perimenopause: the key role of ovarian function. Menopause 2008;15:603–12.

35. Hale GE, Zhao X, Hughes CL, et al. Endocrine features of menstrual cycles in middle and late reproductive age and the menopausal transition classified according to the Staging of Reproductive Aging Workshop (STRAW) staging system. J Clin Endocrinol Metab 2007;92:3060–7.

36. Landgren BM, Collins A, Csemiczky G, et al. Menopause transition: annual changes in serum hormonal patterns over the menstrual cycle in women during a nine-year period prior to menopause. J Clin Endocrinol Metab 2004;89:2763–9.

37. Burger HG, Dudley E, Mamers P, et al. Early follicular phase serum FSH as a function of age: the roles of inhibin B, inhibin A and estradiol. Climacteric 2000;3:17–24.

38. Robertson DM. Anti-Mullerian hormone as a marker of ovarian reserve: an update. Womens Health (Lond Engl) 2008;4:137–41.
39. Freeman EW, Sammel MD, Lin H, et al. Obesity and reproductive hormone levels in the transition to menopause. Menopause 2010;17:718–26.
40. Gracia CR, Freeman EW, Sammel MD, et al. The relationship between obesity and race on inhibin B during the menopause transition. Menopause 2005;12:559–66.
41. Huddleston HG, Cedars MI, Sohn SH, et al. Racial and ethnic disparities in reproductive endocrinology and infertility. Am J Obstet Gynecol 2010;202:413–9.
42. Randolph JF Jr, Sowers M, Bondarenko IV, et al. Change in estradiol and follicle-stimulating hormone across the early menopausal transition: effects of ethnicity and age. J Clin Endocrinol Metab 2004;89:1555–61.
43. Santoro N, Lasley B, McConnell D, et al. Body size and ethnicity are associated with menstrual cycle alterations in women in the early menopausal transition: the Study of Women's Health across the Nation (SWAN) Daily Hormone Study. J Clin Endocrinol Metab 2004;89:2622–31.
44. Su HI, Sammel MD, Freeman EW, et al. Body size affects measures of ovarian reserve in late reproductive age women. Menopause 2008;15:857–61.
45. Johnson BD, Merz CN, Braunstein GD, et al. Determination of menopausal status in women: the NHLBI-sponsored Women's Ischemia Syndrome Evaluation (WISE) Study. J Womens Health (Larchmt) 2004;13:872–87.
46. Hudecova M, Holte J, Olovsson M, et al. Long-term follow-up of patients with polycystic ovary syndrome: reproductive outcome and ovarian reserve. Hum Reprod 2009;24:1176–83.
47. Tehrani FR, Solaymani-Dodaran M, Hedayati M, et al. Is polycystic ovary syndrome an exception for reproductive aging? Hum Reprod 2010;25:1775–81.
48. Santoro N, Arnsten JH, Buono D, et al. Impact of street drug use, HIV infection, and highly active antiretroviral therapy on reproductive hormones in middle-aged women. J Womens Health (Larchmt) 2005;14:898–905.
49. Harlow SD, Crawford SL, Sommer B, et al. Self-defined menopausal status in a multi-ethnic sample of midlife women. Maturitas 2000;36:93–112.
50. Taffe J, Dennerstein L. Time to the final menstrual period. Fertil Steril 2002;78:397–403.
51. Ballinger CB, Browning MC, Smith AH. Hormone profiles and psychological symptoms in peri-menopausal women. Maturitas 1987;9:235–51.
52. Hale GE, Manconi F, Luscombe G, et al. Quantitative measurements of menstrual blood loss in ovulatory and anovulatory cycles in middle- and late-reproductive age and the menopausal transition. Obstet Gynecol 2010;115:249–56.
53. Mitchell ES, Woods NF. Symptom experiences of midlife women: observations from the Seattle Midlife Women's Health Study. Maturitas 1996;25:1–10.
54. Hallberg L, Hogdahl AM, Nilsson L, et al. Menstrual blood loss: a population study. Variation at different ages and attempts to define normality. Acta Obstet Gynecol Scand 1966;45:320–51.
55. Sowers MR, Zheng H, McConnell D, et al. Estradiol rates of change in relation to the final menstrual period in a population-based cohort of women. J Clin Endocrinol Metab 2008;93:3847–52.
56. Astrup K, Olivarius Nde F, Moller S, et al. Menstrual bleeding patterns in pre- and perimenopausal women: a population-based prospective diary study. Acta Obstet Gynecol Scand 2004;83:197–202.
57. Harlow SD, Ephross SA. Epidemiology of menstruation and its relevance to women's health. Epidemiol Rev 1995;17:265–86.

58. Harlow SD, Campbell B. Ethnic differences in the duration and amount of menstrual bleeding during the postmenarcheal period. Am J Epidemiol 1996;144:980–8.
59. Harlow SD, Campbell B, Lin X, et al. Ethnic differences in the length of the menstrual cycle during the postmenarcheal period. Am J Epidemiol 1997;146:572–80.
60. Liu Y, Gold EB, Lasley BL, et al. Factors affecting menstrual cycle characteristics. Am J Epidemiol 2004;160:131–40.
61. Waller K, Swan SH, Windham GC, et al. Use of urine biomarkers to evaluate menstrual function in healthy premenopausal women. Am J Epidemiol 1998;147:1071–80.
62. Kato I, Toniolo P, Koenig KL, et al. Epidemiologic correlates with menstrual cycle length in middle aged women. Eur J Epidemiol 1999;15:809–14.
63. Wise LA, Krieger N, Zierler S, et al. Lifetime socioeconomic position in relation to onset of perimenopause. J Epidemiol Community Health 2002;56:851–60.
64. Sammel MD, Freeman EW, Liu Z, et al. Factors that influence entry into stages of the menopausal transition. Menopause 2009;16:1218–27.
65. Cooper GS, Sandler DP, Whelan EA, et al. Association of physical and behavioral characteristics with menstrual cycle patterns in women age 29–31 years. Epidemiology 1996;7:624–8.
66. Symons JP, Sowers MF, Harlow SD. Relationship of body composition measures and menstrual cycle length. Ann Hum Biol 1997;24:107–16.
67. Harlow SD, Matanoski GM. The association between weight, physical activity, and stress and variation in the length of the menstrual cycle. Am J Epidemiol 1991;133: 38–49.
68. Rowland AS, Baird DD, Long S, et al. Influence of medical conditions and lifestyle factors on the menstrual cycle. Epidemiology 2002;13:668–74.
69. Cooper GS, Klebanoff MA, Promislow J, et al. Polychlorinated biphenyls and menstrual cycle characteristics. Epidemiology 2005;16:191–200.
70. Harlow SD, Campbell BC. Host factors that influence the duration of menstrual bleeding. Epidemiology 1994;5:352–5.
71. Belsey EM, d'Arcangues C, Carlson N. Determinants of menstrual bleeding patterns among women using natural and hormonal methods of contraception. II. The influence of individual characteristics. Contraception 1988;38:243–57.
72. Lin HT, Lin LC, Shiao JS. The impact of self-perceived job stress on menstrual patterns among Taiwanese nurses. Ind Health 2007;45:709–14.
73. Sternfeld B, Jacobs MK, Quesenberry CP Jr, et al. Physical activity and menstrual cycle characteristics in two prospective cohorts. Am J Epidemiol 2002;156:402–9.
74. Gold EB, Bromberger J, Crawford S, et al. Factors associated with age at natural menopause in a multiethnic sample of midlife women. Am J Epidemiol 2001;153: 865–74.
75. Dorman JS, Steenkiste AR, Foley TP, et al. Menopause in type 1 diabetic women: is it premature? Diabetes 2001;50:1857–62.
76. Luborsky JL, Meyer P, Sowers MF, et al. Premature menopause in a multi-ethnic population study of the menopause transition. Hum Reprod 2003;18:199–206.
77. Strotmeyer ES, Steenkiste AR, Foley TP Jr, et al. Menstrual cycle differences between women with type 1 diabetes and women without diabetes. Diabetes Care 2003;26: 1016–21.
78. Benson RC, Dailey ME. The menstrual pattern in hyperthyroidism and subsequent posttherapy hypothyroidism. Surg Gynecol Obstet 1955;100:19–26.
79. Sowers M, Luborsky J, Perdue C, et al. Thyroid stimulating hormone (TSH) concentrations and menopausal status in women at the mid-life: SWAN. Clin Endocrinol (Oxf) 2003;58:340–7.

80. Chen CR, Buck GM, Courey NG, et al. Risk factors for uterine fibroids among women undergoing tubal sterilization. Am J Epidemiol 2001;153:20–6.
81. Clevenger-Hoeft M, Syrop CH, Stovall DW, et al. Sonohysterography in premeno-pausal women with and without abnormal bleeding. Obstet Gynecol 1999;94: 516–20.
82. DeWaay DJ, Syrop CH, Nygaard IE, et al. Natural history of uterine polyps and leiomyomata. Obstet Gynecol 2002;100:3–7.
83. Marino JL, Eskenazi B, Warner M, et al. Uterine leiomyoma and menstrual cycle characteristics in a population-based cohort study. Hum Reprod 2004;19:2350–5.
84. Wegienka G, Baird DD, Hertz-Picciotto I, et al. Self-reported heavy bleeding associ-ated with uterine leiomyomata. Obstet Gynecol 2003;101:431–7.
85. Sjalander A, Friberg B, Svensson P, et al. Menorrhagia and minor bleeding symptoms in women on oral anticoagulation. J Thromb Thrombolysis 2007;24:39–41.
86. Windham GC, Elkin EP, Swan SH, et al. Cigarette smoking and effects on menstrual function. Obstet Gynecol 1999;93:59–65.
87. Hornsby PP, Wilcox AJ, Weinberg CR. Cigarette smoking and disturbance of men-strual function. Epidemiology 1998;9:193–8.

Mood and Menopause: Findings from the Study of Women's Health Across the Nation (SWAN) over 10 Years

Joyce T. Bromberger, PhD[a],*, Howard M. Kravitz, DO, MPH[b]

KEYWORDS

- Menopause • Mood • Depression • Risk factors

Depression exacts great emotional, social, and economic costs in the form of treatment expenses, lost productivity, and emotional and social impairment. This is particularly consequential for women because the lifetime prevalence of major depression (MD) alone is more than 20%.[1,2] Women have a 2-fold greater risk for depression than men. These gender differences have been found for both major depressive disorder as well as depressive symptoms in a large European study (the Depressive Research in European Society[3]). Considerable research has focused on the physiologic and psychosocial differences between men and women as sources of depression. An important target of study has been the periods of reproductive changes and events that occur at puberty, postpartum, and menopause.

For decades, a controversy has existed regarding the extent to which, if at all, the menopausal transition or postmenopause increases the risk for elevated depressive symptoms and/or disorders. In 1995, when the Study of Women's Health Across the Nation (SWAN) began, the state of knowledge about this issue was unclear and

The Study of Women's Health Across the Nation (SWAN) has grant support from the National Institutes of Health (NIH), DHHS, through the National Institute on Aging (NIA), the National Institute of Nursing Research (NINR) and the NIH Office of Research on Women's Health (ORWH) (Grants NR004061; AG012505, AG012535, AG012531, AG012539, AG012546, AG012553, AG012554, AG012495). The content of this manuscript is solely the responsibility of the authors and does not necessarily represent the official views of the NIA, NINR, ORWH or the NIH.

Supplemental funding from The National Institute of Mental Health is also gratefully acknowledged. University of Pittsburgh, Pittsburgh, PA — Joyce T. Bromberger, PI (R01 MH59689); Rush University, Medical Center, Chicago, IL — Howard M. Kravitz, PI (R01 MH59770); New Jersey Medical School, Newark, NJ — Adriana Cordal, PI (R01 MH59688).

[a] Departments of Epidemiology and Psychiatry, University of Pittsburgh, 3811 O'Hara Street, Pittsburgh, PA 15213, USA

[b] Departments of Psychiatry and Preventive Medicine, Rush University Medical Center, 2150 West Harrison Street – Room 275, Chicago, IL 60612, USA

* Corresponding author.

E-mail address: brombergerjt@upmc.edu

confusing, based largely on a cycle of "beliefs" and inconsistent findings from predominantly cross-sectional and small clinical studies that used varied measures of depressive symptoms. At that time, the most recent epidemiologic studies of menopause had found no relationship between depressive symptoms and menopausal status or in some cases, higher levels of symptoms during perimenopause (see Matthews et al[4] for a review). SWAN provided an opportunity to address the issue with the largest, most representative, diverse cohort until that time.

The current paper presents findings relevant to 4 important questions regarding depression, menopause, and aging: (1) Does the menopausal transition or postmenopause render women more vulnerable to depression than does the premenopause? (2) Does the risk for depression vary by race/ethnicity or by differing influences on risk by menopausal status among different ethnic groups? (3) If depression is more prevalent during or after the transition, is this owing to hormonal alterations, psychological, developmental, and/or somatic changes associated with the transition, midlife (more generally) or genetic vulnerability? and (4) What are the risk factors for depression during midlife and what is the impact of menopausal status on depression relative to these other factors? We also examined these questions for negative mood symptoms including irritability, nervousness, and frequent mood changes (also comprising psychological distress or dysphoric mood).

Depression has been variously defined across a spectrum ranging from a relatively brief negative mood state that includes feeling sad or being "blue" to a medically defined syndrome called Major Depressive Disorder/Minor Depression (a subthreshold depressive disorder that has fewer symptoms than major) or "clinical depression." The criteria for clinical depression include the duration of symptoms for a minimum of 2 weeks and symptoms that cause significant distress or impairment in functioning. Depressive symptom measures are useful for estimating symptom level or severity, and, in some cases, as a screen for clinical depression. However, the presence of depressive symptoms measured by a variety of scales usually focus on a prescribed period of time (usually the previous 1–2 weeks), does not have a duration or impairment criterion nor does it inquire about past symptoms.

SWAN included a standard measure of depressive symptom levels in its baseline and annual assessments at all sites. With funding from the National Institute of Mental Health, 3 of the SWAN sites (Chicago, Newark, and Pittsburgh) conducted at baseline the Structured Clinical Interview for DSM-IV Axis I Disorders (SCID),[5,6] a semi structured psychiatric assessment to ascertain diagnoses of multiple psychiatric disorders, including clinical depression. Pittsburgh has continued to conduct these assessments annually, and now has collected 11 years of annual follow-up data to chart the course of depression as these women have transitioned to early postmenopause. This paper presents what we have learned about depression from women participating in Core SWAN as well as the ancillary Mental Health Study over the past 16 years. For comparison purposes, we review other recent large longitudinal epidemiologic studies of menopause and depression conducted during this period.[7–10] These recent studies had larger or more diverse samples, longer and more frequent follow-up, more careful definitions of menopausal status, and conducted analyses that utilized more fully the longitudinal data than did earlier studies. Published SWAN findings are presented separately for negative mood and depressive symptoms and clinical disorder (major and minor depressive disorders) outcomes. We also describe briefly our analyses showing that depression is a risk factor for physical health outcomes.

Table 1		
SWAN studies examining menopausal status and risk factors for negative mood and depressive symptoms and disorder		
Reference	**Design/Sample**	**Outcome: Symptoms**
Bromberger et al[19]	Cross-sectional/n = 10,374 women, aged 40–55 years, screened	Psychological distress, feeling blue, irritable and tense
Brombergeret al[20]	Cross-sectional/baseline cohort[a]	Frequent mood symptoms occurring ≥6 days/2 wks (3 above and mood change)
Bromberger et al[21]	Cross-sectional/baseline cohort[a]	Depressive symptoms, CES-D ≥ 16
Bromberger et al[22]	Longitudinal/baseline through V5	CES-D ≥ 16
Bromberger et al[24]	Longitudinal/baseline through V8; n = 3015–3302	CES-D ≥ 16
Reference	**Design/Sample**	**Outcome: MD**
Bromberger et al[37]	Longitudinal/baseline through V7; n = 266	MD
Bromberger et al[23]	Longitudinal/baseline through V9; n = 221	MD

[a] Cohort, aged 42–52 years.

DEPRESSIVE SYMPTOMS AND MENOPAUSE
How Do We Measure Depression in SWAN at All 7 Sites?

All sites have been using the Center for Epidemiological Studies Depression Scale (CES-D)[11] to assess depressive symptom levels. The CES-D was designed to be used as a screen for depression in epidemiologic studies, not for making diagnoses.[12] We chose to use this self-report scale for its minimal cost and burden, its wide use in epidemiologic and clinical studies including those of menopause, the evidence that it would provide reliable estimates of depressive symptom levels, and because it has been validated for administration in different ethnic groups.[13–17] The CES-D asks about the frequency of being bothered by 20 depressive symptoms during the previous week on a 4-point scale of 0 (rarely) to 3 (most or all of the time).[11] A total score of 16 or higher is commonly used to identify potential clinical depression[12,18] and was used to indicate clinically relevant depressive symptoms in SWAN.

At baseline, 23% of the sample scored 16 or higher on the CES-D. Baseline characteristics varied significantly between women with a CES-D of 16 or higher ("high CES-D") and those with a CES-D of less than 16. Women with high CES-D were less well educated and more likely to be younger, had a negative attitude toward aging and menopause, and reported greater financial strain. They were also more likely to be African American or Hispanic, less likely to be Chinese or Japanese, and more likely to be early perimenopausal than those with low CES-D (*P*<.0001).

What Have We Learned about Depressive Symptoms/Negative Mood and the Menopausal Transition in SWAN?

Does the risk for high depressive symptom levels vary by menopausal status and is it independent of known risk factors for depression?
We have published 5 papers on depressive or negative mood symptoms (3 baseline cross-sectional and 2 longitudinal) relevant to the transition to menopause (**Table 1**).

(1) The initial cross-sectional paper was based on data from 10,374 women who completed the screening questionnaire at baseline. Psychologic distress was defined as feeling blue, irritable, and tense. We compared presence of distress in women who were premenopausal with those who were early perimenopausal, late perimenopausal, or postmenopausal.[19] (2) In the baseline cohort, we compared the prevalence of persistent mood symptoms and overall dysphoric mood between premenopause and early perimenopause women, adjusted for multiple covariates.[20] (3) We examined the race/ethnic differences in the prevalence of depressive symptoms (CES-D≥16) adjusted for multiple covariates including menopausal status at baseline.[21] (4) Annual data from baseline through visit 5 were used to examine the longitudinal relationship between menopausal status and risk of elevated depressive symptoms (CES-D≥ 16).[22,23] (5) Annual data from baseline through visit 8 were used to extend the previous analyses to evaluate the relationship between serum hormone levels and high depressive symptoms and whether hormone levels or their changes might explain the association of menopausal status with depressive symptoms.[24]

The first 3 papers reported that prevalences of psychologic distress, dysphoric mood, and a CES-D of 16 or greater were lowest in the premenopausal women (20.9%, 9%, and 20.9%, respectively); prevalences in the early perimenopausal women were 28.9%, 15%, and 27.8%, respectively. Dysphoric mood consisted of the total score for 4 mood symptoms that ranged from 0 to 16; we defined dysphoric mood as the top 10% of the distribution, which is why the prevalences are much lower than those for psychologic distress (top 24%) and CES-D of 16 or higher (top 23%). In the cross-sectional screening study sample,[19] prevalences of psychological distress in late perimenopause and postmenopause were 25.6% and 22%, respectively. Compared with premenopause, the adjusted risk of psychological distress, dysphoric mood, or high CES-D, was 20% to 62% higher in early perimenopause.

Results of the longitudinal analyses for depressive symptoms were consistent with those from the cross-sectional analyses.[22,24] In multivariable random effects logistic regression models using data from 5 years and 8 years of annual assessments, being perimenopausal or postmenopausal compared with being premenopausal remained significantly associated with CES-D of 16 or higher in all analyses. For example, across 5 years, women were significantly more likely to report a high CES-D when early perimenopausal (odds ratio [OR], 1.30), late perimenopausal (OR, 1.71), and postmenopausal (OR, 1.57) relative to when they were premenopausal and when they were late perimenopausal (OR, 1.32) compared with when early perimenopausal. In these analyses, we also reported on the risk of depression among women who had ever used exogenous hormones (OR, 1.43). These results were independent of education, race/ethnicity, vasomotor symptoms (VMS), stressful life events, and low social support at each visit.[22] The 8-year findings extended and were consistent with those from the first 5 years[24] (**Fig. 1**).

Does the risk for elevated depressive symptoms vary across race/ethnic groups or by differing relationships between symptoms and menopausal status among the different groups?

At baseline, there were race/ethnic differences in the prevalence of negative mood symptoms and high CES-D as well as in the relationship of menopausal status with odds of high CES-D. The differences varied depending on the outcomes. In baseline unadjusted analyses, Caucasian, African-American, and Hispanic women had the highest rates of CES-D of 16 or greater, frequent irritability, nervousness, and psychological distress; Chinese and Japanese women had the lowest (**Fig. 2**). Adjustments for sociodemographic, psychosocial, and health factors attenuated the

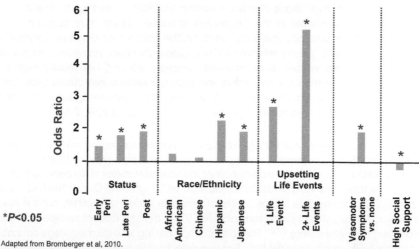

*P<0.05

Adapted from Bromberger et al, 2010.

Note: Referent for early peri, late peri, and post was premenopausal; referent for 1 and 2+ life events was no life events.
Adjusted for education, concurrent testosterone, age, smoking status, psychotropic medications, body mass index, and site.

Fig. 1. Fully adjusted random effects logistic regression model examining the odds of high depressive symptoms (CES-D≥16). (*Data from* Bromberger JT, Schott LL, Kravitz HM, et al. Longitudinal change in reproductive hormones and depressive symptoms across the menopausal transition: results from the Study of Women's Health Across the Nation (SWAN). Arch Gen Psychiatry 2010;67:598–607.)

effects of race/ethnicity. These results suggest that psychosocial and health related factors accounted for higher odds of depressive symptoms among African-American and Hispanic.[21]

The multivariable longitudinal analyses for race/ethnicity were not entirely consistent with the cross-sectional analyses. Over the first 8 years of the study, the odds of high depressive symptoms significantly increased in Hispanic and Japanese compared with the Caucasian women. The odds of the African-American and Chinese women were not

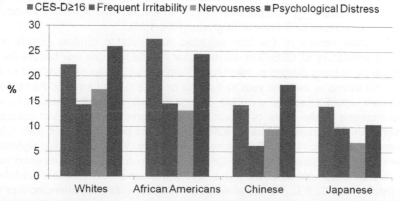

Fig. 2. Prevalence of CES-D of 16 or higher, frequent irritability, nervousness, and psychological distress at baseline by race/ethnicity.

significantly different than those of the Caucasian women[24] (see **Fig. 1**). The 2 sets of analyses differed somewhat in the covariates included, which may account for the different findings. It is also possible that, over time, the risk for high depressive symptoms among the race/ethnic groups relative to Caucasians changed. However, the elevated risk for the Japanese women over time was unexpected and not readily explained. Associations between menopausal status and high depressive symptoms were similar among 4 of the 5 ethnic groups. Among Hispanic women, perimenopause was associated with more than a 2-fold risk of high depressive symptoms (OR, 2.45).[21]

What factors contribute to risk for high depressive symptoms among midlife women, what is the relative importance of menopausal status, and do hormone levels or changes or VMS account for the association of menopausal status with depression?
Numerous factors were independently associated with high CES-D over the first 5 and 8 years of SWAN. The models for the 2 sets of analyses varied somewhat, but the results were similar. The significant predictors included VMS, being a current smoker, low social support, very stressful events,[22,24] financial strain,[22] having less than a college education, and a higher body mass index (BMI).[24] For example, having less than a college education was associated with an increased odds ratios of 1.5 to 2 times compared with having a college education or more; VMS increased the odds by 62% to 77% and reporting 2 or more life events increase the odds by more than 5 times. For every 1 unit increase in BMI, the odds of high depressive symptoms increased by 1%. High social support was protective and reduced the odds by nearly 20%[24] (see **Fig. 1**).

A key question is the role of reproductive hormones in the development of depression and negative mood during the menopausal transition or shortly after. Neurobiological data have indicated that gonadal steroids affect a wide range of neuromodulator processes, including the neuromodulators serotonin and norepinephrine, which are implicated in the development of depression.[25,26] However, epidemiologic and clinical studies that have examined associations between reproductive hormones and depression have yielded inconsistent results.[10,27] Using 8 years of follow-up data, we assessed whether reproductive hormones were related to risk of high depressive symptoms (CES-D$\geq$16).[24] Specifically, we examined the association between serum levels and changes in follicle-stimulating hormone, estradiol (E2), and testosterone (T) and odds of high depressive symptoms. Multivariable random effects logistic regression models showed that log transformed T ($_{log}$T) was significantly positively associated with higher odds of CES-D of 16 or higher (OR, 1.15) across 8 years and a larger increase in $_{log}$T from baseline to each annual visit was significantly associated with increased odds of CES-D of 16 or greater (OR, 1.23).[24]

Fig. 1 shows results of the fully adjusted multivariable random effects model examining predictors of CES-D of 16 or higher.[24] The multiple risk factors for high depressive symptoms ranged in magnitude from an odds ratio of 5.13 for 2 or more stressful life events in the past year to 1.42 for being a current smoker. As noted, the independent effect of status on odds of high CES-D was substantial, showing a graded increase in the odds of reporting high depression symptoms across the transition from early perimenopause (OR, 1.35) to late perimenopause (OR, 1.68) to postmenopause (OR, 1.83). Furthermore, reporting VMS was also significantly independently associated with high CES-D in these analyses. Thus, each menopause-related factor (menopausal status, T, VMS) made an independent contribution to the risk for high CES-D. Nevertheless, it is noteworthy that experiencing 2 or more upsetting life events in the previous year was the strongest predictor of risk, increasing it by more than 5 times.

Table 2 Criteria for MDE
A. Five (or more) of the following symptoms have been present during the same 2-week period and represent a change from previous functioning; at least 1 of the symptoms is either (1) depressed mood or (2) loss of interest or pleasure.
1. Depressed, sad mood
2. Decreased interest/pleasure in activities
3. Significant weight loss/gain or decreased/increased appetite
4. Insomnia or hypersomnia
5. Psychomotor agitation or retardation
6. Fatigue
7. Feelings of worthlessness or excessive guilt
8. Decreased ability to think or concentrate, or indecisiveness
9. Recurrent thoughts of death, suicidal ideation with or without a plan or suicide attempt
B. The symptoms do not meet criteria for a mixed episode (manic and depressive symptoms together).
C. The symptoms cause clinically significant distress or impairment in social, occupational, or other important areas of functioning.
D. The symptoms are not due to the direct physiologic effects of a substance (e.g., a drug of abuse, a medication) or a general medical condition (e.g., hypothyroidism).
E. The symptoms are not better accounted for by bereavement, i.e., after the loss of a loved one.
Criteria for Minor Depression
2–4 symptoms lasting for ≥2 weeks.
Criteria B–E for MD above

Data from Diagnostic and Statistical Manual of Mental Disorders, Fourth Edition. American Psychiatric Association 1994.

Finally, being perimenopausal or postmenopausal remained significantly associated with risk for CES-D of 16 or greater in all analyses. These results suggest that neither hormones nor VMS accounted for the association of menopausal status defined by bleeding patterns with elevated depressive symptoms.

MAJOR DEPRESSIVE DISORDER AND MENOPAUSE
How Is MD Defined and How Was It Assessed in the Chicago, Newark, and Pittsburgh SWAN?

MD is defined as the presence of at least 5 depressive symptoms with impaired functioning for at least most of 2 weeks[28] (**Table 2**). It is a highly prevalent major health problem and the leading cause of health-related disability in women.[29] About 22% of women in midlife have a history of MD[1] and 5% have current MD.[30] Similar findings were reported in the NCS Replication study.[2] Of individuals who have a first episode, 50% to 80% experience another.[31] MD is associated with a worse course and outcome of physical illness and can complicate its treatment; it also has a major impact on a woman's functioning in her various roles.[32,33]

As noted, diagnoses of lifetime and current major depressive disorders were determined from interviews conducted by trained clinicians utilizing the SCID.[6] The SCID has been used with many different ethnic groups and extensive field testing has demonstrated its suitability for research purposes; adequate reliability has been demonstrated in numerous studies,[5] including SWAN's Mental Health Study. The SCID was administered at baseline by all 3 sites and annually in Pittsburgh only.

At baseline, 35% of the cohort had a lifetime history of MD; 17% had a history of recurrent MD. Prevalence of current MD (past month) was 3%. Our lifetime prevalence was higher than those reported in epidemiologic studies such as the National Comorbidity Survey (NCS),[1] and its replication (NCS-R).[1,2] On the other hand, MD rates in the Virginia Twin Study[34,35] were considerably higher than the NCS, at 30% to 35% for women based on same-gender twins. The methods used in the latter study involved extensive training procedures and clinically trained interviewers, and are similar to those we used. It is also possible that women who participate in a longitudinal study of menopause may be more likely to have had previous emotional problems or be more willing to discuss these. Baseline characteristics between women with and without a history of MD varied significantly. Women with a history were less well educated and were more likely to report greater financial strain, be unemployed, smoke currently, and report low social support. Prevalence of history of MD did not vary by race/ethnicity. Among the middle-aged overall[36] and women specifically aged 45 to 54 years,[30] the prevalence rates for 30-day, 12-month, and lifetime major depressive episodes (MDEs) are similar between or higher in Caucasians than African Americans. However, in the NCS, there were few women in this age group.[30] Importantly, to our knowledge, other than the Penn Ovarian Aging Study (POAS),[27] no studies have examined the occurrence of MDEs during and soon after the menopausal transition in substantial numbers of African Americans.

What Have We Learned About MD and the Menopausal Transition in SWAN?

Does the risk for MD vary by menopausal status and is it independent of known risk factors for depression?

We have published 2 papers on MD relevant to menopause (**Table 1**). Both used the longitudinal data and therefore included only the data from the Pittsburgh cohort. To examine whether women were more likely to experience a MDE during perimenopause or postmenopause compared with when they were premenopausal, we analyzed data from the baseline and the first 8 annual assessments of 221 women who were premenopausal at study entry.[23] Using repeated measures logistic regression, we found that women were 2 to 4 times more likely to experience a MDE when they were perimenopausal (OR, 2.27) or postmenopausal (OR, 3.57), even after controlling for a variety of factors associated with depression, including a history of MD at baseline, annual psychotropic medication use, BMI, very upsetting life events, and frequent VMS. These data also were analyzed separately for African-American and Caucasian women, and both had similar odds for onset of a depressive episode during the transition.

The second paper reported on the determinants of a first onset of MD during midlife.[37] We were particularly interested in the role of menopausal factors in first onsets. The subcohort included in this analysis was comprised of the 266 women without past or current MD at baseline. Cox proportional hazards analyses of data from 8 annual assessments identified predictors of first onsets. Forty-two (15.8%) of the 266 women met criteria for a first onset MDE during the transition. In contrast with the results of the analyses in the full sample described, menopausal status was not significant in univariate or multivariate analyses.

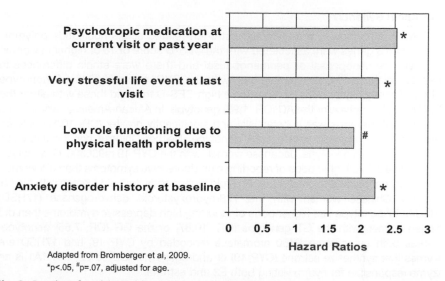

Fig. 3. Results of multivariable model predicting first depression onset. (*Data from* Bromberger JT, Kravitz HM, Matthews K, et al. Predictors of first lifetime episodes of major depression in midlife women. Psychol Med 2009;39:55–64.)

What factors contribute to risk for MD among midlife women, what is the relative importance of menopausal status, and do hormone levels or changes or VMS account for the association of menopausal status with risk for MD?

As noted, MD is multifactorially determined. It is well-known that the strongest predictor of an episode of MD is having a history of MD,[38] which tripled the odds in our analysis. Higher BMI was also marginally significantly associated with MD over the study. In both sets of analyses, we found that experiencing very upsetting life events was a consistently strong predictor of MD. In the case of predictors of first onset MD, whereas menopausal status and frequent VMS were nonsignificant, very upsetting life events doubled the odds of experiencing a new MDE. VMS were significant in the univariate analysis only, suggesting that upsetting life events were more important for first onset MD than frequent VMS. In addition to menopausal status and upsetting life events, we examined health-related risk factors as predictors of first MD because of their salience for midlife women. Although higher baseline social and role functioning and previous annual BMI and frequent VMS were each significantly associated with odds of first onset MD in univariate analyses, they did not retain their significance in the multivariate analyses. Indeed, as shown in **Fig. 3**, the results of Cox regression multivariable analyses indicated that a history of an anxiety disorder (hazard ratio [HR], 2.20) at baseline, and psychotropic medication use (HR, 2.53) and at least 1 very stressful event (HR, 2.25) at the last visit before meeting criteria for a depressive episode currently or in the year since prior visit, were significant independent predictors of first MD onset. Low role functioning owing to physical health was marginally significant.

Neither baseline reproductive hormone levels nor changes over time were significantly associated with MD in any of the analyses. Similar to findings for high depressive symptoms, we observed that neither endogenous hormones nor VMS attenuated the menopausal status–MD associations, suggesting that they did not account for the association of menopausal status defined by bleeding patterns with MD.

What About Genetics?

The SWAN data showed that selected estrogen-related single nucleotide polymorphisms from 3 genes were associated with the CES-D score of 16 or higher in women who were premenopausal or perimenopausal and there were ethnic differences in these associations.[39] Caucasian women with the CYP1A1 rs2606345 CC genotype had significantly higher odds of reporting a high CES-D than did those with either the AA (OR, 2.49) genotype or the AC (OR, 1.98) genotype. In African-American women, the magnitude of the odds was substantially and significantly greater (OR, 10.17) only for those with CC compared with the AA genotype. Neither Chinese nor the Japanese women had the AA genotype. Japanese women with the CYP 19 rs936306 TT genotype had almost a 5-fold higher odds of reporting high depressive symptoms than did women with the CC genotype and greater than 9.6-fold higher odds than did women with the CT genotype. Chinese women with the 17β-hydroxysteroid dehydrogenase (17HSD) rs615942 TT genotype had higher odds of reporting high depressive symptoms than did Chinese women with the GT genotype (OR, 10.87) or the GG (OR, 7.65) genotype. Whereas both cytochrome P450 aromatase (encoded by CYP 19) and 17HSD are enzymes that synthesize estrone (CYP 19) or androgens (17HSD) to E2, CYP1A1 is an enzyme responsible for hydroxylating both E2 and estrone.

Although these are findings are only preliminary and observed in relatively small samples, they do suggest that variation in these 3 estrogen-related genes may be associated with depressive symptoms in women. Moreover, for each of these 3 polymorphisms, the results remained significant after controlling for psychosocial factors that we have shown to be associated with depressive symptoms in different ethnic groups.[21] Our findings lend support to notions that genes together with psychosocial factors may influence risk for depressive symptoms and that estrogen may contribute to the development of these symptoms in midlife women.

OTHER LONGITUDINAL EPIDEMIOLOGIC STUDIES OF MENOPAUSE AND DEPRESSION

Four recent longitudinal studies have examined the relationship between menopausal status and depressive symptoms[7–10] and/or clinical or severe depression (**Tables 3 and 4**).[7,8,27] Despite using different sampling frames, sizes, and compositions and varying designs and analyses, the results were consistent—they all reported that risk for depression (symptoms or disorder) increased during the perimenopause. Moreover, with the exception of Maartens et al,[9] in which 2103 women provided data 3 years apart via mailed questionnaires, these studies did not find an increased risk for depressive symptoms in the postmenopause compared with premenopause. The null findings may have been due to insufficient power to detect a difference because of relatively small numbers of women followed through postmenopause. For example, the POAS[8] reported that depressive symptoms but not disorder increased in the perimenopause and subsequently declined in the postmenopause over 4 years of follow-up. However, in this study 73% of the 332 participants remained premenopausal over the 4 years of follow-up and only 3% completed the transition, making the numbers for postmenopause and MD too small to determine significance.

Also in the POAS, Freeman et al[27] found a significantly increased adjusted odds ratio (AOR, 5.44) for the first onset of high depressive symptoms during perimenopause compared with premenopause. In the Harvard Study of Moods and Cycles, Cohen et al[7] reported that women who became perimenopausal had only a marginally significant higher odds of first onset high depressive symptoms (AOR, 1.9) after adjustment for age and stressful life events than did those who remained premeno-

Table 3

Depression by menopause transition: recent longitudinal studies of midlife women

Study	Design	Sample	Covariates/Predictors	Outcome(s)	Results
University of Tilburg, The Netherlands (Maartens et al[9])	Postal Quest. 2 waves of data 3.5 years apart	n = 2103, aged 47–53 years	Demographics, life events, ↑ depressive symptoms at T1.	EDS symptom score > 12	Peri- and post, financial prob significant
POA (Freeman et al[8])	In-home visits. 6 assessments over 4 years	n = 436, aged 35–47 years		CES-D symptom score ≥16 in past week. Primary Care Evaluation of Mental Disorders in past month	Peri-, African American, VMS, PMS, poor sleep significant
Seattle Midlife Women's Health Study (Woods et al[10])	9 years apart	n = 508, aged 35–55		CES-D symptom score ≥ 16	Late peri-, greater BMI, postpartum blues, no children, stressor significant

Abbreviations: EDS, edinburgh depression scale; PMS, premenstrual syndrome.

Table 4				
First onset depression by menopause transition: longitudinal studies				
Study	**Design**	**Sample**	**Outcome**	**Results**
The Harvard Study of Moods and Cycles (Cohen et al[7])	8 years apart	n = 460, no history of depression	First onset high depressive symptoms: CES-D, CES-D+ (severe symptoms)	Perimenopause marginally significant overall Significant in women with VMS and stressful event
POAS (Freeman et al[27])	8 years apart	n = 231 women, no history of depression	First onset high depressive symptoms CES-D and depressive disorder	Perimenopause significant for symptoms, not for depressive disorder greater BMI, E2, greater SD significant

Abbreviation: SD, standard deviation.

pausal across 8 years. For depressive disorder, the POAS also found that, in unadjusted analysis, perimenopause doubled the odds compared with premenopause, but perimenopause was no longer a significant predictor in multivariable analyses. Importantly, neither study included women who were postmenopausal and each only examined a subset of women.

The longitudinal studies examined multiple and varying potential risk factors for depression in addition to menopausal status. Freeman et al[8] reported that African Americans had nearly twice the odds of high depressive symptoms relative to Caucasians. However, their analyses did not adjust for socioeconomic and psychosocial factors that have been shown in other studies[21,40] to account for the higher risk for depression among African Americans. Other significant predictors included a history of depression at study entry, lack of employment, severe premenstrual syndrome (PMS), poor sleep, and hot flashes. Although postpartum depression was significant in bivariate analyses, it did not remain significant in the multivariable analysis possibly because of the high correlation between severe PMS and postpartum depression. Woods et al[10] reported that the number of undesirable events in the previous year, self-reported BMI, postpartum blues, and no live births each increased the odds of high depressive symptoms by 1.5 to 2 times. Hot flashes were significant in bivariate analyses, but not in multivariable ones. Maartens et al[9] found that being unemployed, prior depression (at T1, Edinburgh Postnatal Depression Scale (EPDS ≥ 12), financial problems, and death of partner were significant predictors of an increase in depressive symptoms over 3.5 years. This study did not include hot flashes.

Factors associated with first onset high depressive symptoms in the POAS included BMI, hot flashes, severe PMS, current smoking, and E2. Higher BMI, presence of hot flashes and greater variability of E2 at 2 consecutive follicular phase blood draws increased the odds, whereas current PMS and smoking significantly decreased them.[27] Cohen et al[7] did not present the odds of VMS or adverse life events in the full model, but their data suggest that only perimenopausal women with VMS or adverse life events had a significantly increased risk of first onset depression. Freeman et al[27] reported results that contrasted with those from SWAN.[24] They found that only BMI and variability of E2 measured in 2 consecutive follicular phase blood draws were associated with significant odds of depressive disorders. Hot flashes, PMS, and smoking were nonsignificant. In their analysis, perimenopause was not a significant predictor, which may have been due to the confounding of E2 variability and hot flashes with perimenopause or the small number of women with a depressive disorder.

CLINICAL IMPLICATIONS

Thus far, we have presented SWAN data about the magnitude of negative mood and depressive symptoms and disorder during the perimenopause and early postmenopause and associated risk factors for depression during this stage of a woman's life. However, depression can affect a woman's psychological well-being and pose a risk for her health. Depressive symptoms and disorder are associated with multiple medical conditions and symptoms, including cardiovascular disease (CVD), diabetes, and pain,[41–45] and can be both a risk factor for and a consequence of illness.[46,47] For example, depression has been associated with morbidity and subsequent coronary events in patients with CVD.[45] Further, concurrent physical illness can have synergistic effects on worsening physical functioning.[48] We have shown in SWAN that depressive symptoms are associated longitudinally with a 3-year increase in diabetes risk in 2662 women with baseline glucose levels above 126 mg/dL,[49] inflammatory and hemostatic factors,[50] and progression of coronary calcification.[51] Further, independent of standard CVD risk factors, past recurrent MD doubled the odds of early predictors of clinical disease, including carotid plaque,[52] coronary and aortic calcification,[53] and incident metabolic syndrome over 2 to 5 years.[54] Recurrent MD was also associated with progression of coronary calcification.[55] Past recurrent MD increased the odds at baseline of bodily pain (OR, 2.3), treatment for back pain (OR, 4.2), and low social functioning (OR, 2.1) in women without current depression.[56]

SWAN is not a treatment study. Nevertheless, the findings from SWAN are important and contribute to our knowledge about depression in women during the menopausal transition. The increased risk of depression during the transition and its implications for women's health and functioning suggest that women may benefit from close monitoring of mood and functioning as well as an assessment of their situational and environmental circumstances. Such monitoring could lead to earlier interventions designed to interrupt the progression from dysphoric mood to minor or MD. These could include interventions indicated at other times in the life cycle, such as behavioral therapy, antidepressants, and psychotherapy.

Early interventions can include brief counseling on coping with changes in mood and symptoms associated with perimenopause. Behavioral interventions, such as regular exercise or relaxation, can reduce depression.[57,58] Treatment approaches might also target symptoms that may exacerbate or be associated with depression and are unique to this period in a woman's life, such as VMS and genitourinary symptoms and sleep difficulties.[59] Because the potential consequences of underrecognized and untreated depression are considerable, clinicians need to be cognizant that depression can be present with physical as well as mood symptoms in women during this transition. Frey and Soares[60] have reviewed the potential therapeutic benefits of pharmacotherapies, both hormonal and nonhormonal, for perimenopausal depression.

SUMMARY

Data from SWAN as well as from other prospective epidemiologic studies and those reviewed by Freeman et al[61] and Soares and Frey[62] clearly indicate that perimenopause is a period of heightened risk for depressive symptoms as well as clinical and subclinical depressive disorders. As we and others[62,63] have described, vulnerability to depression during the perimenopause can be attributed to a number of factors, including discomfort from somatic symptoms associated with the transition (particularly VMS), psychosocial stressors, inadequate social support, health behaviors, lifestyle, sociodemographic characteristics, and a history of clinical depression. Given the changes in reproductive hormone dynamics during the menopausal transition, it is likely that the altered estrogen and progesterone milieu contribute to the risk for depression at this time, although the data supporting this are largely indirect and sparse. Our findings are similar to those of the recent large longitudinal studies,[7–10] although, except for Maartens et al, these studies did not find an increased risk postmenopause possibly owing to insufficient postmenopausal data. In our sample, the increased vulnerability to depression during or after the menopausal transition was not accounted for by frequent VMS or by levels of or changes in reproductive hormones. Thus, although we have evidence that the period of transition from the late reproductive years to postmenopause is a time of increased risk for depression, we still do not fully understand why this is the case. In our future work, we plan to evaluate further the characteristics of women at risk for depression during the menopausal transition and postmenopause and whether there are subgroups of women at greater or lesser risk. We also hope to continue the work we have begun to look at depression as a risk factor for other health outcomes as women age.

REFERENCES

1. Kessler RC, McGonagle KA, Zhao S, et al. Lifetime and 12-month prevalence of DSM-III-R psychiatric disorders in the United States. Results from the National Comorbidity Survey. Arch Gen Psychiatry 1994;51:8–19.
2. Kessler RC, Berglund P, Demler O, et al. The epidemiology of major depressive disorder: results from the National Comorbidity Survey Replication (NCS-R). JAMA 2003;289:3095–105.
3. Angst J, Gamma A, Gastpar M, et al. Gender differences in depression. Epidemiological findings from the European DEPRES I and II studies. Eur Arch Psychiatry Clin Neurosci 2002;252:201–9.
4. Matthews KA, Bromberger JT, Egland G. Behavioral antecedents and consequences of the menopause. In: Korenman SG, editor. The menopause. Norwell (MA): Serono Symposia; 1990.
5. Williams JB, Gibbon M, First MB, et al.The Structured Clinical Interview for DSM-III-R (SCID). II. Multisite test-retest reliability. Arch Gen Psychiatry 1992;49:630–6.
6. Spitzer RL, Williams JB, Gibbon M, et al. The Structured Clinical Interview for DSM-III-R (SCID). I: History, rationale, and description. Arch Gen Psychiatry 1992;49: 624–9.
7. Cohen LS, Soares CN, Vitonis AF, et al. Risk for new onset of depression during the menopausal transition: the Harvard study of moods and cycles. Arch Gen Psychiatry 2006;63:385–90.
8. Freeman EW, Sammel MD, Liu L, et al. Hormones and menopausal status as predictors of depression in women in transition to menopause. Arch Gen Psychiatry 2004;61:62–70.
9. Maartens LW, Knottnerus JA, Pop VJ. Menopausal transition and increased depressive symptomatology: a community based prospective study. Maturitas 2002;42: 195–200.
10. Woods NF, Smith-DiJulio K, Percival DB, et al. Depressed mood during the menopausal transition and early postmenopause: observations from the Seattle Midlife Women's Health Study. Menopause 2008;15:223–32.

11. Radloff LS. The CES-D Scale: a self-report depression scale for research in the general population. Applied Psychological Measurement 1977;1:385–401.
12. Boyd JH, Weissman MM, Thompson WD, et al. Screening for depression in a community sample. Understanding the discrepancies between depression symptom and diagnostic sales. Arch Gen Psychiatry 1982;39:1195–200.
13. Jones-Webb RJ, Snowden LR. Symptoms of depression among blacks and whites. Am J Public Health 1993;83:240–4.
14. Potter LB, Rogler LH, Moscicki EK. Depression among Puerto Ricans in New York City: the Hispanic Health and Nutrition Examination Survey. Soc Psychiatry Psychiatr Epidemiol 1995;30:185–93.
15. Roberts RE. Reliability of the CES-D Scale in different ethnic contexts. Psychiatry Res 1980;2:125–34.
16. Salgado-de Snyder VN, Maldonado M. [The psychometric characteristics of the Depression Scale of the Centro de Estudios Epidemiologicos in adult Mexican women from rural areas]. Salud Publica Mex 1994;36:200–9.
17. Ying YW. Depressive symptomatology among Chinese-Americans as measured by the CES-D. J Clin Psychol 1988;44:739–46.
18. Comstock GW, Helsing KJ. Symptoms of depression in two communities. Psychol Med 1976;6:551–63.
19. Bromberger JT, Meyer PM, Kravitz HM, et al. Psychologic distress and natural menopause: a multiethnic community study. Am J Public Health 2001;91:1435–42.
20. Bromberger JT, Assmann SF, Avis NE, et al. Persistent mood symptoms in a multiethnic community cohort of pre- and perimenopausal women. Am J Epidemiol 2003;158:347–56.
21. Bromberger JT, Harlow S, Avis N, et al. Racial/ethnic differences in the prevalence of depressive symptoms among middle-aged women: The Study of Women's Health Across the Nation (SWAN). Am J Public Health 2004;94:1378–85.
22. Bromberger JT, Matthews KA, Schott LL, et al. Depressive symptoms during the menopausal transition: the Study of Women's Health Across the Nation (SWAN). J Affect Disord 2007;103:267–72.
23. Bromberger JT, Kravitz HM, Chang YF, et al. Major depression during and after the menopausal transition: Study of Women's Health Across the Nation (SWAN). Psychol Med 2011;9:1–10.
24. Bromberger JT, Schott LL, Kravitz HM, et al. Longitudinal change in reproductive hormones and depressive symptoms across the menopausal transition: results from the Study of Women's Health Across the Nation (SWAN). Arch Gen Psychiatry 2010;67:598–607.
25. Golden R, Gilmore J. Serotonin and mood disorders. Psychiatr Ann 1990;20:580–6.
26. Janowsky H, Halbreich U, Rausch J. Association among ovarian hormones, other hormones, emotional disorders, and neurotransmitters. In: Jensvold M, Halbreich U, Hamilton J, editors. Psychopharmacology and women: sex, gender, and hormones. Washington (DC): American Psychiatric Press;1996. p. 85–106.
27. Freeman EW, Sammel MD, Lin H, et al. Associations of hormones and menopausal status with depressed mood in women with no history of depression. Arch Gen Psychiatry 2006;63:375–82.
28. Diagnostic and Statistical Manual of Mental Disorders. 4th ed. Washington (DC): American Psychiatric Association; 1994.
29. Murray C, Lopez A. The global burden of disease. Cambridge (MA): Harvard University Press; 1996.

30. Blazer DG, Kessler RC, McGonagle KA, et al. The prevalence and distribution of major depression in a national community sample: the National Comorbidity Survey. Am J Psychiatry 1994;151:979–86.

31. Kessler RC, Zhao S, Blazer DG, et al. Prevalence, correlates, and course of minor depression and major depression in the National Comorbidity Survey. J Affect Disord 1997;45:19–30.

32. Beekman AT, Deeg DJ, Geerlings SW, et al. Emergence and persistence of late life depression: a 3-year follow-up of the Longitudinal Aging Study Amsterdam. J Affect Disord 2001;65:131–8.

33. Hybels CF, Blazer DG. Epidemiology of late-life mental disorders. Clin Geriatr Med 2003;19:663–96.

34. Kendler KS, Prescott CA. A population-based twin study of lifetime major depression in men and women. Arch Gen Psychiatry 1999;56:39–44.

35. Kendler KS, Prescott CA. Genes, environment, and psychopathology: understanding the causes of psychiatric and substance use disorders. New York: The Guilford Press; 2006.

36. Dunlop DD, Song J, Lyons JS, et al. Racial/ethnic differences in rates of depression among preretirement adults. Am J Public Health 2003;93:1945–52.

37. Bromberger JT, Kravitz HM, Matthews K, et al. Predictors of first lifetime episodes of major depression in midlife women. Psychol Med 2009;39:55–64.

38. Mueller TI, Leon AC, Keller MB, et al. Recurrence after recovery from major depressive disorder during 15 years of observational follow-up. Am J Psychiatry 1999;156:1000–6.

39. Kravitz HM, Janssen I, Lotrich FE, et al. Sex steroid hormone gene polymorphisms and depressive symptoms in women at midlife. Am J Med 2006;119:S87–S93.

40. Holzer CE, Swanson JW, Shea BM. Ethnicity, social status, and psychiatric disorder in the Epidemiologic Catchment Area Survey. In: Price RK, Shea BM, Mookherjee HN, editors. Social psychiatry across cultures: studies from North America, Asia, Europe, and Africa. New York: Plenum Press; 1995. p. 93–104.

41. Dew M. Disorder in the context of physical illness. In: Dohrenwend B, editor. Adversity, stress, and psychopathology. New York: Oxford University Press; 1998. p. 219–32.

42. Hotopf M, Mayou R, Wadsworth M, et al. Temporal relationships between physical symptoms and psychiatric disorder. Results from a national birth cohort. Br J Psychiatry 1998;173:255–61.

43. Krishnan KR, Delong M, Kraemer H, et al. Comorbidity of depression with other medical diseases in the elderly. Biol Psychiatry 2002;52:559–88.

44. Mojtabai R, Olfson M. Major depression in community-dwelling middle-aged and older adults: prevalence and 2- and 4-year follow-up symptoms. Psychol Med 2004;34:623–34.

45. Rugulies R. Depression as a predictor for coronary heart disease. A review and meta-analysis. Am J Prev Med 2002;23:51–61.

46. Bruce ML. Psychosocial risk factors for depressive disorders in late life. Biol Psychiatry 2002;52:175–84.

47. Matthews KA, Schott LL, Bromberger JT, et al. Are there bi-directional associations between depressive symptoms and C-reactive protein in mid-life women? Brain Behav Immun 2010;24:96–101.

48. Schmitz N, Wang J, Malla A, et al. Joint effect of depression and chronic conditions on disability: results from a population-based study. Psychosom Med 2007;69:332–8.

49. Everson-Rose SA, Meyer PM, Powell LH, et al. Depressive symptoms, insulin resistance, and risk of diabetes in women at midlife. Diabetes Care 2004;27:2856–62.

50. Matthews KA, Schott LL, Bromberger J, et al. Associations between depressive symptoms and inflammatory/hemostatic markers in women during the menopausal transition. Psychosom Med 2007;69:124–30.
51. Janssen I, Powell LH, Matthews KA, et al. Depressive symptoms are related to progression of coronary calcium in midlife women: The Study of Women's Health Across the Nation (SWAN) Heart Study. Am Heart J 2011;1186–91.
52. Jones DJ, Bromberger JT, Sutton-Tyrrell K, et al. Lifetime history of depression and carotid atherosclerosis in middle-aged women. Arch Gen Psychiatry 2003;60:153–60.
53. Agatisa PK, Matthews KA, Bromberger JT, et al. Coronary and aortic calcification in women with a history of major depression. Arch Intern Med 2005;165:1229–36.
54. Goldbacher EM, Matthews KA. Are psychological characteristics related to risk of the metabolic syndrome? A review of the literature. Ann Behav Med 2007;34:240–52.
55. Matthews KA, Chang YF, Sutton-Tyrrell K, et al. Recurrent major depression predicts progression of coronary calcification in healthy women: Study of Women's Health Across the Nation. Psychosom Med 2010;72:742–7.
56. Bromberger JT, Kravitz HM, Wei HL, et al. History of depression and women's current health and functioning during midlife. Gen Hosp Psychiatry 2005;27:200–8.
57. Blumenthal JA, Babyak MA, Moore KA, et al. Effects of exercise training on older patients with major depression. Arch Intern Med 1999;159:2349–56.
58. Ernst E, Rand JI, Stevinson C. Complementary therapies for depression: an overview. Arch Gen Psychiatry 1998;55:1026–32.
59. Stewart DE, Khalid MJ. Menopause and mental health. In: Romans SE, Seeman MV, editors. Women's mental health: a life-cycle approach. Philadelphia: Lippincott Williams & Wilkins; 2006. p. 297–309.
60. Frey BN, Lord C, Soares CN. Depression during menopausal transition: a review of treatment strategies and pathophysiological correlates. Menopause Int 2008;14:123–8.
61. Freeman EW. Associations of depression with the transition to menopause. Menopause 2010;17:823–7.
62. Soares CN, Frey BN. Is there a role for estrogen in treating depression during menopause? J Psychiatry Neurosci 2010;35:E6–E7.
63. Schmidt PJ, Rubinow DR. Sex hormones and mood in the perimenopause. Ann N Y Acad Sci 2009;1179:70–85.

Index

Note: Page numbers of article titles are in **boldface** type.

A

B

Obstet Gynecol Clin N Am 38 (2011) 627–637
doi:10.1016/S0889-8545(11)00089-1
0889-8545/11/$ – see front matter © 2011 Elsevier Inc. All rights reserved.

Printed and bound by CPI Group (UK) Ltd, Croydon, CR0 4YY

03/10/2024

01040452-0008